iHealth

An Interactive Framework

D0061132

iHealth
3rd Edition
An Interactive Framework

Phillip B. Sparling
Georgia Institute of Technology

Kerry J. Redican
Virginia Tech
and
Virginia Tech Carilion School of Medicine

IHEALTH: AN INTERACTIVE FRAMEWORK, THIRD EDITION

Published by McGraw-Hill Education, 2 Penn Plaza, New York, NY 10121. Copyright © 2017 by McGraw-Hill Education. All rights reserved. Printed in the United States of America. Previous editions © 2013 and 2011. No part of this publication may be reproduced or distributed in any form or by any means, or stored in a database or retrieval system, without the prior written consent of McGraw-Hill Education, including, but not limited to, in any network or other electronic storage or transmission, or broadcast for distance learning.

Some ancillaries, including electronic and print components, may not be available to customers outside the United States.

This book is printed on acid-free paper.

1 2 3 4 5 6 7 8 9 DOC 21 20 19 18 17 16

ISBN: 978-0-07-802858-8
MHID: 0-07-802858-2

Chief Product Officer, SVP Products &
  Markets: *G. Scott Virkler*
Vice President, General Manager,
  Products & Markets: *Michael Ryan*
Vice President, Content Design & Delivery:
  Kimberly Meriwether David
Managing Director: *Gina Boedeker*
Director: *Gina Boedeker*
Brand Manager: *Penina Braffman*
Product Developer: *Anthony McHugh*
Marketing Manager: *Meredith Leo*
Director, Content Design & Delivery:
  Terri Schiesl

Program Manager: *Marianne Musni*
Content Project Managers: *Sandra Schnee,*
  George Theofanopoulos, Susan Trentacosti
Buyer: *Sandy Ludovissy*
Design: *Debra Kubiak*
Content Licensing Specialists: *Ann Marie*
  Jannette, Lori Slattery
Cover Image: *fStop/PunchStock*
Compositor: *Aptara®, Inc.*
Printer: *R. R. Donnelley*

All credits appearing on page or at the end of the book are considered to be an extension of the copyright page.

Library of Congress Cataloging-in-Publication Data

Names: Sparling, Phillip B. (Phillip Belton), 1949- author. I Redican, Kerry J., author.
Title: ihealth : an interactive framework / Phillip B. Sparling, Georgia Institute of Technology, Kerry J. Redican, Virginia Tech and Virginia Tech Carilion School of Medicine.
Description: 3rd edition. I New York, NY : McGraw-Hill, [2017] I Includes bibliographical references and index.
Identifiers: LCCN 2016019906 I ISBN 9780078028588 (alk. paper) I ISBN 0078028582 (alk. paper)
Subjects: LCSH: Health—Textbooks. I Health—Electronic information resources.
Classification: LCC RA776 .S6959 2017 I DDC 613.0285—dc23 LC record available at https://lccn.loc.gov/2016019906

The Internet addresses listed in the text were accurate at the time of publication. The inclusion of a website does not indicate an endorsement by the authors or McGraw-Hill Education, and McGraw-Hill Education does not guarantee the accuracy of the information presented at these sites.

Contents in Brief

Contents in Detail

Part II

iHealth is dedicated to our students and colleagues, who inspire us to be better teachers, and to our wives, Phyllis and Barbara, for their support of our efforts to provide a new approach.

Information overload is real—especially when it comes to personal health. Adding to the overload is the rapid pace at which scientific advances revolutionize medical treatments and health recommendations. Achieving good health is not a one-course deal. If only it was as straightforward as arithmetic. Memorize the multiplication tables once and count on them for life! For health education, mastering core content is simply phase one. Critical analysis and implementing behavior change are the lasting skills we aim to instill.

iHealth was developed to help students navigate the changing sea of medical research and recommendations—to help you reach a higher level of health literacy and personal well-being. By presenting only the most essential topics, less time is spent memorizing and more time discussing and evaluating. Focusing on critical thinking and communication skills provides carryover value for making smart health decisions long into the future.

Using a conversational writing style, we have distilled each topic into small sections. Brief content coverage translates into more time to explore special aspects or issues during class sessions. Carefully selected articles from diverse publications reinforce and expand the essential material. By tackling controversies, presenting possible solutions, and raising new questions, these articles lead readers to consider different perspectives.

Health topics are often complex with many perspectives. After all, health-related issues occur within the broader context of our lifestyle, health care system, and society. *iHealth* functions well for courses using a traditional topics approach or a more interactive issues-based approach.

iHealth is an integrated digital product in sync with today's instructional technology. Opportunities to practice critical thinking and develop healthier lifestyle skills are available through an assortment of assessments and readings. With each edition, we've incorporated feedback from instructors and students as well as updated content. We are excited to offer *iHealth* 3e.

Phillip B. Sparling
Kerry J. Redican

iHealth
An Interactive Framework

The *iHealth* Story

iHealth started with instructors like you. Through extensive research, ranging from online surveys and reviews to focus groups and symposia, McGraw-Hill learned that personal health instructors were looking for a new kind of teaching tool—one that provides a framework for efficiently covering the subject's key topics, that offers the flexibility to meet personal instructional goals and student needs, and that effectively engages their students. Phillip Sparling and Kerry Redican, themselves participants in this research, were so enthusiastic about this new type of tool that they decided to build it themselves. The result is *iHealth*, an integrated print–digital learning system that is engaging, flexible, and innovative to meet the needs of today's students and educators.

You Made *iHealth* Even Better . . .

iHealth improved because of instructors like you. The new edition of *iHealth* is better because we watched how you use *iHealth* and listened to what you said about it.

- The **SmartBook** adaptive reading and study experience guides students to master and remember key concepts, giving them a tool that is shown to improve grades. The new *iHealth* test bank is aligned with the SmartBook objectives to help drive students toward full comprehension and mastery of the content.

- Updated online articles and health assessments provide students with a relevant, balanced look at a variety of important health issues. These additional assessment features are now easier for instructors to assign and grade.

- The **Connect** platform offers full integration with Blackboard, and through McGraw-Hill Campus, quick and easy integration with *any* course management system. Connect also provides a platform for the easy uploading of your own course or assignment files, new social networking tools, and improved online performance.

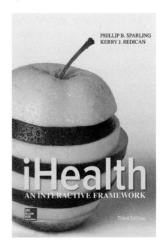

Why *iHealth* Works

iHealth is used by hundreds of instructors and thousands of students because it provides a foundation for building solid research skills, critical thinking skills, and behavior change skills that will enable students to make good decisions and live a more fulfilling life.

iHealth Gives Students What They Want

McGraw-Hill listened to students, who said they want:

- **A concise, accessible book.** *iHealth* presents essential health concepts in a clear, concise, portable text that is available in print, eBook, and SmartBook formats. *iHealth* is a personal health handbook that is both carefully documented and practical.
- **Relevant multimedia content.** Connect for *iHealth* includes updated online articles and health risk assessments to put concepts in a real-world context, motivating students to think critically, build research skills, and apply what they learn to their own lives.
- **Dynamic personalized learning plans.** SmartBook for *iHealth* is an unparalleled adaptive study tool that helps students identify and close knowledge gaps through a continually adaptive reading experience. With SmartBook, students are able to study more efficiently and effectively, be more informed participants in class discussions, and perform better on quizzes and exams.

iHealth Gives Instructors What They Need

McGraw-Hill listened to instructors, who said they want:

- **More time.** *iHealth*'s concise 13-chapter framework and auto-graded assignments enable instructors to maximize limited class hours while also providing the flexibility to cover additional topics and themes to fit the needs of their course.
- **Tools to build critical thinking and research skills.** *iHealth*'s rich library of interactive assignments—including online articles and health risk assessments—are designed to give instructors the resources to teach their students research skills, critical thinking skills, and behavior change skills that will last a lifetime.

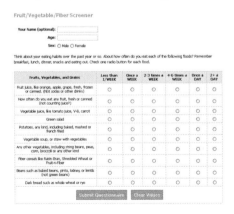

- **Flexibility.** The online components that accompany *iHealth*, powered by the Connect platform, allow instructors the flexibility to design the course that they want and that best suits their students' needs. Using Connect, instructors can now upload and create an assignment around any article, video, or podcast of their choice, further enhancing the flexibility of *iHealth* and providing more opportunities for customization.

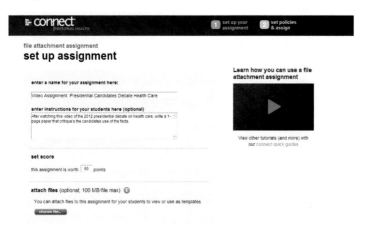

- **Seamless integration with Blackboard.** Through a partnership between McGraw-Hill and Blackboard, the *iHealth* online components can now be easily and seamlessly integrated with the Blackboard course management system. Among other things, this integration enables Connect activities, assessments, grades, and other content to appear within your university's Blackboard system. Setup is fast, easy, and flexible, and students can access Connect using their university logins.

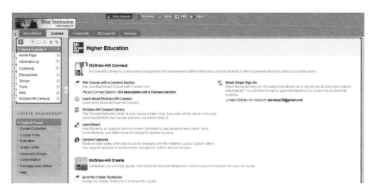

- **McGraw-Hill Campus.** Regardless of what course management system your school uses, McGraw-Hill now makes it quick and easy for *all* faculty to find just the right online and digital resources, at no additional cost. McGraw-Hill Campus will provide all faculty and students streamlined access to unlimited digital resources at no additional costs and will enable quick, simple connections between McGraw-Hill Connect and multiple learning management systems.

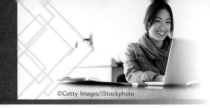

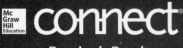

Required=Results

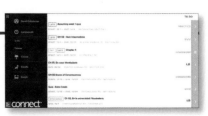

©Getty Images/iStockphoto

McGraw-Hill Connect®
Learn Without Limits

Connect is a teaching and learning platform that is proven to deliver better results for students and instructors.

Connect empowers students by continually adapting to deliver precisely what they need, when they need it, and how they need it, so your class time is more engaging and effective.

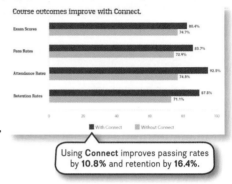

Course outcomes improve with Connect.

Using **Connect** improves passing rates by **10.8%** and retention by **16.4%**.

> 88% of instructors who use **Connect** require it; instructor satisfaction **increases** by 38% when **Connect** is required.

Analytics ────

Connect Insight®

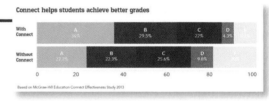

Connect helps students achieve better grades

Based on McGraw-Hill Education Connect Effectiveness Study 2013

Connect Insight is Connect's new one-of-a-kind visual analytics dashboard—now available for both instructors and students—that provides at-a-glance information regarding student performance, which is immediately actionable. By presenting assignment, assessment, and topical performance results together with a time metric that is easily visible for aggregate or individual results, Connect Insight gives the user the ability to take a just-in-time approach to teaching and learning, which was never before available. Connect Insight presents data that empowers students and helps instructors improve class performance in a way that is efficient and effective.

> Students can view their results for any **Connect** course.

Mobile ────

Connect's new, intuitive mobile interface gives students and instructors flexible and convenient, anytime–anywhere access to all components of the Connect platform.

Adaptive

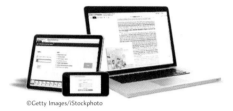

THE ONLY **ADAPTIVE READING EXPERIENCE** DESIGNED TO TRANSFORM THE WAY STUDENTS READ

More students earn **A's** and **B's** when they use McGraw-Hill Education **Adaptive** products.

SmartBook®

Proven to help students improve grades and study more efficiently, SmartBook contains the same content within the print book, but actively tailors that content to the needs of the individual. SmartBook's adaptive technology provides precise, personalized instruction on what the student should do next, guiding the student to master and remember key concepts, targeting gaps in knowledge and offering customized feedback, and driving the student toward comprehension and retention of the subject matter. Available on smartphones and tablets, SmartBook puts learning at the student's fingertips—anywhere, anytime.

Over **4 billion questions** have been answered, making McGraw-Hill Education products more intelligent, reliable, and precise.

www.mheducation.com

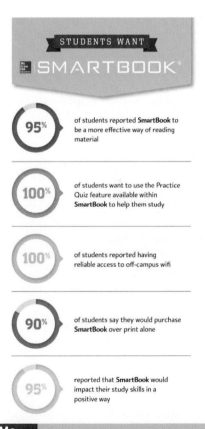

STUDENTS WANT

SMARTBOOK®

95% of students reported **SmartBook** to be a more effective way of reading material

100% of students want to use the Practice Quiz feature available within **SmartBook** to help them study

100% of students reported having reliable access to off-campus wifi

90% of students say they would purchase **SmartBook** over print alone

95% reported that **SmartBook** would impact their study skills in a positive way

Mc Graw Hill Education

*Findings based on a 2015 focus group survey at Pellissippi State Community College administered by McGraw-Hill Education

Acknowledgments

Many people at McGraw-Hill made *iHealth* possible. A few folks deserve special mention:

Nick Barrett, who shared our vision and began the project in 2004; Chris Johnson, who shepherded the project from infancy to graduation; and development editors Erin Strathmann and Emily Pecora, who showed finesse and patience from start to finish.

We also gratefully acknowledge Lydia Kim, Briana Porco, Kate Engelberg, Rhona Robbin, Margaret Young, Melanie Field, Jennifer Gordon, Bill Glass, Julie Bickar, Mike Ryan, and Steve Debow. Each helped in different ways, at different points— but all as a team toward our shared goal of seeing *iHealth* and *iHealth* 2e become a reality. Many others unnamed also contributed. Our thanks to all.

Our excellent team for the *iHealth* 3e included Penina Braffman, Erin Guendelsberger, Ann Marie Jannette, Debra Kubiak, Sandy Ludovissy, Anthony McHugh, Marianne Musni, Sandy Schnee, Lori Slattery, George Theofanopoulos, and Susan Trentacosti. Among these outstanding professionals, a special thanks goes to three individuals—Erin Guendelsberger, Anthony McHugh, and Susan Trentacosti—for their accessibility, timely follow-up, collegiality, and patience.

Last, it's our pleasure to thank dozens of fellow college teachers from across the nation for feedback and insights during the development and production of *iHealth* through three editions. Those who reviewed the 3rd edition are cited below. Your contributions are sincerely appreciated.

Phillip B. Sparling
Kerry J. Redican

Academic Reviewers

Claire Belles
Central Piedmont Community College

Lynne Edmondson
Alabama A&M University

Julie Feeny
Illinois Central College

Paul Finnicum
Arkansas State University

Caroline Fuller
Virginia Union University

Kathie Garbe
University of North Carolina–Asheville

Tarin Hampton
Norfolk State University

Ann Maria Klinkenborg
Columbus State University

Janie Leary
Fairmont State University

Fern Lucero
College of San Mateo

Darlene Marie Martin
Liberty University

Mitch Mathis
Arkansas State University

Teresa K. Snow
Georgia Institute of Technology

Natalie Stickney
Georgia Perimeter College

Steven Terry
Hartnell Community College

Jane Vatchev
College of DuPage

Contributors

iHealth

An Interactive Framework

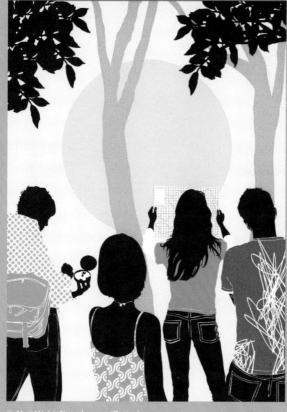

Learning is like rowing upstream. Not to advance is to fall backward.

—Chinese Proverb

© Neil Webb/Ikon Images/Getty Images

Chapter 1

FOUNDATIONS OF PERSONAL HEALTH

In Chapter 1, we provide a framework for understanding fundamental health topics, from health behaviors and medical conditions to health care considerations. This orientation can guide you in optimizing your health. We review the modern concept of health followed by the crosscutting themes of health literacy, health risk, impact of health advances, and health behavior change.

Modern Concept of Health

DEFINITION OF HEALTH

DIMENSIONS OF HEALTH

DIVERSITY AND HEALTH

Health Literacy

SELF-DIRECTED LEARNING

EFFECTIVE COMMUNICATION

CRITICAL THINKING

Concept of Risk

RISK PERCEPTION

RELATIVE RISK

Advances in Public Health

ADVANCES IN THE 20TH CENTURY

CHALLENGE OF THE 21ST CENTURY

HEALTHY PEOPLE 2020

WHAT LIES AHEAD?

Understanding Health Behaviors

SOCIAL COGNITIVE THEORY

HEALTH BELIEF MODEL

STAGES OF CHANGE MODEL

LIFE EXPECTANCY rose dramatically in the United States during the 20th century. Life expectancy for Americans born in 1900 was 47 years, whereas for those born in 2015, life expectancy is 79 years. Thirty-two years is a phenomenal gain in average lifespan. Yet, researchers who study the biology of human aging believe that most of us are still dying prematurely. They contend that with prudent lifestyles, young people in America today can expect to live to an average age of 90 years.

The trends are evident. In 2010, the year of the last national census, over 11 million Americans were 80 years or older, and nearly 80,000 were centenarians—100 years or older. Lizzie Brown of Fayetteville, Georgia, took everything in stride and lived to 111. At 110 she was still tending her garden at the house in which she had lived for 62 years. Among long-lived celebrities, Bob Hope reached 100 and was still performing in his mid-90s, UCLA basketball coach John Wooden lived to 99 and remained active giving talks until his last year, and Les Paul, inventor of the steel guitar, gave a concert the week before his death—at age 94. Yet, we also know of older folks in assisted care or nursing homes who are only in their 70s. Most will reside there for years or even decades. This thought gives us pause.

Undeniably, a full life is what we long for, not merely a long life. If we invest the time and effort to truly improve our health, are there immediate paybacks, or are the benefits only to be gained in middle age and beyond? How much control do we have in living a life that is full today *and* promising for the future? Our aim in writing *iHealth: An Interactive Framework* is to address these fundamental questions.

➤ Modern Concept of Health

Health is a universal term used widely in everyday language. We all have a general sense about what the term means but are unsure about specific definitions. Has the definition of *health* changed over time? How should the term *health* be used today? Let's take a closer look. We'll begin by defining health and then discuss its dimensions and how the meaning of health is influenced by social and cultural factors.

DEFINITION OF HEALTH

For over 50 years, the World Health Organization (WHO) has defined health as a state of complete physical, mental, and social well-being and not merely the absence of disease or infirmity. Yet, for most of us, the importance of health becomes clear only when we are sick or injured. Consequently, a natural response is to dichotomize health. That is, one is either healthy or unhealthy. A continuum exists only on the unhealthy side depending on the severity of the illness. This lopsided and mistaken view has a serious unintended consequence—it limits human development and potential. This narrow view overlooks the existence of the broad continuum on the positive side of health. With little conscious intention, many of us simply drift along

Health is a dynamic human condition with multiple but intertwined dimensions—physical, emotional, social, intellectual, spiritual, and environmental. Health can be viewed as a continuum with positive and negative poles. Positive health is associated with a capacity to enjoy life and to withstand challenges. Negative health is associated with illness and disease and, in the extreme, with premature death.

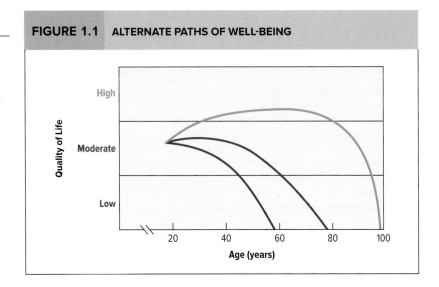

FIGURE 1.1 ALTERNATE PATHS OF WELL-BEING

on the positive side of the continuum. The good news is that by becoming more aware of what it means to be healthy, we can take steps to improve our well being—in significant ways.

Quality of life is an important related concept. In a nutshell, *quality of life* refers to our overall sense of well-being. **Quality of life** is a subjective rating of the difference between our hopes and expectations and our present experience. Health professionals sometimes have patients rate their quality of life to measure the effects of disorders and disabilities as well as medical treatments. These ratings are used to help guide medical decisions. For most young adults, quality of life is synonymous with overall enjoyment of life and is, in fact, highly dependent on current and expected health.

The relationship between quality of life and longevity is illustrated in Figure 1.1. From adolescence into young adulthood, we have increasing control over lifestyle choices and set the trajectory for our quality of life. The lower curve and the upper curve represent two hypothetical boundaries within which individual lifespan curves can be drawn. The upper curve reflects an individual who maximizes lifestyle choices and healthy behaviors. This leads to *both* a full life and a long life, reaching the 90-year potential and perhaps beyond. Ideally, the end of life is preceded by a sharp decline of short duration, with only a few weeks or months of deteriorating function and loss of independence, as in the case of Lizzie Brown.

In contrast, the lower curve represents a person who is unaware of or uninterested in a healthy life and adopts unhealthy behaviors. This compromises quality of life and substantially shortens a normal biological lifespan. Death at 60 rather than 90 is life truly cut short. Sadly, we all have firsthand knowledge of premature deaths

Quality of life is one's overall sense of well-being or enjoyment of life. It's a subjective rating of the difference between a person's hopes and expectations and his or her present experience, and it is sometimes used in medical settings to help assess the effects of disease, disability, and treatments.

FIGURE 1.2 TWO VIEWS OF HEALTH

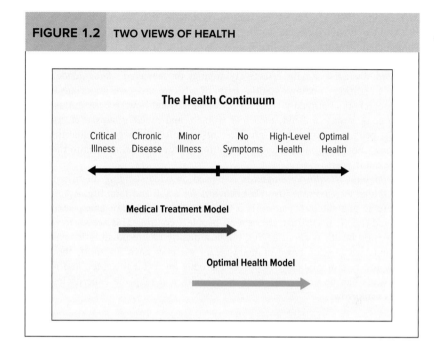

and incomplete lives. In this scenario, many years of disability and a poor quality of life may precede a person's early death.

The middle curve depicts the path of many Americans who are aware of key health issues but unsuccessful in effectively translating their knowledge into better lifestyle behaviors. Note that the area between the lower and upper curves is large—it is high (along the Quality of Life axis) and wide (along the Age axis). Within these broad bounds, we have enormous control on setting our own course. This is the potential area for growth available to us.

As in the WHO definition, health is often referred to as a state of optimal functioning, which implies the highest achievable level physically, mentally, and socially. A more contemporary perspective views health not as a state of being but as a goal that people continually work toward throughout their life. In Figure 1.2, health is depicted as a continuum extending from critical illness to optimal health. The traditional "medical treatment model" focuses on the left side of the continuum, and its emphasis is on freedom from sickness and disease. The proactive "optimal health model" focuses more on the right side of the continuum and the challenge of maximizing potential and improving quality of life.

Humans are goal-oriented creatures. We like to set goals and then work to achieve them. The goal of better health is no exception. To craft a plan, we need to know what factors influence movement along the health continuum, especially those we can control or modify. As it turns out, the most important factors are those associated with lifestyle—for example, factors related to eating, exercising, sleeping, drug use (including alcohol and tobacco), and stress. To a great extent, we are in charge on these matters. By choosing which behaviors to develop and which to avoid, each of us sets the course for moving forward (or falling back) along the health continuum.

Certainly, factors beyond our control (nonmodifiable factors) also influence health; namely, heredity, age, gender, and race. Occasionally unfavorable genetic combinations result in hereditary diseases such as cystic fibrosis, sickle cell anemia, and type 1 (juvenile) diabetes. Fortunately, in today's world, many inherited diseases can be effectively treated or managed. Age, gender, and race—in addition to being essential parts of who we are—are important factors that researchers continually study to better understand how risk for disease may vary among young and old, men and women, and racial groups. Yet, as individuals, gender and race have no inherently positive or negative qualities that limit one's ability to move along the continuum toward optimal health throughout the adult years.

Throughout *iHealth* an emphasis is placed on understanding modifiable factors and how to maximize lifestyle behaviors for a full and long life. Admittedly, there are no guarantees because life is unpredictable. Every day, unexpected accidents and deaths occur that are beyond people's control. This serves to remind us that good health is about having the best quality of life possible for whatever conditions we face or however many years we may have. In short, though, a healthy lifestyle dramatically improves the odds for a full life. Men and women of all races can be proactive about their health and reap the benefits today as well as tomorrow.

DIMENSIONS OF HEALTH

The modern view is that health is multidimensional. This characteristic is of fundamental importance in truly understanding health. The view counters the popular notion that health is simply physical well-being. Expanding on the three dimensions (physical, mental, social) cited in the WHO definition, the modern view encompasses six dimensions of health: physical, emotional, social, intellectual, spiritual, and environmental. A brief description of each dimension follows.

Physical Dimension of Health

The physical dimension of health encompasses the functional operation and soundness of the body. How well are you able to perform activities of daily living such as dressing, cooking, walking, and driving? Can you perform routine tasks efficiently without becoming overly fatigued? Do you get regular medical checkups? Do you follow preventive health practices known to optimize physical health—such as eating prudently, exercising regularly, avoiding substance abuse, wearing seat belts, minimizing sun exposure, and getting immunizations? For centuries, health was equated only with physical health. Today, physical health, although the predominant dimension at times, is recognized as only one of six dimensions that underlie our health.

Emotional Dimension of Health

The emotional dimension is associated with the ability to deal with personal feelings in a positive and constructive manner, to cope with stress, and to live independently. How is your outlook on life? Could your outlook be improved? Positive approaches to our emotions characterized by flexibility, balance, and resiliency help us deal effectively with feelings such as anger, happiness, fear, guilt, and love. A strong emotional dimension is a key to greater life satisfaction.

Social Dimension of Health

Closely tied to emotional health, the social dimension is the ability to interact effectively with other people, to develop satisfying interpersonal relationships, and to fulfill social roles. Do you have friends in whom you can confide? Do you have friends who feel comfortable confiding in you? Do you get along well with others and show respect regardless of your differences? Hallmarks of social health are the capacity for intimacy, meaningful relationships with family and friends, and participation in community activities. Young adulthood is a particularly important time for developing and broadening social skills.

Intellectual Dimension of Health

The intellectual dimension is reflected in our ability to question and evaluate information, to think and learn from a variety of experiences, and to be open to new ideas. Do you enjoy solving problems, learning new skills, and exploring new ideas? The academic challenges of college emphasize the development of intellectual health. Make the most of these opportunities. Critical thinking and problem solving are fundamental lifelong pursuits that enable us to continue learning new material and master new skills.

Spiritual Dimension of Health

Being spiritual doesn't necessarily mean belonging to a formal religion, although religion is a fundamental part of this dimension for many. The essential component of spiritual health is a commitment to a set of values or principles that guide our actions. The commitment is often but not always based on a belief in a greater force. This greater force may be a supreme being or an acknowledgment of a higher power or order in the universe. Atheists can have sacred sets of values to live by just as Christians, Muslims, and Jews have divine beliefs to guide them. Spiritual health often involves a dedication to nurture all living beings out of respect for the interrelatedness of all life. The basis for leading a moral and ethical life is rooted in spiritual health.

Environmental Dimension of Health

The importance of the environmental dimension of health is highlighted by the immense growth in the field of ecology (interactions between organisms and their environment) and, in particular, knowledge about environmental risks to human and animal health. This dimension focuses on the state of the environment and the conditions in which we live. Primary environmental concerns include air and water quality and management of wastes and harmful substances, as well as unsustainable use of natural resources and the steady rise in human population. Our health is dependent on understanding that we are part of the natural world, not separate from it. Our challenge is to be good stewards of the earth and to find solutions that are ecologically sound. Many think we will fail to save the planet. Do you?

The dimensions of health do not exist as separate elements. Rather, each dimension relates to all others. As one dimension is affected, so too are the others. Just as individual threads are braided together to form a single cord, so too are the dimensions of health. Each thread or dimension contributes to the overall balance, quality, and strength of the whole.

Self
Assessment
1.1

During the first decade of the 21st century, the issue of diversity has come to the forefront. The changing demographics of America are illustrated with the following examples from the U.S. Census of 2010:

- Over one-third of the population reported their race/ethnicity as other than non-Hispanic White (i.e., "minority"), representing a growth of 29 percent over the decade.
- The Hispanic, African American, and Asian populations now comprise 16, 13, and 5 percent, respectively, of the total population.
- Texas joined California, the District of Columbia, Hawaii, and New Mexico in having a "majority–minority" population, where more than 50 percent of the population is a minority group.
- Fifty-seven percent of college students are women, and over 60 percent of adult women are in the workforce.
- Family structures continue to change. As an example, the proportion of young adults (aged 25–34) never married (46 percent) is now higher than the proportion married (45 percent).
- Immigration to the United States from over the past decade (2000–2009) was at an all-time high, averaging over 1 million per year.

We see diversity in ordinary encounters with individuals and groups who may differ widely in values, beliefs, and experiences—cumulatively referred to as *culture*. Diversity is sometimes criticized as a form of political correctness. That is an unfortunate and shortsighted view. The following quote from Sara Corbett's *New York Times* article "The Long Road from Sudan to America" introduces us to three young refugees from Sudan:

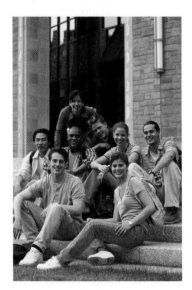

Colleges and universities are among the most ethnically diverse places in America.

© Comstock Images/JupiterImages

One evening in late January, Peter Dut, 21, leads his two teenage brothers through the brightly lit corridors of the Minneapolis airport, trying to mask his confusion. Two days earlier, the brothers, refugees from Africa, had encountered their first light switch and their first set of stairs. An aid worker in Nairobi had demonstrated the flush toilet to them—also the seat belt, the shoelace, the fork. And now they find themselves alone in Minneapolis, three bone-thin African boys confronted by a swirling river of white faces and rolling suitcases.

This description sets a sharp contrast between the lives of these African refugees and those of the Americans who walked by them in the airport. What is ordinary and routine for many may indeed be novel and wondrous for others. Most of us can hardly imagine the environment and circumstances from which these three brothers escaped. Should it be surprising that cultural background and life experiences invariably shape how we perceive one another and the world in which we live?

Of all the places in America, colleges and universities are among the most diverse. A large lecture class may have students who are urban and rural, wealthy and poor, straight and gay, religious and nonreligious. A military veteran juggling jobs or raising children may be sitting next to an 18-year-old first-year college student. Students from both developed and developing countries and various ethnic groups will likely be present. Some will speak English as a second language. Far-ranging human experiences in a classroom provide an opportunity to learn from each other.

Discussing diversity is important because many health topics such as stress, mental health, nutrition, drug use, chronic diseases, and infectious diseases are strongly related to culture. Examples include social stressors (prejudice, economic oppression), mental health disorders (depression, suicidal behavior), food choices (ethnic diets), and drug-use patterns (tobacco, alcohol, other drugs). Gaining insight into how the concept of health varies among different religious, ethnic, and cultural groups helps each of us better define the meaning of health in our own lives. This theme will be followed throughout *iHealth* and highlighted in selected readings.

The diversity of the American population is an asset. It is also one of our nation's greatest challenges because profound health disparities exist between the mainstream population and subpopulations such as African Americans, Hispanics, American Indians, and residents of Appalachia. Health disparities are a reality faced daily by employers, educators, and health professionals. A primary goal of public health is to reduce health disparities through research, education, and improved access to health care. In the wealthiest and most technologically advanced country in the world, affordable and equitable health care should be available to everyone.

NEED TO KNOW

The concept of health is much more than simply not being sick. Health is multidimensional, dynamic, and influenced by social and cultural norms. Our overall health status and the associated quality of life are largely determined by our lifestyle choices and behaviors.

➤ Health Literacy

Health literacy can be defined as the degree to which individuals have the capacity to obtain, process, and understand basic health information and services needed to make appropriate health decisions. Health literacy programs are traditionally targeted to those who are poor, elderly, and with little education. Yet, health literacy is not solely a matter of formal education or access to health information. The National Academy of Medicine estimates that nearly half of all American adults have difficulty understanding and using health information. The challenge

Health literacy is the ability to obtain, process, and understand basic health information and services needed to make appropriate health decisions.

of becoming health literate becomes clearer when considered within the context of our consumer-driven society. More than ever before, consumption defines who we are and what we do.

We are immersed in advertising throughout our waking hours. American children and adolescents are spending an average of seven hours a day on entertainment media, including TVs, computers, phones, and other electronic devices. Yes, that's right—seven hours! Young children recall Ronald McDonald and Tony the Tiger as easily as Santa Claus and Mickey Mouse. Beyond the screen, advertising in other forms from signage to apparel is increasingly found throughout schools. The American Academy of Pediatrics points out that excessive or uncontrolled exposure to TV, movies, music, video games, and the Internet is associated with an array of health problems from obesity and eating disorders to substance abuse, promiscuity, and bullying.

Article
1.1

Advertisers shape our consumer desires and create values in products by portraying them as having the power to change us into "more desirable" people. Commercials feature adults who are attractive, happy, energetic, and often hip and sensuous too. The underlying message is we can be like them if we use those products. Mega shopping malls—real and virtual—have become a cultural primer for telling us how we should dress, furnish our homes, and spend leisure time. Luxuries have become necessities and lifestyles can be purchased. As a side note, psychologist Barry Schwartz, a professor at Swarthmore College, suggests our nearly unlimited choices have resulted in additional stress for the 21st-century consumer—the paradox of choice.

In the health marketplace, frauds and hoaxes remain commonplace. For any ailment or disease, there exist literally hundreds of products, most of which are bogus. Regardless of the source—the Internet, television, social media, newspapers, magazines, radio, neighbors, colleagues—the best advice remains "buyer beware." It is tempting to assume that being college educated ensures the ability to sort out confounding influences and misleading claims from science-based information. But this is true only if we remain health literate. Health literacy is dependent on self-directed learning, effective communication, and critical thinking.

SELF-DIRECTED LEARNING

Self-directed learning is a process in which the individual controls both the learning objectives and the means of learning, with or without the help of others. You are in charge—you determine what should be learned, what resources and methods should be used, and how the success of the effort should be measured. This is in contrast to most college courses and workplace training classes, in which the learning objectives, methods, and evaluation are set by the teacher or employer.

To a large degree, most adult learning is self-directed. A person's objective may be to improve family life, enjoy the arts, participate in a hobby, or to research a medical question. For many people, however, the extent of self-directed learning is quite limited. They may not engage in self-directed learning because they lack the confidence, resources, independence, or some combination of the three. Thankfully, these barriers can be overcome with motivation and guidance.

First and foremost, the Internet is a rich resource for the self-directed learner who is savvy about the effective use the Internet. Here are a few tips to help you expand on and update material presented in *iHealth*. Recognize that you need to

Health & the Media Public Service Announcements

Advertising, a major industry in itself, is adept at creating messages to sell products. In the 1940s, the nonprofit Ad Council created a new type of advertising known as public service announcements (PSAs) to bring about positive social change, including better health. The Ad Council remains active today **(www.adcouncil.org).**

Another approach to communicating messages that promote health is to dispel the illusion of advertising with spoof ads. Cigarette and alcohol ads are especially ripe targets. Adbusters, a Canadian advocacy group and publisher of *Adbusters* magazine, has produced several memorable ones. Its "Absolute on Ice" parody ad evokes a stark contrast to the original ad and makes one think twice about the downsides of excessive drinking. (The product being parodied is Absolut, a vodka.) See other spoof ads such as Joe Chemo, a takeoff on Joe Camel, at **adbusters.org/spoofads.**

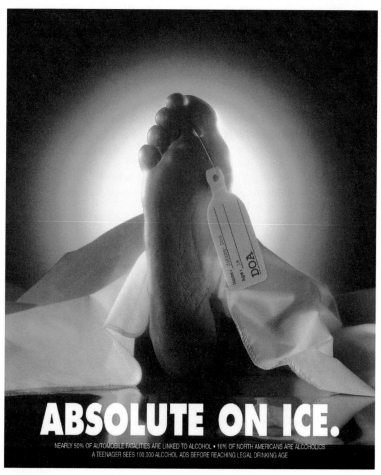

© Adbusters

carefully and critically evaluate all material on the Internet because anyone can post information. Reference books and refereed journal articles are reviewed and evaluated by experts prior to publishing. No such oversight exists for the vast majority of material found on the Internet. Cyberspace remains a Wild West where hearsay and bravado dominate.

As an initial screening procedure, note that certain web addresses (or URLs)—namely, those with the ".org" (nonprofit organization), ".gov" (federal government), and ".edu" (college/university) extensions—are more likely than the ".com" (commercial business) websites to lead to authoritative information. As health decision makers, our primary aim is to find credible and reliable information—not to buy a product! We should look for information that is factual, current, written in everyday language, and sponsored by a reputable group.

The following websites are excellent resources for health information and all abide by the Health on the Net (HON) Code of Conduct, a set of ethical principles to guide the presentation of health and medical information (Figure 1.3). While WebMD is the most popular, all others are cited as "top health websites" by the Medical Library Association. Websites are listed alphabetically. Even with reputable sites, a good practice is to read your desired topic at more than one source and to cross-check information:

1. Centers for Disease Control and Prevention (CDC) **www.cdc.gov** Leading federal agency for preventing and controlling disease, injury, and disability
2. Family Doctor **www.familydoctor.org** Sponsored by the American Academy of Family Physicians, the nation's largest association of family doctors
3. Health Finder **www.healthfinder.gov** Sponsored by the National Health Information Center, U.S. Department of Health and Human Services
4. Kids Health **www.kidshealth.org** The most-visited site for information on health, behavior, and development in children and teenagers
5. Mayo Clinic **www.mayoclinic.org** Sponsored by the renowned Mayo Clinic, the world's first and largest not-for-profit medical practice
6. Medline Plus **medlineplus.gov** Sponsored by the National Library of Medicine and National Institutes of Health
7. NIH Senior Health **www.nihseniorhealth.gov** Information on health for older adults, sponsored by the National Institutes of Health
8. WebMD **www.webmd.com** A leading, for-profit provider of health information, recognized for accurate medical journalism and effective health communication

A few carefully selected websites will be presented in each chapter. Since web addresses sometimes change, occasionally there may be a link that no longer works. If that happens, refer to the *iHealth* web page for updates.

EFFECTIVE COMMUNICATION

The importance of developing written and oral communication skills cannot be overstated, especially in today's world of smartphones and social media. Every day we communicate with many people in many ways and settings. Yet, good communication skills are not routinely learned in school so it's left to each of us to master them as self-directed learners. Regular investments of time and effort to improve communication skills will yield great returns. The likelihood for miscommunication when dealing with medical or health issues is enormous. Let's consider three different scenarios.

FIGURE 1.3	THE HON CODE ICON INDICATES TRUSTWORTHY MEDICAL INFORMATION ONLINE

Created in 1995, Health on the Net Foundation—a nonprofit, non-governmental organization—reviews and certifies websites to protect consumers from misleading health information. Look for the HON icon on the opening page of a website as a sign of credibility and trustworthiness. This seal of approval is based on the following principles:

1. **Authoritative:** Any medical or health advice provided or hosted on the site comes from medically trained and qualified professionals. In the event a piece of advice comes from a nonmedically qualified source or organization, that is also made clear.

2. **Complementarity:** Information provided supports, but does not replace, the doctor–patient relationship.

3. **Privacy:** Data regarding individual patients or visitors to the health-related website remain confidential.

4. **Attribution:** When appropriate, the site contains clear references to source data and, where possible, specific HTML links to that data. The date when a clinical page was last modified is clearly displayed.

5. **Justifiability:** Any claims related to benefits or performance of a specific treatment, product, or service are supported by appropriately balanced evidence in the manner outlined above in Principle 4.

6. **Transparency:** The site designers seek to provide information in the clearest possible manner and provide contact addresses for visitors who seek further information or support. The Webmaster displays his/her email clearly throughout the site.

7. **Financial Disclosure:** The site identifies its funding sources clearly.

8. **Advertising Policy:** The site clearly distinguishes editorial content from advertising.

Source: Reprinted by permission of HON, Health on the Net Foundation. www.hon.ch.

Scenario One

You are waiting in the exam room to see a physician. You have been told to take off your clothes and put on an exam gown. You have an odd illness you have never experienced before. Or you may have a hunch about what's going on but hope it's not true. You know your time with the doctor will be short, perhaps 5–10 minutes. And on top of that, you are feeling really lousy—that's why you've come to the doctor in the first place! This situation is predictably stressful and not conducive to

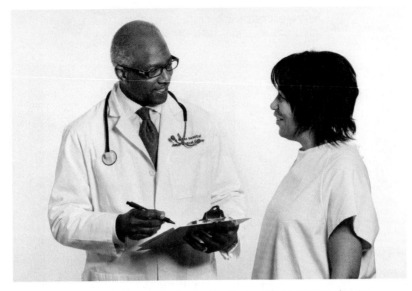

Many people struggle to communicate effectively with physicians due to embarrassment, fear, or time constraints.

© Allison Michael Orenstein/Photodisc/Getty Images

good communication. Common barriers are intimidation, embarrassment, and fear. Many people are intimidated by the medical setting, being half-clothed, and the status of the doctor. They may be embarrassed due to the personal nature of the condition they need to reveal. Some are fearful they may have a serious condition. It's no wonder we often cannot recall exactly what the doctor said or we forget to ask a question. How to prepare for a doctor's appointment and how to get your questions answered are discussed in Chapter 13.

Scenario Two

Your elderly neighbor has asked you to drive her to her doctor's appointment. As you take her home, she tells you that she has diabetes. But she is confused. She relates, "I think some of the words . . . [during the office visit and in brochures], they ought to explain in simple English. Everybody hasn't graduated from high school or college. They should just speak or put them down in plain English." Like millions of Americans, she is struggling with "medspeak," the specialized language of health professionals. The overuse of medical jargon has created a communication barrier for the public. As health professionals work to minimize their use of medspeak with patients, we as health consumers should increase our understanding of basic health and medical terms.

Scenario Three

You are in the pharmacy line at the drugstore and hear a disjointed conversation between the pharmacist and a Hispanic man in front of you. Although he has a heavy accent, his English is understandable. But it is unclear if he completely comprehends the pharmacist's instructions about how the medication should be taken. Communication problems are not limited to obvious language differences between

Breaking It Down   Does Listening to Classical Music Make You Smarter?

In the 1990s the "Mozart effect"—an alleged increase in brain development in children when they listen to the music of Mozart—received wide coverage in the popular print and broadcast media. Since that time, the Mozart effect has taken on a life of its own. It's featured in publications offering parenting advice and educational goals, as well as music appreciation. Governors of several states started programs that give a Mozart CD to every newborn. Dozens of toys suddenly appeared proclaiming themselves "educational" because they played snippets of Mozart's "Rondo Alla Turca" rather than "Mary Had a Little Lamb." The Mozart effect has also been used to sell music lessons and music products. Moreover, claims have expanded: Classical music can not only increase a child's intelligence but also aid an adult's healing process. What caused this Mozart love fest?

The Mozart effect is an example of how the media can flub a science story. It can happen like this. First, scientists publish a new and potentially important finding in a prestigious journal. The scientific study receives attention from the media, as it should. But next comes the oversimplification of the science. Sometimes reporters innocently misstate facts due to poor scientific understanding. Other times, businesses may intentionally exaggerate a study's findings to promote their products and boost sales. Regardless of the cause, once these misstatements are embraced by the general public, what started as a trickle of misinformation can become a river of baloney.

In this case, Frances Rauscher and two colleagues from the Center for Neurobiology of Learning and Memory at the University of California–Irvine reported in *Nature* that listening to a composition of Mozart briefly increased scores among college students on a paper-folding task that measures spatial abilities. The increase in scores lasted only about 10 minutes. Nonspatial tasks measured on the same IQ test were unaffected by listening to the music. The boost in scores was widely reported, but the short-lived effect and narrow nature of the improvement received a lot less attention. The accuracy of the original findings was lost over the years as the Mozart effect morphed into the popular notion that "Mozart makes you smarter." This notion is, of course, a gross oversimplification. Does it really make sense to talk about being "smarter" if it lasts only 10 minutes?

Accuracy is needed in science *and* in the media. Too often, important research is trivialized and misrepresented in the popular media. The case of the Mozart effect can teach us several lessons. First, we should be careful not to abandon common sense when we read health-related news. If a claim seems a bit extreme or too good to be true, then this ought to be a warning flag that the news might be incomplete or distorted. Second, we should allow the data to speak for themselves. When findings are controversial, explore reputable websites for summaries, read the original report and the opinions of experts, and reach your own conclusions. Apply those critical thinking skills!

patients and health care providers. They may also exist between people who come from different regions of the country or who have different values or expectations about health care. It is important to remember that one's customs and beliefs should be considered when communicating health messages.

CRITICAL THINKING

The term *critical thinking* is widely used but not well understood. Most would say it has something to do with logic or analysis, but these terms provide only a partial description. Essentially, critical thinking is careful and deliberate determination of whether to accept, reject, or suspend judgment. These are often the *why* questions. Critical thinking has two components: first, a set of skills to process and generate information and beliefs, and second, the habit—based on intellectual commitment—of using those skills to guide behavior. This is in contrast to the mere acquisition of information, the simple possession of skills, or the use of those skills as an exercise without giving any thought to their results.

Critical thinking is driven by asking the *right* questions. Critical thinking is *not* involved when teachers feed students endless facts for simple recall or when students sit in silence except for superficial or ill-informed questions. Both examples are dead ends. In contrast, good teaching and good questions lead to more questions and eventually to true learning. Overcome lifeless classrooms by asking thought-provoking questions. Learn the skills and establish the habit of critical thinking. From time to time, we are all subject to undisciplined and irrational thought. But is it the norm or the exception? The practice of critical thinking can be developed and refined during the college years but doesn't stop on graduation. Critical thinking can serve us well in all endeavors and should be a lifelong pursuit.

Consider critical thinking as a process that stresses an attitude of suspended judgment, incorporates logical inquiry and problem solving, and leads to an evaluative decision or action. In today's information age, critical thinking is more important than ever before. In addition to being an essential part of our intellectual health, critical thinking allows us to filter and analyze the maze of facts, claims, and hoaxes that surround health and medical issues. Critical thinking is what we must rely on if we are to successfully separate science from marketing and find solutions to complex questions.

✓ NEED TO KNOW

Health literacy is the knowledge and skills that enable us to successfully access, analyze, and interpret relevant information; to answer personal health questions; to provide guidance in dealing with a health condition; and to change a health behavior. Key aspects of health literacy include self-directed learning, effective communication, and critical thinking. These characteristics require related skills that must be developed. Health literacy also assumes a mindfulness and inquisitiveness that motivates continual learning.

➤ Concept of Risk

To fully appreciate the impact of our behaviors on our health, it's essential to understand what a health risk is and how to interpret it. Simply stated, a **health risk** or **risk factor** is the probability that an adverse event (an outcome) will occur if one

A **health risk** or **risk factor** is any factor that increases susceptibility or has a strong association with the occurrence, onset, or progression of a disease or injury.

engages in a certain behavior (exposure). For example, those who do not buckle up when riding in a car are at greater risk for a serious injury should an accident occur than those who do buckle up. The negative behavior (exposure) is not using a seat belt, and serious injury is the likely outcome if an accident occurs. The risk factors (behaviors and other factors) that are associated with specific diseases or injuries are established primarily by epidemiological studies.

Epidemiology is the study of the causes, distribution, and control of diseases in populations. Many medical findings reported in the popular media are based on epidemiological studies in which large numbers of people (hundreds or thousands) have been evaluated repeatedly over many years or decades. The goal of these studies is to investigate the links (associations) between the characteristics (including health behaviors) of the participants and the occurrence of specific outcomes across time (e.g., onset of diseases or death). Epidemiological studies help scientists sort through many, many factors and eventually identify those that are most highly related to a given disease.

Statistical correlations in population studies are based on observational data. That is, changes over time are observed and measured but no experimental treatment or intervention is being tested. As such, epidemiological findings by themselves cannot prove cause and effect. Just because variable A is highly related to variable B does not prove that A causes B. For example, smoking is highly correlated with cirrhosis of the liver. Does smoking cause cirrhosis of the liver? Probably not. Excessive consumption of alcohol is the likely culprit. Yet, since heavy drinkers tend to be heavy smokers, the statistical association is there. More often than not, evidence from experimental research, such as controlled laboratory studies or clinical trials, is used in conjunction with epidemiological findings to support or refute potential causal relationships.

RISK PERCEPTION

David Ropeik, a recognized expert on the subject of risk, has shown that risk perception is not a straightforward, logical process based on the best science. How we decide what to be afraid of and to what degree to be afraid is heavily influenced by psychological factors. Here are three examples of how we decide what's safe and what's risky:

1. People tend to be less afraid of risks that are natural than those that are human-made. There is greater fear of radiation from cell phones or power lines than from the sun, which presents a much greater risk.
2. People are less afraid of a risk they choose to take than one imposed on them. Smokers are less fearful of smoking than they are of asbestos or other indoor air pollutants in the workplace, over which they may have little control.
3. Most of us are less afraid of a risk that comes from people or organizations that we trust and more afraid if the risk comes from a source that we don't trust. We are more likely to accept the risk assessment of a drug's safety from a trusted physician than from the pharmaceutical company that makes it.

Epidemiology is the scientific discipline of studying the occurrence, distribution, control, and prevention of disease, infection, injury, and other health-related events in a defined human population. It includes the study of factors affecting the progress of an illness and, in the case of many chronic diseases, their natural history.

In his book *How Risky Is It, Really?* (2010) Ropeik provides evidence-based information to help put the risks in life in perspective. Researchers have found that Americans tend to overestimate small risks and underestimate large risks, regardless of age, race, or socioeconomic status. When you are making decisions about health risks, be aware that perceptions can be shaped by emotions and feelings. Consider taking a step back and relying on a careful, objective analysis when a major health risk must be evaluated.

RELATIVE RISK

Health risks are generally discussed in the language of medical statistics. **Relative risk** is a common way to quantify and report a health risk. Although statistics can be complex, relative risk is a straightforward concept and one we should know as medical consumers. Relative risk is the "times-greater chance" a person has of acquiring a specific negative health effect (e.g., a disease) based on the extent to which a certain variable (e.g., a characteristic or behavior) is present. Relative risk is the ratio of the rate of disease among those exposed to a variable compared to those not exposed or having limited exposure.

To illustrate, the American Cancer Society reports that the annual death rate from lung cancer among people who smoke is approximately 50 deaths per 100,000 people per year while the death rate of people who don't smoke is only 2.5 deaths per 100,000 people per year. In this case, the relative risk—the ratio of the lung cancer death rates of those exposed (smokers) to those not exposed (nonsmokers)— is 20 (50 divided by 2.5). Put another way, relative risk is the ratio of two absolute risks: The numerator is the absolute risk among those with the risk factor (50 deaths from lung cancer per 100,000 smokers), and the denominator is the absolute risk among those without the risk factor (2.5 deaths from lung cancer per 100,000 nonsmokers). A relative risk of 20 means that those who smoke have a 20-times-greater chance of dying from lung cancer than those who don't smoke. (Relative risk for smoking versus not smoking and death from lung cancer varies between 10 and 20 primarily depending on the amount of smoking.)

Often a relative risk is reported by itself. A relative risk of 10 to 20 (as with smoking) is extremely high. Most relative risks are in the range of 1.5 to 3.0. Let's assume the absolute risk for developing a disease is 4 in 100 among people who exercise regularly, and the risk is increased 50 percent in those who do not exercise. The 50 percent relates to the absolute risk number, 4, so the increase in the risk is 50 percent of 4, or 2. Consequently, nonexercisers' absolute risk of developing the disease is 6 out of 100, and the relative risk is 1.5 for the nonexercisers compared to the exercisers (6 divided by 4). On the one hand, a 50 percent increase sounds alarming, but on the other, because the absolute risk is small, a 50 percent increase is not that significant overall—the risk increased from only 4 out of 100 to 6 out of 100. Consequently, when possible, find out both relative and absolute risks, and do your own calculation to determine the overall risk.

We believe that "knowing the numbers" is important. The trend in public health, however, is to not report any numbers when communicating risk, but simply to rate

Relative risk is a measure of the comparative risk of a health-related event such as disease or death between two groups. It is the chance that a person receiving an exposure will develop a condition compared to the chance that a nonexposed person will develop the same condition.

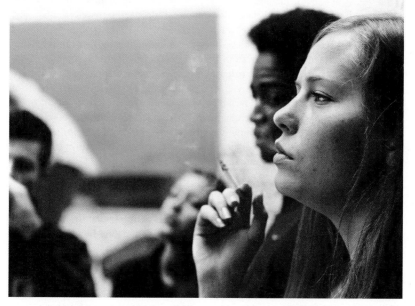

Smokers have a very high relative risk for developing lung cancer.
© BananaStock/PunchStock

the risk of a behavior as low, moderate, or high. This may be fine for some risks but not for others. You must be the judge. When in doubt, continue to ask or research your questions until you completely understand the risks associated with a specific behavior, intervention, or treatment. From the examples presented, the value of using the concepts of absolute and relative risk should be evident. Interpreting results from epidemiological and clinical studies and applying them to individual situations will enable you to make more informed decisions.

NEED TO KNOW

Health risk is the concept that relates specific health-compromising factors (exposures) to increased likelihood of developing diseases or higher death rates (outcomes). Conversely, from a proactive viewpoint, adopting health-enhancing or health-protective behaviors can reduce the probability of unwanted outcomes. Epidemiologists study the disease process in populations and quantify health risk in terms of absolute risk and relative risk.

➤ Advances in Public Health

The health concerns and health care services available when Lizzie Brown, the centenarian mentioned at the beginning of the chapter, was born in 1892 are vastly different from those that exist for a baby born today. A century ago, America was in the midst of the Industrial Revolution. Large numbers of people were migrating to the cities for jobs in factories. City housing was crowded, dirty, unheated, and unventilated. Clean water and proper sanitation (waste disposal) were limited, and food supplies were unreliable and often contaminated. These conditions allowed **infectious diseases** such as influenza, pneumonia, and tuberculosis to thrive.

Death rates fluctuated widely from year to year depending on disease (epidemics), severe weather (snowstorms, floods, hurricanes), and the harvest (varying from poor to bountiful). Infant mortality was high. In some cities, up to 30 percent of babies did not live to their first birthday. Many women died during childbirth. In short, life was hard. Under these conditions, it's understandable that good health would be thought of as being simply one step beyond the necessities for survival— that is, having adequate food and shelter and not being ill. Life expectancy for an American born in 1900 was less than 50.

ADVANCES IN THE 20TH CENTURY

During the 20th century, particularly the first half, amazing public health advances were made: provision of clean water, improved sanitation (the building of sewer systems), and the development of vaccines and antibiotics. Today, we take all of these for granted, but then these engineering and medical feats were major breakthroughs in the control of infectious diseases. These advances saved lives and markedly improved day-to-day living. Other public health achievements were safer and healthier foods, reduction in injuries and accidents, and greater access to health care along with improved technology.

There are many notable examples. Since 1900, infant mortality has decreased 90 percent and maternal mortality 99 percent. Substantial reductions in disability (morbidity) and death (mortality) have resulted from improvements in workplace safety (e.g., regulations in mining, manufacturing, and construction) and motor vehicle safety (e.g., better-engineered vehicles and highways and seat belt use). Most public health advances have been translated into public policy, such as school immunization policies and seat belt laws. Today we can hardly imagine the difficulties our ancestors faced only four or five generations ago.

As infectious diseases were controlled, the leading causes of death and disability in America shifted. In 1900 the three leading causes of death were pneumonia, tuberculosis, and diarrheal diseases. Today the three leading causes of death are not infectious diseases but chronic diseases—heart disease, cancer, and chronic lower respiratory disease. **Chronic diseases** are medical conditions that are prolonged, do not resolve spontaneously, and are rarely cured completely. And, just as with infectious diseases, chronic diseases impose huge human and economic costs.

An **infectious disease** is a medical condition typically resulting from a disease-causing organism—usually a bacterium, virus, or parasitic worm—known as a pathogen. Most infectious diseases are short-term or highly treatable illnesses, such as the common cold and strep throat. Other infectious diseases such as AIDS are long-term diseases for which no medical cure has yet been developed.

A **chronic disease** is a medical condition that is permanent, leaves a residual disability, is caused by a nonreversible pathological condition, and requires special training of the patient for rehabilitation or is expected to require a long period of supervision or care. Coronary heart disease and cancer are two common examples.

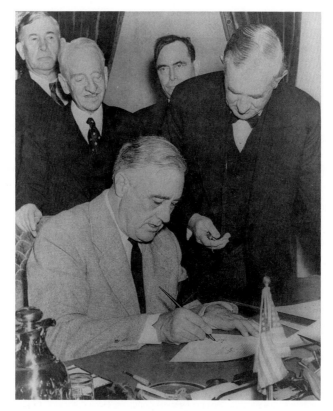

President Franklin Delano Roosevelt contracted polio as an adult and was paralyzed from the waist down for the rest of his life. Polio epidemics are now practically unheard of in the developed world thanks to the discovery of vaccines.

Source: Library of Congress [LC-USZ62-15185]

The terms *heart disease* and *cancer* are familiar, but *chronic lower respiratory disease* may not be. Also known as chronic obstructive pulmonary disease, **chronic lower respiratory disease** is a progressive disease that makes it hard to breathe; emphysema and chronic bronchitis are the two main conditions.

CHALLENGE OF THE 21ST CENTURY

The 10 leading causes of death in 2013 are shown in Figure 1.4. As we once faced the scourge of infectious diseases, we now face a different challenge to our health, one that won't be met by breakthroughs in medical technology or new drugs. We've learned that the rise of chronic diseases over the past several generations is due

Chronic lower respiratory disease is a progressive disease that makes it hard to breathe; also known as chronic obstructive pulmonary disease, emphysema and chronic bronchitis are the two main conditions and the leading cause is cigarette smoking.

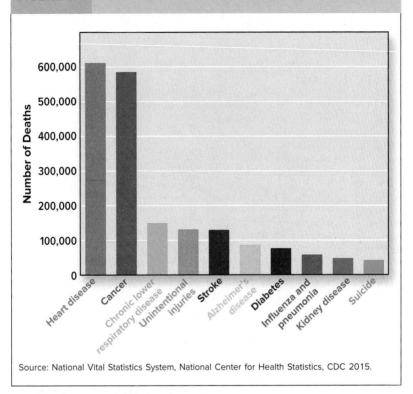

FIGURE 1.4 LEADING CAUSES OF DEATH

Source: National Vital Statistics System, National Center for Health Statistics, CDC 2015.

primarily to changes in our day-to-day habits. Accordingly, we refer to these medical conditions as "lifestyle diseases." Six of the first nine are chronic diseases: the first three in addition to stroke (#5), diabetes (#7), and kidney disease (#9) are tied to what we eat, how physically active we are, and whether or not we smoke. National estimates indicate that about 50 percent of disease and premature deaths (i.e., death before age 65) are due to unhealthy lifestyles. Heart disease, cancer, stroke, and diabetes will be discussed in Part 3.

When considering lifestyle diseases, another approach is to consider deaths by actual causes—the root causes—as opposed to the medical conditions listed on death certificates. In Figure 1.5, poor diet leads the list, resulting in an estimated 680,000 deaths annually; these are deaths whose official causes end up being heart disease, cancer, stroke, diabetes, or kidney disease among others. Tobacco use is number two, responsible for an estimated 466,000 deaths per year. Tobacco-attributed deaths cut across several chronic diseases, including 90 percent of deaths from lung cancer and chronic lower respiratory disease (chronic bronchitis and emphysema) and lower percentages of deaths from heart disease, stroke, and other cancers. Deaths due to low physical activity (234,000) is number three and accounts for more deaths than the next three causes combined. These life-shortening behaviors impact measures of disability in similar fashion. Clearly, our habits regarding eating, tobacco, exercise, and alcohol have a major impact on individual and population health.

FIGURE 1.5 ACTUAL CAUSES OF DEATH

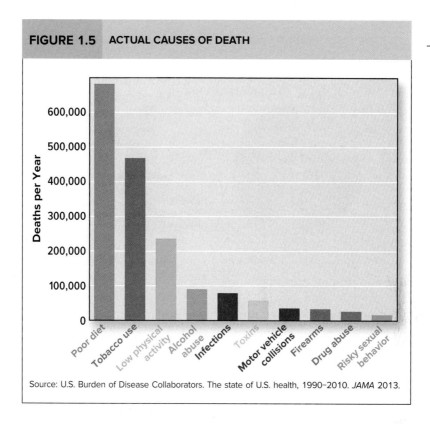

Source: U.S. Burden of Disease Collaborators. The state of U.S. health, 1990–2010. *JAMA* 2013.

Because most of you are young adults, let's consider the leading causes of death for your age group. Since death among young people is unusual, it should come as no surprise that for those aged 20–29 (Figure 1.6), the leading cause of death is unintentional injury, primarily motor vehicle accidents. The second and third leading causes of death are homicide and suicide. Causes of death remain similar for the age group 30–39. However, by early middle age—the 40–49 age group—cancer and heart disease are the first and second leading causes of deaths, a stark reminder that these diseases are not just diseases of older adults.

These statistics highlight the importance of using seat belts; being alert to thoughts of suicide; considering consequences regarding use of alcohol, drugs, and firearms; and screening for cancer (particularly melanoma) and heart disease. In addition to personally minimizing these risks, consider the positive influence you might have with your peers. A few words of concern and caution from a friend can make a big difference.

While leading causes of deaths are important to discuss, it's equally important to step back and acknowledge that risky behaviors more often lead to serious injury than to death. The incidence of permanent injuries resulting from accidents such as car crashes is often overlooked. The ratio of fatal to nonfatal but significant injuries is about 1 to 4. We all know of someone who survived a terrible accident yet sustained a life-changing injury such as brain damage or paralysis. The risk of death among young adults in America is low; the risk of disability, somewhat higher. Both are tragic—especially when preventable. Most serious accidents are linked to alcohol and drug abuse. Simply taking the time to consider the possible dire consequences

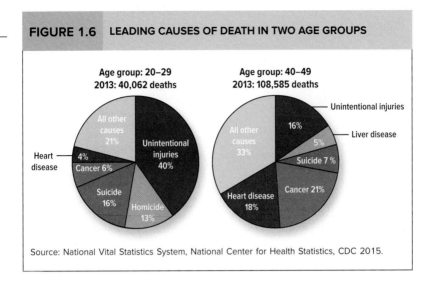

FIGURE 1.6   LEADING CAUSES OF DEATH IN TWO AGE GROUPS

Age group: 20–29
2013: 40,062 deaths

Age group: 40–49
2013: 108,585 deaths

All other causes 21%

Unintentional injuries 40%

Heart disease 4%

Cancer 6%

Suicide 16%

Homicide 13%

All other causes 33%

Unintentional injuries 16%

Liver disease 5%

Suicide 7%

Cancer 21%

Heart disease 18%

Source: National Vital Statistics System, National Center for Health Statistics, CDC 2015.

goes a long way in preventing dangerous situations. As my grandmother used to say, "Have fun but be careful!"

HEALTHY PEOPLE 2020

Every 10 years, the U.S. Department of Health and Human Services releases new national goals and objectives for health promotion and disease prevention. The most recent version, *Healthy People 2020* (**www.healthypeople.gov**), was released in December 2010. This comprehensive document is based on updated scientific and medical evidence as well as feedback from a wide range of government agencies, dozens of organizations, and the public. *Healthy People 2020* identifies the most significant preventable threats to public health and sets specific goals to reduce those risks. For example, health experts point out that the chronic diseases of heart disease, cancer, and diabetes are responsible for 7 of every 10 deaths among Americans each year and account for 75 percent of the nation's health spending. Since many of the risk factors contributing to the development of these diseases are preventable, a major challenge is to help people take specific actions to reduce risk and improve health.

The overarching goals of *Healthy People 2020* are:

1. Attain high-quality, longer lives free of preventable disease and premature death.
2. Achieve health equity, eliminate disparities, and improve the health of all groups.
3. Create social and physical environments that promote good health for all.
4. Promote quality of life, healthy development, and healthy behaviors across life stages.

The second goal is in response to known inequities due to race/ethnicity, socioeconomic status, gender, age, disability status, sexual orientation, and geographic location. The third and fourth goals are new and reflect a broader, more collaborative approach to improving the nation's health.

To progress toward these goals, the national plan uses an ecological approach focusing on both individual-level and population-level factors that influence health. This approach recognizes that health and health behaviors are determined

TABLE 1.1 DETERMINANTS OF HEALTH: TYPES AND EXAMPLES

INDIVIDUAL BEHAVIORS

- Diet
- Physical activity
- Alcohol, tobacco, and other drug use
- Hand washing

BIOLOGY AND GENETICS

- Age and gender
- Family history of heart disease
- Inherited conditions (e.g., hemophilia, cystic fibrosis)
- *BRCA1* or *BRCA2* mutation (higher risk for breast/ovarian cancer)

HEALTH SERVICES

- Lack of availability
- High cost
- Lack of insurance coverage
- Limited language access

PHYSICAL ENVIRONMENT DETERMINANTS

- Natural environment such as green space, weather, climate
- Worksites, schools, and recreational settings
- Housing, homes, and neighborhoods
- Exposure to toxic substances and other physical hazards

SOCIAL ENVIRONMENT DETERMINANTS

- Availability of quality schools
- Exposure to crime and violence
- Social support and social interactions
- Social norms and attitudes including discrimination

POLICYMAKING

- Food labeling laws
- Smoking bans in public places
- Gun control laws
- Auto safety standards (e.g., seat belts and air bags)

Source: *Healthy People 2020* (**www.healthypeople.gov**).

by influences at multiple levels, including personal (biological and psychological), organizational/institutional, environmental (social and physical), and policy levels. In the past, individual-level health approaches were the mainstay. With *Healthy People 2020,* though, an emphasis is placed on making our social and physical environments healthier. In Table 1.1, determinants of health are categorized and specific examples are provided for each category.

It's the interplay among factors such as those listed in Table 1.1 that determine individual and population health. Interventions that involve multiple determinants are most likely to be effective. The lesson here is that our health is influenced by a combination of factors beyond the boundaries of standard health care and public

TABLE 1.2 — *HEALTHY PEOPLE 2020:* HEALTH INDICATORS AND TOPIC AREAS

LEADING HEALTH INDICATORS

1. Healthy behaviors
2. Tobacco use
3. Substance abuse
4. Responsible sexual behavior
5. Mental health
6. Chronic disease
7. Injury and violence
8. Environmental determinants
9. Social determinants
10. Maternal and infant health
11. Access to care
12. Quality of care

TOPIC AREAS (LISTED ALPHABETICALLY)

1. Access to health services
2. Adolescent health*
3. Arthritis, osteoporosis, chronic back conditions
4. Blood disorders and blood safety*
5. Cancer
6. Chronic kidney disease
7. Dementias including Alzheimer's disease*
8. Diabetes
9. Disability and health
10. Early and middle childhood*
11. Educational and community-based programs
12. Environmental health
13. Family planning
14. Food safety
15. Genomics*
16. Global health*
17. Health communication and health information technology
18. Health care–associated infections*
19. Health-related quality of life*
20. Hearing and related disorders
21. Heart disease and stroke
22. HIV
23. Immunization and infectious diseases
24. Injury and violence prevention
25. Lesbian, gay, bisexual, and transgender health*
26. Maternal, infant, and child health
27. Medical product safety
28. Mental health and disorders
29. Nutrition and weight status
30. Occupational safety and health
31. Older adults*
32. Oral health
33. Physical activity
34. Preparedness*
35. Public health infrastructure
36. Respiratory diseases
37. Sexually transmitted diseases
38. Sleep health*
39. Social determinants of health*
40. Substance abuse
41. Tobacco use
42. Vision

*Indicates new topic area in *Healthy People 2020*.

Sources: Institute of Medicine (**www.iom.edu**); *Healthy People 2020* (**www.healthypeople.gov**).

health. For example, harmful aspects of social and physical environments negatively impact us individually and collectively. Over the next decade, public health experts believe that establishing effective partnerships among different sectors of a community (e.g., education, housing, transportation, agriculture, business) will be instrumental to improving population health.

The 12 leading health indicators and 42 topic areas for *Healthy People 2020* are presented in Table 1.2. The leading health indicators represent the nation's most pressing public health issues. They are intended to help Americans—health professionals *and* consumers—understand which areas we need to focus on to improve our health and the health of our families and communities. The 42 topic areas provide a comprehensive framework for goal setting across the spectrum of public health issues. Be sure to notice the 13 new topic areas—for example, genomics, global health, preparedness, and sleep health. Also, the health communication area has been expanded and now includes an emphasis on information technology to improve population health outcomes and health care quality. As society and the world change, so too do our public health needs. Both the priority health indicators and wide-ranging topic areas underscore our role in making healthy choices—for ourselves and those close to us—about doctors, health insurance, health information, and a healthy lifestyle.

In *iHealth* you will find chapters, chapter sections, or selected articles on all 12 of the leading health indicators. As *iHealth* is purposely concise, all indicators do not have their own chapter. Rather, discussions on selected indicators—including injury and violence, environmental determinants, social determinants, and maternal and infant health—are featured in articles and intertwined as appropriate within related chapters.

The public health goal reflected by indicator 7 (and topic 24) is to reduce injuries, disabilities, and deaths due to injuries and violence. Most people sustain a significant injury at some time during their lives. Some mistakenly believe that injuries happen by chance and are the result of unpreventable accidents. On reflection, though, most of us know that is not the case. Most injuries are predictable and preventable. As noted previously, the leading cause of death among young adults is injury. Most injuries—unintentional and intentional—are associated with motor vehicle crashes, firearms, poisoning, falls, fires, and drowning, and the vast majority of these occur under the influence of alcohol or drugs.

Violence is also sometimes a factor in injuries. Date rape, spousal abuse, gang violence, and the mass murders at Virginia Tech in 2007 are examples, from the more common to the rare. We all agree that such grievous incidents must be prevented whenever possible. Yet, what can we do? As you study the chapters on drugs, sexuality, stress, mental disorders, and personal health care, thoughtfully weigh the injury and violence issues and consider preventive actions you can take.

For public health indicators 8 and 9 (and topics 12 and 39), the goal is to promote well-being for all through healthy physical and social environments. The quality of the physical environment in which we live is a crucial factor. Examples include preventing or managing exposure to hazardous agents (biological, chemical, physical) in the air, water, soil, and food. Concerns about our physical environment also relate to our broader social environment and a range of diverse issues—from carpooling to city planning to the homeless. Our social and physical environments overlap and interact in many areas such as housing, land use, transportation, agriculture, manufacturing, and public safety. How can we give higher priority to protecting our living spaces and providing social networks and services that support healthy living?

Global environmental health issues also need to be faced. For instance, the effects of pathogens (disease-causing microbes) on food supplies and health are an increasing concern as world markets and international travel continue to expand. Then there are the calamities of natural disasters and the ever-present threat of bioterrorism. Less sensational but perhaps even more serious is the impact of over-population on health. Can we avert planetary overload and environmental degradation by controlling population growth and managing environmental resources? On these global issues, is multinational cooperation possible? Although it may be difficult to think of ourselves as members of a world community, it's becoming more of a reality every day and warrants our attention and action. Consider how our

Article
1.3

environment—both social and physical aspects—influences individual, community, and population health as you read the chapters on diet, stress, mental health, cancers, infections, and health care.

WHAT LIES AHEAD?

Descriptions of today's achievements in science, technology, and medicine read like the science fiction of your grandparents' generation. What medical advances are on the horizon over the next decade? And, importantly, what are the implications for such progress? Selected health trends associated with key scientific concepts provide examples of what the future holds:

- Based on human genome research, the ability to screen for genetically based diseases and to tailor interventions will be greatly expanded. Issues associated with genetic counseling, patient privacy, and insurability will continue to be debated.
- Major advances will continue to be made in noninvasive medical imaging designed to screen for and diagnose cancers, heart disease, and neurological disorders such as depression and Alzheimer's disease. Next-generation scanners will be faster, more accurate, and less burdensome on patients.
- The concept of racial blending will begin to replace the traditional racial-categories paradigm. Reducing health disparities among groups will no longer be based on race per se, but rather on economic, educational, and cultural factors.
- A grand melding of molecular biology, genetic engineering, and nanotechnology will strengthen the drug discovery and delivery process. Pharmacological research will develop drugs to treat every major disease.
- Advances in biomedical engineering will yield a new generation of tissue and organ replacements and improve the transplantation process. Growing and harvesting tissues in the laboratory will become a reality.

These examples give a sense of the wondrous medical advances that are being made. Yet, such scientific and technological developments must be seriously considered and debated in light of ethical, social, and economic implications before translation into public policy.

Article 1.4

Our health will continue to be influenced by a wide array of scientific advances, public health goals, changing societal expectations, and new and revised governmental policies. Yet, at the level of the individual and the family, it's ironic that the greatest potential benefit for the future health of Americans is not biomedical research. Rather, as prominent scientific and medical experts increasingly agree, the greatest promise for improved health lies with preventive medicine and a focus on understanding health as a consequence of human behavior.

✓ NEED TO KNOW

Over the past century, tremendous gains have been made in lifespan and quality of life due largely to major advances in public health, drug discovery, and medical technology. Today the major causes of death are chronic diseases, not infectious diseases. Chronic diseases—such as heart disease, cancer, and diabetes (type 2)—are strongly tied to how we choose to live, to our daily habits. The nation's high-priority health issues are summarized in *Healthy People 2020*. They remind us that environmental factors (social and physical) also influence our health.

Textbooks on personal health focus primarily on knowledge and secondarily on contextual factors that influence our views and behaviors. Perhaps it is time to switch the emphasis and focus more on behavior change, as *knowledge by itself does not ensure good decision making.* If it did, we would not see physicians who smoke or dietitians who are overweight. Attitudes, beliefs, and values as well as knowledge underlie our decisions about health. This mix of influences makes it unlikely that a single factor is the basis of any given health decision. How can knowledge be separated from attitudes? Or attitudes from values? Decision making is clearly dependent on multiple factors.

The presentation of content is never done in a vacuum. Attitudes, beliefs, and values are shaped by our environment. The influence of family, friends, school, workplace, the media, and societal customs is substantial. Both formal and informal learning occur within these social and societal contexts. No individual makes decisions that are truly independent of all other persons and the society in which we live. The process by which we learn a new behavior or modify a current one is multifaceted. An appreciation of this is a prerequisite to understanding behavior.

Many of us have good intentions about changing an unhealthy habit (e.g., quitting smoking) or adopting a healthier behavior (e.g., eating more fruits and vegetables). The challenge is *how* to do it. As pointed out, our behaviors are complex, and from personal experience we know habits are not changed easily. So if we wish to change a behavior, we need a well-grounded plan. But before we can make a plan, we must first have a basic understanding of how people change.

To better understand health habits and behavior change, psychologists have developed **health behavior theories.** Dissecting a behavior into its components and seeing the logic that connects the pieces can provide insights to our behaviors. Briefly reviewing several theories can be instructive because each takes a different approach to analyzing and explaining behavior changes. Three of the most practical theories are social cognitive theory, the health belief model, and the stages of change model. A brief overview of each is presented; more complete explanations are available in the online booklet *Theory at a Glance.*

SOCIAL COGNITIVE THEORY

Albert Bandura's social cognitive theory is based on the principle that behavior is dynamic, depending on individual and environmental factors, all of which influence one another simultaneously. As illustrated in Figure 1.7, there is an ongoing interaction among a person's characteristics (biological, psychological, experiential), the environment within which the behavior is performed (social influences, physical environment, societal norms), and the specific behavior's characteristics.

A **health behavior theory** is a conceptual framework of key factors or variables hypothesized to influence health behavior. An established theory is logical, supported by evidence, and underpins behavior change plans and strategies.

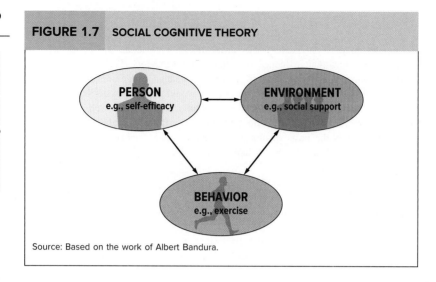

FIGURE 1.7 SOCIAL COGNITIVE THEORY

Source: Based on the work of Albert Bandura.

A change in one component of the model will affect the others. To see how this works, let's use exercise as a behavior we wish to increase (target behavior). A personal characteristic such as confidence in being able to exercise for 30 minutes on a treadmill (an example of self-efficacy) will influence whether the person does, in fact, perform that behavior. Characteristics of the environment include available facilities (e.g., fitness center or exercise equipment) and associated factors such as affordability, convenience, and safety. The environment also includes the social environment (e.g., the degree to which family and friends encourage and support the person's new exercise routine). Finally, the positive and negative characteristics of the behavior itself must be considered (e.g., whether the exercise was invigorating, challenging, and completed with a sense of accomplishment or exhausting, boring, and frustrating).

Social cognitive theory holds that the interactions among the individual, the environment, and the specific behavior are subtle and complex, but it provides a framework for understanding them. This ecological approach attempts to encompass all possible determinants of health behavior for individuals in their everyday lives. A key point is that success in changing a health behavior is just not a matter of self-determination. In addition to intention and commitment, an awareness of other potential intervening factors is necessary. The ecological framework for understanding population health (inclusion of environmental determinants, both social and physical) adopted by *Healthy People 2020* can be seen as an expansion of social cognitive theory.

HEALTH BELIEF MODEL

Irwin Rosenstock's health belief model, one of the first theories of health behavior, was developed in the 1950s to explain why so few people participated in a national chest X-ray screening program for tuberculosis. The hypothesis was that

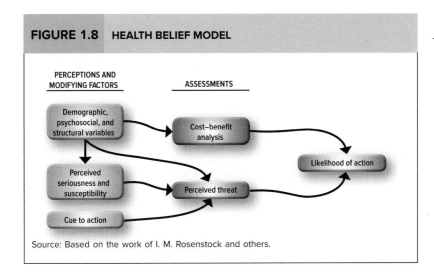

FIGURE 1.8   **HEALTH BELIEF MODEL**

Source: Based on the work of I. M. Rosenstock and others.

many people hold mistaken beliefs about a disease or the screening process and that this keeps them from taking advantage of beneficial screening. In recent years, the health belief model has been used to improve participation in mammogram screening and to prevent the spread of sexually transmitted infections (STIs) and HIV.

The premise of the health belief model is that health-seeking behavior is influenced by a person's perception of a threat posed by a health problem and the value associated with actions aimed at reducing that threat. This involves a sequence from perception to assessment to action (or inaction). As seen in Figure 1.8, a person first forms a belief about the seriousness of and susceptibility to a medical condition. How dangerous is it? Will I get it? Cues to action (e.g., media campaigns, advice from others, illness of family member, doctor's explanation) can influence the person's perceived threat. A host of factors—both individual (e.g., age, gender, personality, personal experience) and socioeconomic (e.g., peer pressure, ethnicity, education, income)—play a role in the perception of risk and the person's cost−benefit analysis (barriers to action versus benefits of action).

The model predicts that individuals will take action (e.g., screening, treatment) if (1) they perceive themselves to be susceptible and that the condition will have serious consequences (high perceived threat), and (2) they believe a successful course of action to reduce susceptibility or minimize consequences is available and the benefits of taking action outweigh the barriers (positive cost−benefit analysis). The final step to take action is then dependent on the person's confidence to follow through (self-efficacy). The health belief model has been applied to sex education programs that aim to prevent STIs and HIV by increasing condom use, as well as in secondary prevention efforts to aid early detection of STIs or HIV. This model provides a framework for individuals, health care workers, and educators to use in understanding and intervening in the spread of these conditions.

STAGES OF CHANGE MODEL

James Prochaska and Carlo DiClemente's stages of change model—technically known as the transtheoretical model—is often integrated with other theories (hence *trans-* or "across"). The central premise is that behavior change is a process, not an event, and that individuals have varying levels of motivation or readiness to change. For most health behaviors, there appear to be five stages of change: (1) precontemplation—not thinking about change, (2) contemplation—thinking about change, (3) preparation—making small changes toward the desired behavior, (4) action—actually engaging in the desired behavior, and (5) maintenance—sustaining the new behavior over a prolonged period (Figure 1.9). The model predicts that individuals progress through these stages, but it also recognizes that setbacks occur. People can and do relapse to previous stages. This is accepted as a normal part of the change process.

The stages of change model was initially developed as a framework to understand smoking cessation programs. Over the years, the model has been adapted and used with a number of other health behaviors including eating and physical activity. The conceptual appeal of the stages of change model is that specific behavior-change strategies can be matched to specific stages. The type of information, counseling, incentives, or reinforcement can be tailored to an individual's level of readiness or motivation (stage of change). Time frames may be associated with specific stages; for example, the "action stage" typically refers to the first six months of change, and the "maintenance stage" refers to continuing the behavior beyond six months. After several years, the target behavior becomes an established habit and part of one's lifestyle.

Across many different behavior-change theories, four factors appear to be necessary for successful change to occur: a *knowledge* or awareness of the benefit of the change, the *motivation* to take action, the *opportunity* in terms of resources and

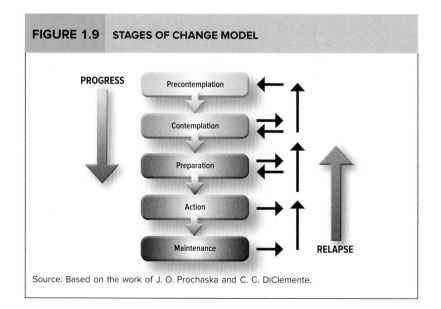

FIGURE 1.9 STAGES OF CHANGE MODEL

Source: Based on the work of J. O. Prochaska and C. C. DiClemente.

time, and the necessary *behavioral skills.* Your personal health course and *iHealth* are oriented toward increasing knowledge and assisting you in developing the requisite skill set (planning, organizational, and behavior-specific skills) to modify or adopt a target behavior. Increased motivation may be a byproduct of the class experience as well. When thinking about changing a health behavior, use the behavior-change models and keep the four common factors in mind: *knowledge, motivation, opportunity,* and *skills.*

NEED TO KNOW

Behavior change is a complex process and often difficult to sustain. Developing healthy behaviors sometimes means competing against ingrained social and environmental practices. Information by itself is typically not enough. The benefits of behavior change must be compelling and outweigh the barriers. Three widely used health behavior models are social cognitive theory, the health belief model, and the stages of change model. Across models, four factors appear to be necessary for successful behavior change: knowledge, motivation, opportunity, and skills. Use conceptual frameworks and these four factors to guide you in making healthful lifestyle changes.

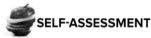

ARTICLES

1.1 "No Truth to the Fountain of Youth." *Scientific American*. While no anti-aging product has been proven to be a true cure, some products have been proven dangerous.
1.2 "Simple Tools for Understanding Risks: From Innumeracy to Insight." *British Medical Journal*. A psychologist and a medical professor discuss common pitfalls in medical decision making related to not understanding statistics.
1.3 "Global Warming: No Big Deal?" *The Atlantic*. How personal risk perception colors a person's worldview on broad issues such as global warming.
1.4 "Getting Serious about the Prevention of Chronic Diseases." *Preventing Chronic Disease*. Two public health experts talk about key strategies to include in the health reform movement.

SELF-ASSESSMENT

1.1 Consider the Six Dimensions of Health

Website Resources

Centers for Disease Control and Prevention **www.cdc.gov**
Family Doctor **www.familydoctor.org**
Health Finder **www.healthfinder.gov**
Health Literacy & Communication **www.health.gov/communication**
Healthy People 2020 **www.healthypeople.gov**
Kids Health **kidshealth.org**
Mayo Clinic **www.mayoclinic.com**
Medical Library Association **www.mlanet.org/for-health-consumers**
Medline Plus **medlineplus.gov**
NIH Senior Health **nihseniorhealth.gov/**
Office of Minority Health **minorityhealth.hhs.gov/**
Theory at a Glance **www.sneb.org/2014/Theory**
U.S. Census Bureau **www.census.gov**
WebMD **www.webmd.com**
World Health Organization **www.who.int/en/**

Knowing the Language

1. Contrast the medical treatment model and the optimal health model.
2. What is meant by *health literacy*? What are the underlying factors that contribute to a person's health literacy?
3. What is epidemiology? Contrast the terms *absolute risk* and *relative risk*. As a young adult, what are your greatest risks for injury or illness and death?
4. Contrast the terms *infectious disease* and *chronic disease*. What is meant by the term *lifestyle disease*? What are the leading *actual* causes of disease in the United States?
5. Describe two behavior-change theories and how they could be used to help a person improve a health behavior.

Exploring Ideas

1. Why should health be thought of as having different dimensions? How can this be helpful in improving our health or achieving personal goals?
2. To what degree do you have control over your current quality of life? Is it determined by your conscious decision making or by factors beyond your control?
3. How should one go about gathering information on a health topic? Select a health question, investigate it, and report on the process and your findings.

Selected References

Atlanta Journal Constitution. Lizzie Brown, 111, calm, kind, centenarian. Obituary section, January 6, 2003.

Bandura A. *Self-efficacy: The Exercise of Control.* New York: W. H. Freeman, 1997.

Centers for Disease Control and Prevention. Mortality Data, National Vital Statistics System, National Center for Health Statistics, 2015.

Centers for Disease Control and Prevention. Ten great public health achievements—United States, 1900–1999. *MMWR* 48: 241–243, 1999.

Corbett S. The long road from Sudan to America. *New York Times,* April 1, 2001.

Glanz K, Rimer BK, Viswanath K. *Health Behavior and Health Education: Theory, Research, and Practice* (5th ed.). San Francisco: Jossey-Bass, 2015.

Institute of Medicine. *Health Literacy: Past, Present, and Future.* Washington, DC: National Academies Press, 2015.

Institute of Medicine. *Leading Health Indicators for Healthy People 2020.* Washington, DC: National Academies Press, 2011.

McMichael AJ. *Planetary Overload: Global Environmental Change and the Health of the Human Species.* New York: Cambridge University Press, 1993.

National Institute of Aging. Understanding Risk: What Do Those Headlines Really Mean? **www.nia.nih.gov/health/publication/understanding-risk**

Prochaska JO, DiClemente CC. Stages and processes of self-change of smoking: Toward an integrated model of change. *Journal of Consulting and Clinical Psychology* 51: 390–395, 1983.

Rauscher FH, Shaw GL, Ky KN. Music and spatial task performance. *Nature* 365: 611, 1993.

Ropeik D. *How Risky Is It, Really? Why Our Fears Don't Always Match the Facts.* New York: McGraw-Hill, 2010.

Rosenstock IM, Strecher VJ, Becker MH. Social learning theory and the health belief model. *Health Education Quarterly* 15: 175–183, 1988.

Schwartz B. *The Paradox of Choice: Why More Is Less.* New York: HarperCollins, 2004.

U.S. Burden of Disease Collaborators. The state of U.S. health, 1990–2010. *JAMA* 310: 591–606, 2013.

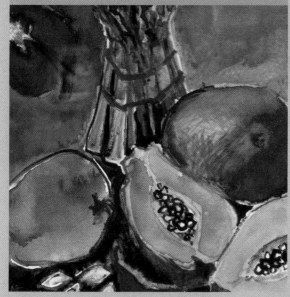

*It's difficult to think
anything but pleasant
thoughts while eating a
homegrown tomato.*

—Lewis Grizzard

© Marilyn Simler/Illustration Works/Getty Images

Chapter 2

CHOOSE A HEALTHY DIET

In Chapter 2 we discuss food, a subject near and dear to all.
We present the basic vocabulary of nutrition and current recommendations for a healthy diet, and we discuss steps and strategies to improve our eating habits. We give special attention to
the topic of weight control because it is of particular interest
and relevance. Our aim is to separate the science from the
advertising and show you how to navigate the gray areas.

A CENTURY AGO, the majority of Americans lived on farms and raised their own food. Nearly every family had a vegetable garden and kept chickens for eggs. Working the garden and canning (and later freezing) the "produce" (vegetables and fruits) was standard practice. It was essential to stock the pantry to provide for food throughout the winter and into the spring. Many homesteads had a milk cow. Some also raised hogs or cattle for meat. Sausage and ham or beef cuts were bartered in exchange for other goods. Grains were taken to a central stone mill to be ground into flour. The food supply was direct and simple; food was minimally processed. Agribusiness and the food industry were in their infancy.

Life was physically demanding, whether working on the farm or in a mill, mine, or factory. And the way people ate reflected the physical demands of how they lived. Breakfast, a hearty hot meal, included meat and eggs, not cereal out of a box. Dinner—the midday meal—was the largest meal of the day, with meats, vegetables, and bread or biscuits, made from scratch every day. Lunch was a meal that evolved in the cities. The evening meal, known as supper, was a lighter meal, often leftovers from dinner.

Unlike today, an ample food supply was not a given. There were good years and lean years, depending on the weather, crop infestations, natural disasters, and human and animal epidemics. A plentiful harvest was celebrated, and hard times were endured. Think of the changes your great-grandparents lived through and how those changes affected their eating patterns. Examples include transitioning from rural to city life, the development of refrigeration and modern appliances, new job opportunities not dependent on manual labor, and the ever-expanding grocery store.

Over the past century, dramatic changes have occurred in nearly every aspect of American life, including how and what we eat. Thanks to the scientific research of the past 30 to 40 years, we have an excellent understanding of the connections between nutrition and health. Without question, food resources and nutrition knowledge are far more extensive today than when your grandparents were your age. By considering the historical perspective, you can better appreciate the current food environment and understand the origins of the diet-related health challenges we now face. Your generation can share in the bounty of food choices available today but also must face pressing contemporary issues such as obesity, eating disorders, and dietary supplements. Keep this in mind as you study this chapter and learn to eat healthier.

➤ Nutrition Basics

Nutrition is the science of food and how the body uses it in health and disease. A nutrient is simply a substance found in food that is used by the body to support normal growth, maintenance, and repair. The six nutrient classes are carbohydrates, fats, protein, vitamins, minerals, and water.

Nutrients can be broadly categorized based on the quantity that should be consumed. The **macronutrients**—carbohydrates, fats, protein, and water—are the main

---

Macronutrients are nutrients that are the main constituents of our food—carbohydrates, fats, proteins, and water.

TABLE 2.1	MACRONUTRIENTS: ENERGY DENSITY AND RANGES FOR DAILY ENERGY INTAKE	
	ENERGY DENSITY	**ENERGY INTAKE**
Carbohydrates	4 Cal/gram	45–65%
Emphasize complex carbohydrates		Minimize added sugars to ≤10%
Fats	9 Cal/gram	20–35%
Emphasize unsaturated fats		Minimize saturated & *trans* fats to ≤10%
Protein	4 Cal/gram	10–35%

Sources: *Dietary Guidelines;* Academy of Nutrition and Dietetics.

constituents of our food and form the bulk of what we eat every day. In contrast, the **micronutrients**—vitamins and minerals—are needed only in small quantities, and many are not required daily. Micronutrients occur naturally in many of our unprocessed foods such as fruits, vegetables, and whole grains.

Nutrients are also categorized based on whether they are energy sources. Carbohydrates, fats, and protein are the energy nutrients. Vitamins, minerals, and water do not yield energy, but their presence in the body is necessary to aid in the proper use of the energy nutrients. Consequently, vitamins, minerals, and water are known as regulatory nutrients.

From a biological perspective, good nutrition is about providing both the right blend of nutrients and adequate fuel (energy) for the body's many needs. Balancing energy intake with energy expenditure is fundamental to maintaining a healthy weight. Weight control, a widely debated and often controversial topic, is addressed later in this chapter. In terms of basic nutrition, energy density (energy yield per weight) and recommended ranges for daily energy intake by macronutrient are summarized in Table 2.1.

For the sake of clarity, a comment about energy units is warranted. The common energy unit in the United States is the **Calorie (Cal), or kilocalorie (kcal).** (For the curious, the rest of the world uses the kilojoule, abbreviated kj.) Technically, 1 Cal, or kcal, is the amount of heat needed to raise 1 kg of water 1°Celsius. Yes, a Calorie (with a capital "C") is the same as a kilocalorie. Both terms are widely used: Food labels typically report Calories, while energy expenditure is often expressed in kilocalories. For example, a 12-oz. can of Coca-Cola contains 140 Cal, which is equivalent to the 140 kcal expended in walking 1.5 miles. To remove any confusion, our convention in *iHealth* is to use only Calories (Cal) when reporting energy intake or expenditure values.

Micronutrients are the nutrients needed only in small quantities, the vitamins and minerals.

Calorie (Cal), or alternately the **kilocalorie (kcal),** is the standard unit of energy used in the United States to define and describe human energy intake and energy expenditure.

The main function of **carbohydrates** is to provide energy. They are your body's main energy source, the primary fuel for your cells. Each gram of carbohydrate yields approximately 4 Cal, the same as a gram of protein. Carbohydrates should compose the largest percentage of daily caloric intake, at about 55 percent (within a range of 45–65 percent). Carbohydrates include both starches and sugars. Starches, or complex carbohydrates, are found in bread, rice, pasta, cereals, and vegetables. Sugars, or simple carbohydrates, are natural constituents of fruits and milk, while added sugar is common in processed foods and drinks—such as candy, pastries, desserts, and soft drinks.

In addition to supplying energy, complex carbohydrates and sugars from fruits and milk supply fiber, vitamins, minerals, and water. Consequently, they should be emphasized over sugars from candy, other sweets, and soft drinks. In addition, your body absorbs complex carbohydrates more slowly than it absorbs sugars, providing more energy for a longer period. A key point: sugar-laden snacks and desserts provide many calories but offer negligible amounts of other nutrients. That is why typical junk foods are often referred to as having "empty calories," or as having low nutrient density. In the United States, soft drinks are the top source of added sugars.

Fiber—also referred to as roughage—is the indigestible part of plant-based foods. Nutritionists divide fiber into two types: soluble and insoluble. Soluble fiber may improve your cholesterol and blood sugar (glucose) levels. It's found in oats, dried beans, and some fruits. Insoluble fiber adds bulk to your stool and helps prevent constipation. It also reduces your risk of colorectal cancer. It's found mainly in vegetables, whole grains, and wheat bran. The average American consumes only 10 to 15 g (grams) of total fiber per day. Federal guidelines recommend 25 g per day for women and 38 g per day for men.

Self
Assessment
2.1

What's the best way to increase fiber? Eat a variety of whole grains, vegetables, legumes (peas, beans, lentils), and fruits. When buying bread, look for the word *whole* next to the name of the grain in the list of ingredients (e.g., whole wheat). Select bread with at least 3 g of fiber per slice and cereals with 3 g or more of fiber per serving. Try whole-wheat pasta—it typically has three times the amount of fiber as regular pasta.

To help encourage Americans to eat a variety of fruits and vegetables every day, the Produce for Better Health Foundation administers a web page with interactive features: **fruitsandveggiesmorematters.org.** You can calculate how many fruits and vegetables you need and get tips for adding more servings into your daily routine. The guideline is five or more servings of fruits and vegetables every day. The more the better!

FATS AND CHOLESTEROL

Fats, or lipids, in the diet serve several purposes. They are the most concentrated energy source, yielding about 9 Cal per gram, more than twice that of carbohydrate

Carbohydrates are organic compounds (i.e., they contain carbon, oxygen, hydrogen) divided into two types—simple and complex; they are generally known as sugars and starches.

Fats, or lipids, are organic compounds that provide the most concentrated source of calories in a diet. Saturated fats are found primarily in animal products, and unsaturated fats come from plants.

or protein. The Academy of Nutrition and Dietetics recommend that fats comprise 20–35 percent of daily energy intake. Fats satisfy hunger because of their slow absorption rate from the digestive system. Fats also play a role in many other functions, such as maintenance and function of cell membranes and the absorption of the four fat-soluble vitamins (A, D, E, and K).

Just as there are different types of carbohydrates, there are different types of fats, some to avoid and others to emphasize. Let's discuss those to avoid first—saturated fats and *trans* fats. Saturated fats come primarily from animal sources such as red meats and dairy products (butter, cream, whole milk, cheese), but also from palm and coconut oils, which come from plants. Saturated fats are generally solid at room temperature. *Trans* fats are the other harmful type of fat. They are vegetable oils chemically converted to a solid form; refer to "Breaking It Down" for the full story. Diets high in saturated fats and *trans* fats elevate risk of cardiovascular disease, so limit consumption to no more than 10 percent of total daily calories.

Self
Assessment
2.2

Remember, though, all fats do not get the thumbs down. Unsaturated fats are good for us! These fats are mainly plant-based and are liquid at room temperature. Polyunsaturated fats like corn, safflower, and sunflower oils are healthy choices. And monounsaturated fats like olive, peanut, and canola oils are even better, being the most healthful of the unsaturated fats. Also, substantial evidence indicates that omega-3 fatty acids—found in certain types of fish, such as salmon—bestow a variety of benefits, particularly to cardiovascular health.

Cholesterol is a fatlike substance found throughout cells of the body. It is an essential substance that the body can obtain through diet or by production in the liver. All animal fats contain cholesterol, whereas fats from plant sources do not. Concentrated sources include eggs yolks (about 200 mg per yolk) and meats (60–100 mg per 3-oz. serving). For several decades, a diet high in cholesterol was thought to be a key cause of heart disease. In the last few years, this has been shown to be false. Accordingly, the *2015–2020 Dietary Guidelines* no longer recommends limiting cholesterol. We now know the primary dietary determinant of high blood cholesterol, a major risk factor for heart disease, is high intake of saturated fats and *trans* fats, not cholesterol. Paradoxical but true.

PROTEIN

Protein, which is contained in every cell in your body, is necessary for tissue growth and maintenance. Protein is found in foods from animal and plant sources. Each gram of protein yields about 4 Cal, the same as carbohydrate. However, its role as an energy source is secondary to that of carbohydrate and fat. Poultry, seafood, meat, dairy products, legumes (beans, peas, peanuts, soy products), nuts, and seeds are the richest sources of proteins. About 15 percent of total daily calories should come from protein (range, 10–35 percent). A higher protein intake (20–35 percent) may be beneficial for certain individuals. As more studies are published on this issue, dietary advice will evolve.

The basic components of proteins are amino acids. Of the 22 amino acids used in the body, only 9 are necessary in the diet and thus are known as the

Proteins are complex organic compounds made up of amino acids that perform a wide variety of functions that include serving as structural components, enzymes, and signaling molecules.

The unusual story of *trans* fats deserves mention in any discussion of dietary fats. *Trans* fats are produced when unsaturated oils are partially hydrogenated (through the addition of hydrogen), a process that converts vegetable oils to more solid forms. This conversion increases shelf life and flavor stability. In 1911 Procter & Gamble introduced Crisco, a product of hydrogenation. It was the first solidified shortening product made entirely of vegetable oil. Crisco provided an economical alternative to lard (animal fat) and butter. In the 1940s stick margarines were introduced, followed by tub margarines and vegetable oil spreads in the 1960s. With a growing awareness of the health risks of saturated fats, the scientific community promoted the use of margarine—an unsaturated fat—as the healthy alternative to butter. The resulting increase in the use of *trans* fats occurred not only in our kitchens but also in restaurants and the fast-food and baking industries as hydrogenated vegetable oils replaced lard.

At that time, there was no way to know that the process of hydrogenation chemically altered vegetable oil in a detrimental way. Yet, by the 1990s, substantial evidence had come to light showing that *trans* fats are actually as harmful, or even more harmful, in increasing blood cholesterol levels as the saturated fats they were meant to replace. In recent years, the challenge has been to update the American consumer. In 2003, after further study and careful review, the Food and Drug Administration (FDA) mandated that by 2006 all food labels must report the amount of *trans* fats as well as saturated and unsaturated fats. Many food companies have already reduced or eliminated *trans* fats in their products. The bottom line: Check the food labels and eat as few *trans* fats as possible.

So we have come full circle. Vegetable shortening and margarine (*trans* fats from hydrogenation) were initially hailed as a healthy, practical option to lard and butter and widely accepted by the public. In the ensuing years, the effects of eating the new *trans* fats were studied, and they were found to be as dangerous as or worse than animal-based fats. What's the lesson? Creating new food products can have both upsides and downsides, and sometimes only time will reveal them.

essential amino acids. The body has the ability to manufacture the remaining 13. Animal protein is complete, containing all 9 essential amino acids in sufficient amounts. In contrast, plant proteins are incomplete, lacking one or more of the essential amino acids. However, different plant foods can be eaten together to supply a complete protein, such as beans with rice or peanut butter on whole-grain bread. These complementary plant–protein relationships are especially important to vegetarians.

The amount of protein your body needs depends primarily on your body size. Recommended protein intake is 0.8 g per kg of body weight per day. For example, if you weigh 154 lb. (70 kg), then you should be consuming 56 g of protein per day. Most Americans typically consume far more protein than they need. What happens to those excess calories? If your body does not need the protein, it converts and stores those extra calories as fat. A final tip: Remember to choose your sources of proteins wisely. Many of the high-protein animal-based foods are also high in saturated fat. Emphasize meats that are lean, skinless, and nonfried, and consider obtaining some of your protein from plant sources.

VITAMINS AND MINERALS

Vitamins (organic compounds) and **minerals** (chemical elements) are found only in small quantities in our food, yet these micronutrients have multiple and diverse roles in regulating and maintaining our bodies' functions. Many play special roles in the prevention and treatment of common chronic diseases. Federal standards for good nutrition (known as Dietary Reference Intakes) are available for 13 vitamins and 15 minerals and are organized by age, gender, and special conditions such as pregnancy. A link to these detailed tables is provided under Website Resources at the end of the chapter. Although a complete review of the micronutrients is beyond the scope of *iHealth,* we provide a brief overview to set the stage for further self-directed study.

Vitamins are either fat-soluble or water-soluble. The fat-soluble vitamins—A, D, E, and K—are necessary for the function or structural integrity of specific body tissues and membranes and are retained in the body. Most water-soluble vitamins are catalysts or coenzymes in metabolic processes and energy transfer and are excreted fairly rapidly.

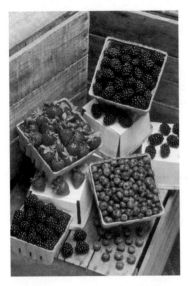

Berries are examples of antioxidant-rich foods.

© Scott Bauer/USDA

It is important to highlight the potential benefits of vitamins A, E, and C as antioxidants; antioxidants counter the harmful oxidative effects of free radicals and in so doing may protect body cells from damage.

Calcium, iron, sodium, and potassium are four minerals familiar to many of us because they are linked to medical conditions. Low calcium intake is related to osteoporosis (brittle bones), a disease that impacts women more than men. Low iron intake can lead to anemia (iron-deficiency anemia), particularly in young women. Conversely, high intakes of some minerals can be problematic. Excess iron intake (iron overload) in men increases risk for heart disease and cancer, and high sodium intake is related to hypertension in both men and women.

Vitamins are a class of diverse organic substances that occur in many foods in small amounts and are necessary in trace amounts for the normal metabolic functioning of the body.

Minerals are a group of inorganic elements that are essential to a variety of physiological processes and are obtained through the foods and beverages we consume.

Temporary deficiencies may lead to acute conditions. For example, the nausea and weakness associated with dehydration and heat illness are due in part to loss of potassium and sodium in sweat, as these minerals regulate water balance and nerve function. Accordingly, these minerals are put in sports drinks to aid recovery. As with vitamins, several minerals including selenium and manganese have been identified as antioxidants.

For additional information on vitamins and minerals, visit the website: **ods.od.nih.gov/factsheets/list-VitaminsMinerals.**

WATER

Water is the most essential nutrient. For many Americans, though, water could just as well be called the forgotten nutrient as sweetened beverages dominate everyday fluid consumption patterns. People can ingest too few (or none) of the other nutrients for days or weeks before problems arise—not so with water. Insufficient water intake can result in symptoms ranging from lethargy to disorientation to death, depending on the degree of dehydration. Loss of water occurs primarily through urination, perspiration, and respiration (water vapor in the air we breathe out).

Women who appear to be adequately hydrated consume an average of about 90 oz. (2.7 liters [L])—from all beverages and foods—each day, while men average about 125 oz. (3.7 L) daily. About 80 percent of people's total water intake comes from drinking water and beverages—including caffeinated drinks—and the other 20 percent comes from food. Based on these estimates, women should be drinking about nine 8-oz. glasses of water and beverages per day (72 oz.), and men about 12–13 glasses (100 oz.). Due attention should be given to *what* we are drinking, however. The Beverage Guidance Panel reports that about 50 percent of Americans' excess calories come from sweetened (nondiet) beverages. The panel recommends that water be the drink of choice and consumption of sweetened beverages be reduced.

Individual water needs may vary widely with body size, environmental conditions, and exercise patterns. Since the body's main method of cooling is by evaporation of perspiration, living in a hot climate or engaging in heavy physical activity can increase the body's water requirement substantially. Individuals can easily lose 1–3 percent of their body weight after several hours of exertion in the heat. Under these conditions, thirst alone may not be a good indicator of dehydration. Other measures for monitoring hydration are recommended: for example, checking body weight on a daily basis to ensure (water) weight is regained by drinking plenty of fluids in the hours following prolonged heat exposure or exercise.

NEED TO KNOW

Nutrition is about understanding what types of and how much food a person needs. To appreciate and apply nutrition principles, we must know that nutrients are composed of macronutrients (carbohydrates, fats, protein, water) and micronutrients (vitamins, minerals), and we must learn the basics about each type of nutrient. This fundamental knowledge serves as the foundation for making wise decisions about what we eat.

➤ Recommendations for Healthy Eating

The American public is under siege from an information blitz about how our diet affects our health. And much of the news is bleak. Obesity is a major public health problem. As a society we eat too much and exercise too little. Many of the foods we eat are high in saturated fat, low in fiber, and stripped of naturally occurring vitamins and minerals. Poor diet increases risk for many chronic diseases.

We live in a fast-paced, affluent society where convenience and competition rule. New food products seem to appear weekly. Supermarkets are open round-the-clock with literally thousands of items on the shelves. Restaurants continually revamp menus and new eateries launch every day. In our food landscape, the choices are plentiful, affordable, and ever changing.

Along with the huge array of packaged processed foods, the options to select fresh produce and wholesome foods are also greater than ever before. The challenge is to make smart choices. To be successful, we must sort the marketing from the science and this can be difficult—as the two often blend together. Should we be surprised that the consumer is confused? Since the connection between what we eat and how we feel and function is indisputable, it's clearly worth the effort to be informed and stay informed.

As part of public health policy, the federal government disseminates science-based dietary guidelines to aid the American consumer. Let's apply the basic terms and concepts reviewed in the previous section to the current guidelines. And let's look below the surface. They deserve more than a superficial glance. These are not simply a list of "rules" to eat by. Our aim is to help you develop a working knowledge of the recommendations—not only the *what* but also the *why* and the *how*.

The U.S. Department of Agriculture (USDA) has provided nutrition information and advice to Americans for over a century. In 1994 the USDA bolstered its role in this regard by creating the Center for Nutrition Policy and Promotion. This came at a time when the consumer was becoming increasingly aware of the importance of diet yet was receiving conflicting nutrition messages. A major role of the center is to serve as a trusted source of nutrition information based on sound research and analysis. At its website **(www.cnpp.usda.gov/)** links are provided to the *Dietary Guidelines for Americans* and the ChooseMyPlate food guidance system.

DIETARY GUIDELINES FOR AMERICANS 2015–2020

The *Dietary Guidelines for Americans* are the cornerstone of federal nutrition policy and nutrition education activities. They are a joint project of the U.S. Department of Health and Human Services (HHS) and the USDA. They were first issued in 1980 and are updated every five years; the most recent version was released in 2016. The following questions and answers provide insight on how they are developed and highlight fundamental recommendations.

What Are the Dietary Guidelines?

The *Dietary Guidelines* are based on what experts have determined to be the best scientific knowledge about diet, physical activity, and other issues related to what we should eat and how much physical activity we need. The *Dietary Guidelines* are designed to help Americans choose diets that meet nutrient requirements, promote health, support active lives, and reduce risks of chronic disease.

Why Are the Dietary Guidelines *Important?*

The *Dietary Guidelines* allow government agencies to speak with one voice when presenting advice about proper dietary habits for healthy Americans. All federal dietary guidance for the public must be consistent with the *Dietary Guidelines*. They also influence the direction of government nutrition programs, including research, labeling, and promotion.

How Are the Dietary Guidelines *Developed?*

The *Dietary Guidelines* are prepared in a three-stage process. In the first, an independent advisory committee of eminent scientists compiles a report based on the best available evidence. In the second, government scientists and officials review the advisory committee's report and, based on the report and agency and public comments, develop the *Dietary Guidelines*. In the third stage, health communication specialists translate the *Dietary Guidelines* into meaningful messages for the public and educators. The latest consumer guide is ChooseMyPlate, presented in the next section.

What Are the Key Points from Current Guidelines?

The *2015–2020 Dietary Guidelines* provides five overarching recommendations. Importantly, these recommendations recognize that individuals will need to make shifts in their food and beverage choices to achieve a healthy pattern, and acknowledge that all segments of our society have a role to play in supporting healthy choices. The *Guidelines* also embody the idea that a healthy eating pattern is not a rigid prescription but, rather, an adaptable framework, one in which individuals can enjoy foods that are affordable and meet their personal and cultural preferences.

- *Follow a healthy eating pattern.* All food and beverage choices matter. Choose a healthy eating pattern at an appropriate calorie level to help achieve and maintain a healthy body weight, and reduce the risk of chronic disease.
- *Focus on variety, nutrient density, and amount.* To meet nutrient needs and stay within calorie limits, choose a variety of nutrient-dense foods across all food groups. Nutrient-dense foods include vegetables, fruits, whole grains, and fat-free or low-fat dairy products.
- *Limit calories from added sugars and saturated fats and reduce sodium.* Follow an eating pattern that is low in added sugars, saturated fats, and sodium.
- *Shift to healthier food and beverage choices.* Choose nutrient-dense foods and beverages across all food groups in place of less healthy choices. Consider cultural and personal preferences to make these shifts easier to accomplish and maintain.
- *Support healthy eating patterns for all.* Everyone has a responsibility to support healthy eating in all settings—home, school, work, or wherever food is available.

Daily limits are recommended for several of our pervasive "problem" nutrients that are overconsumed by kids and adults alike. Less than 10 percent of total calories should come from saturated and *trans* fats combined. The same limit applies to added sugars, no more than 10 percent. Surprising fact: two 12-oz. servings of a typical sugar-sweetened soft drink exceeds the 10 percent limit for children and most adults.

Daily sodium intake should be reduced to less than 2,300 mg (about 1 teaspoon [tsp.] of salt). Among African Americans, sodium should be further reduced to 1,500 mg. The lower intake also applies to those with hypertension, diabetes, or chronic kidney disease and to all over the age of 50. As a result, the 1,500-mg recommendation should be followed by about half of the U.S. population.

Health & the Media The Milk Mustache Ad Campaign

Launched in 1996, the national "Got milk?" campaign, portraying celebrities wearing milk mustaches, has been one of the most enjoyed and recognized of any food product ad campaign. The print ads have featured dozens of celebrities over the years, each with a catchy story line linking his or her persona with the health benefits of drinking milk. Hugh Jackman, Spike Lee, Sheryl Crow, Jackie Chan, and Kermit the Frog are a few notables who have posed with a contented look, sporting the "milk mustache." This one features singer-songwriter Taylor Swift. The ad campaign blends celebrity, creativity, and flair. It has become part of American pop culture. Funded by America's milk processors and dairy farmers, the milk mustache ads continue today. Who is the latest athlete or entertainer urging us to drink our milk?

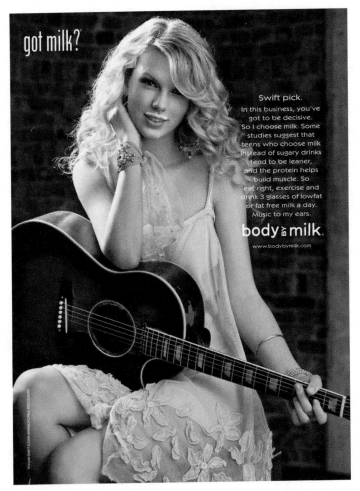

© ZCB WENN Photos/Newscom

Unhealthy fats, added sugars, and sodium are not intended to be reduced in isolation, but as a part of a shift to a healthier dietary pattern. Rather than focusing purely on reduction, emphasis should also be placed on replacements. Butter and margarine (saturated fats) for cooking can be replaced with vegetable oils (unsaturated fats). In lieu of sugar-sweetened beverages, let water become the drink of choice. The use of low-calorie sweeteners is not recommended.

If you drink alcohol, do so in moderation: up to one drink per day for women and two drinks per day for men. Sadly, excessive drinking by some is a reality. Resist peer pressure to overindulge. Also, remember that alcohol should not be consumed by some individuals, including those who cannot restrict their alcohol intake, women who are pregnant or lactating, children and adolescents, and persons taking certain medications. And, of course, drinking and driving can be lethal. Bottom line—if you choose to drink, do so sensibly.

Good news for coffee lovers: moderate consumption of 3 to 5 cups per day or up to 400 mg of caffeine per day is not associated with chronic disease among healthy individuals. In fact, it may reduce risk of heart disease, type 2 diabetes, and Parkinson's disease. A caveat, though: coffee as normally consumed contains added calories from cream, milk, and sugar, so be willing to cut back on the extras. Let the full flavor of java come through.

For the complete set of dietary recommendations, go to **health.gov/dietaryguidelines/2015/**.

USDA CHOOSEMYPLATE

Due to the enormous variability in food preferences and food choices, learning to eat healthier—let alone maintaining the good habits we already have—can be a challenge. In 2011, the USDA unveiled a new approach—ChooseMyPlate.gov—designed to make it easier for people to make better food choices. A plate-shaped image (Figure 2.1) replaces the long-used food guide pyramid (1992−2011). Lauded by nutrition experts as a solid step forward, the MyPlate icon is simple and intuitive. The five groups of fruits, vegetables, grains, protein foods, and dairy are represented using a familiar mealtime visual—a place setting.

The MyPlate website **(choosemyplate.gov)** features practical information on all five food groups with corresponding galleries of food images that depict serving sizes. Under the heading Popular Topics is the 10 Tips Series that provides easy-to-follow tips on diverse subjects—from "Build a Healthy Meal" to "Kid-Friendly Veggies and Fruits"—in a high-quality, printable format (1-page PDFs). These are excellent for posting in the kitchen or sharing with others. Under the heading Interactive Tools, click on Super Tracker to explore different tools **(supertracker.usda.gov)**. Three of particular interest are Food Tracker, Food-A-Pedia, and My Plan.

Food Tracker is a dietary assessment tool. Enter all food and beverage you consume in a day and receive a report that includes total calories and an analysis of macro- and micronutrients. A quality rating based on the types and amounts of foods eaten is also generated. To get a representative picture of eating habits, input at least three days (two weekdays and one weekend day). As with any computerized analysis, accurate output is dependent on accurate input! Become familiar with Food Tracker features, keep detailed written records of everything you eat and drink, and enter data carefully. This will take time, but getting an accurate report is worth the effort. Give it a try and see how you score.

The Food-A-Pedia interactive tool taps into a huge database and provides quick access to basic facts on nearly every food. Input the food (e.g., pizza) and it will

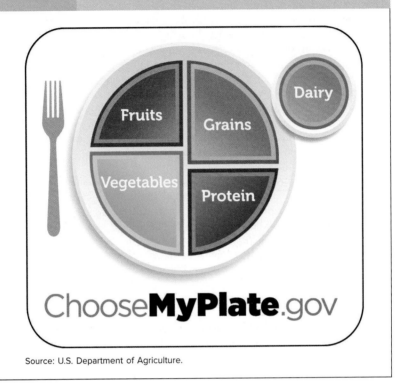

FIGURE 2.1 USDA MYPLATE ICON

Source: U.S. Department of Agriculture.

query you for more information as necessary (e.g., type, condiments, portion size). Results will include the caloric content of the food and its contributions to the food groups. You can easily compare foods too.

Article 2.1

Some of you may want a food plan to get you started on the path to healthier eating. To meet this need, try My Plan (listed under the banner). With this tool, you can personalize a plan based on your age, gender, and physical activity level. After entering this information, a food plan is generated at the appropriate calorie level. The plan will specify daily amounts from each food group and a limit for discretionary calories (saturated fats, added sugars, alcohol). Use the plan to set short-term goals and to compare with current eating patterns.

In closing this section, we should point out that the recommendations reviewed here are for the general adult population. The *Dietary Guidelines* and MyPlate also contain recommendations for specific groups such as infants and young children, women who are pregnant and breastfeeding, and older adults. Since the majority of college students are young women, information on maternal and infant nutrition may be of special interest. With that in mind, a comment on the importance of breastfeeding is apropos.

Healthy People 2020, the American Academy of Nutrition and Dietetics, and the American Academy of Pediatricians advocate the value of breastfeeding for its many health benefits to both the baby (e.g., protects from infections, reduces risk of sudden infant death, developing asthma, or becoming obese) and the mother (e.g., decreased risk of breast and ovarian cancers and type 2 diabetes). Three out of four

FIGURE 2.2 HEALTHY EATING PLATE

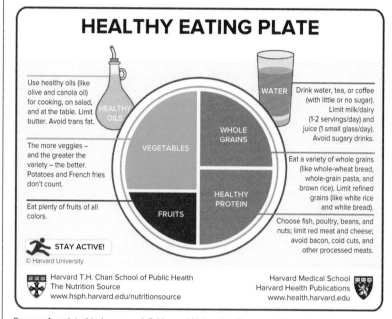

HEALTHY EATING PLATE

Use healthy oils (like olive and canola oil) for cooking, on salad, and at the table. Limit butter. Avoid trans fat.

HEALTHY OILS

The more veggies – and the greater the variety – the better. Potatoes and French fries don't count.

Eat plenty of fruits of all colors.

STAY ACTIVE!

© Harvard University

VEGETABLES

WHOLE GRAINS

HEALTHY PROTEIN

FRUITS

WATER Drink water, tea, or coffee (with little or no sugar). Limit milk/dairy (1-2 servings/day) and juice (1 small glass/day). Avoid sugary drinks.

Eat a variety of whole grains (like whole-wheat bread, whole-grain pasta, and brown rice). Limit refined grains (like white rice and white bread).

Choose fish, poultry, beans, and nuts; limit red meat and cheese; avoid bacon, cold cuts, and other processed meats.

Harvard T.H. Chan School of Public Health
The Nutrition Source
www.hsph.harvard.edu/nutritionsource

Harvard Medical School
Harvard Health Publications
www.health.harvard.edu

Source: As printed in image and © Harvard University. For more information visit: **www.health.harvard.edu.** NOTE: Harvard Health Publications does not endorse any products or medical procedures.

mothers start out breastfeeding (75 percent), but by six months the rate drops to less than 50 percent. Programs are in place to increase these rates. Mother's milk is a perfect nutrition, so encourage breastfeeding.

ALTERNATIVE APPROACHES

Findings from the scientific report of the *2015–2020 Dietary Guidelines* show that a diet higher in plant-based foods, such as vegetables, fruits, whole grains, legumes, nuts, and seeds, and lower in calories and animal-based foods is both healthier and more sustainable than the current U.S diet. A variation of this health-promoting, environmentally conscious approach to eating has been dubbed the "healthy U.S.-style pattern" and is described in detail at the MyPlate website. Other variations include a healthy Mediterranean-style pattern and a healthy vegetarian pattern.

The traditional Mediterranean diet was identified by scientists decades ago as a model to promote lifelong good health. It is based on fresh fruits and vegetables, olive oil, whole grains, and fish, with little red meat and animal products. Features of the Mediterranean diet include reliance on locally grown and harvested food, minimal use of modern processed foods, and the enjoyment of good food with others.

The Healthy Eating Plate, developed by Harvard's Department of Nutrition, modifies the MyPlate pattern to a Mediterranean-style diet (Figure 2.2). Some nutrition

Article 2.2

experts and consumer advocates believe the Healthy Eating Plate better reflects the latest science (e.g., a plant-based diet is healthiest) and is free from corporate influence. A complete description is available online at **hsph.harvard.edu/nutritionsource/ healthy-eating-plate.**

A vegetarian diet, followed by growing numbers of Americans, is a step beyond the Mediterranean diet. Nearly all eat a vegetarian diet to improve overall health, and over half cite concerns about the environment and animal welfare as reasons for their choice. It is estimated that about 16 million Americans follow a vegetarian-based diet with another 25 million on a vegetarian-inclined diet. The American Academy of Nutrition and Dietetics and *Dietary Guidelines* endorse the healthful-ness of vegetarian diets. MyPlate provides guidance for planning a well-balanced vegetarian diet.

FOOD LABELS

Reading food labels is an important step in making sound nutritional choices. By law the "Nutrition Facts" panel on food labels is standardized to give consumers easy access to key information. A sample food label is shown in Figure 2.3. A few of the key facts should be highlighted. Note that "a serving" is defined by the manufacturer—usually by size (e.g., one cup) or pieces (e.g., three cookies). While some manufacturers use the definition of a serving as given by the *Dietary Guidelines,* many do not. What constitutes a single serving can vary, sometimes widely, from one product line to another. Consider how many servings are in the food package, then ask yourself, "How many servings am I consuming?" Is it half a serving, one serving, or more? Note that serving size is always listed first, followed by the calories. In the calorie line (point 2), the fat percentage of the product can be calculated by simply dividing the calories from fat by the total calories. In this macaroni and cheese product, 44 percent (110/250) of the calories are from fat!

Grams for each of the energy nutrients are reported next, with additional information on the types of fat and carbohydrate. Under "Total Fat," a breakdown is given for saturated fat and *trans* fat. Under "Total Carbohydrate," a breakdown is given for dietary fiber and sugars. Saturated fat, *trans* fat, cholesterol, and sodium are nutrients that Americans generally need to limit, whereas dietary fiber, vitamins A and C, calcium, and iron are nutrients that most of us should aim to increase. With practice, using information from the "Nutrition Facts" label along with the list of ingredients will allow you to quickly determine the nutritional characteristics of the food. How healthy would you rate this macaroni and cheese product (Figure 2.3)?

In Figure 2.4, nutrition labels from two brand-name packages of one-serving chicken-pasta-broccoli frozen entrees are presented. Although both are essentially the same size (total weight: 10.5 vs. 9.5 oz.), the meal on the left has 41 percent more calories than the meal on the right (380 vs. 270 Cal). The difference in total energy is due almost entirely to higher fat intake: 15 versus 6 g, more than twice as much. The saturated fat comparison is 6 g versus only 1.5 g—four times as much. Finally, the meal on the left has significantly more sodium, less fiber, and more sugar than the one on the right. It's easy to make the healthy choice between these two meals, especially since the costs are similar and the low-fat, low-calorie entree tastes just as good. In recent years, food scientists have developed many flavorful low-fat food products. Be ready to be surprised.

FIGURE 2.3 **UNDERSTANDING A FOOD LABEL**

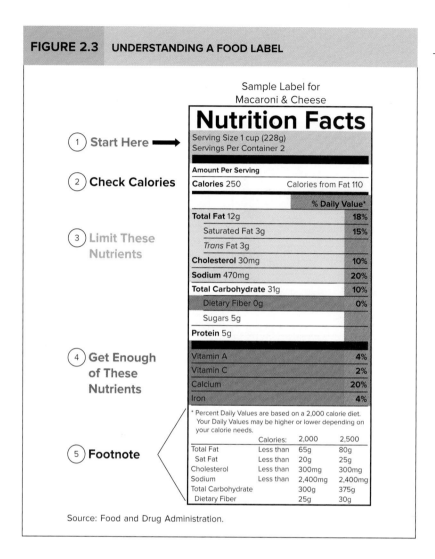

Source: Food and Drug Administration.

In July 2015, the Food and Drug Administration (FDA) proposed two changes to the food label. The first is to include the % Daily Value for added sugars. This would be a new line similar to the lines for sodium and certain fats. It is a necessary addition considering the limit for added sugars (10 percent) recently set by the *Dietary Guidelines*. The second change is to make calories and serving sizes more prominent (enlarge and boldface) to emphasize parts of the label that are important in addressing current health concerns such as obesity, diabetes, and cardiovascular disease. Once label changes are approved, companies will have two years to comply— look for new labels by 2018.

Use food labels to apply your nutrition knowledge and make informed choices. Review and compare the nutrition facts, critically analyze, and make your own judgments.

FIGURE 2.4 COMPARISON OF TWO FROZEN ENTREES*

Nutrition Facts
Serving Size 1 package (10.5 oz)
Servings per Container about 1

Amount per Serving

Calories 380   Calories from Fat 140

	% Daily Value*
Total Fat 15g	23%
Saturated Fat 6g	30%
Cholesterol 40mg	13%
Sodium 1090mg	45%
Total Carbohydrate 37g	12%
Dietary Fiber 3g	12%
Sugars 8g	
Protein 25g	

*Percent Daily Values are based on a 2,000 calorie diet. Your daily values may be higher or lower depending on your calorie needs.

Nutrition Facts
Serving Size 1 package (9.5 oz)
Servings per Container about 1

Amount per Serving

Calories 270   Calories from Fat 50

	% Daily Value*
Total Fat 6g	9%
Saturated Fat 1.5g	8%
Cholesterol 60mg	20%
Sodium 550mg	23%
Total Carbohydrate 34g	11%
Dietary Fiber 5g	20%
Sugars 6g	
Protein 19g	

*Percent Daily Values are based on a 2,000 calorie diet. Your daily values may be higher or lower depending on your calorie needs.

*Stouffer's Chicken Fettuccine versus Lean Cuisine Bow Tie Pasta & Chicken.

Source: **www.foodfacts.com.**

FOOD SAFETY

"I was sick as a dog last night." This phrase conjures up images of a dog vomiting, its entire body convulsing with the effort—generally the result of a dietary indiscretion (eating garbage or worse). Or the saying might prompt a personal memory of a long, sleepless night in the bathroom combating nausea and dealing with gastrointestinal distress while hunched over the toilet. Thankfully, for most of us, these "bad food" experiences—although often intense, with symptoms of nausea, stomach cramps, diarrhea, vomiting, and fever—are generally short-lived.

But the fact remains that we are more likely to experience foodborne illness than nearly any other health risk. About one in four, or roughly 75 million Americans, suffers a bout of food poisoning every year. The consequence for the vast majority of those afflicted is a day or two of distress. However, foodborne illness also kills about 5,000 Americans a year. With prevention in mind, let's consider the primary risk factors and identify those people who are most vulnerable.

Foodborne illness or disease—routinely called "food poisoning"—is caused by consuming contaminated foods or beverages. Many different disease-causing microbes (pathogens) can contaminate foods as can poisonous chemicals. Most foodborne diseases are infections, caused by a variety of bacteria, viruses, and parasites. For

Foodborne illness, or "food poisoning," is an acute gastrointestinal disorder caused by the consumption of food contaminated with harmful microorganisms and, less often, toxic chemicals; it is marked by nausea, vomiting, and diarrhea.

example, *Salmonella* in chicken and eggs and *E. coli* (strain 0157:H7) in ground meat are bacterial pathogens that periodically receive media attention when identified as the "bugs" (microbes) responsible for outbreaks of foodborne illness. In nearly all cases, infections were preventable and resulted from inattention to safe food-handling practices. Unintended poisonings caused by harmful toxins or chemicals—accidentally eating poisonous mushrooms, for example—are less common.

Because it is the immune system that protects the body against pathogens, the most severe effects of foodborne diseases occur in very young individuals, very old individuals, or anyone with a compromised immune system. In newborns and infants, the immune system is not fully developed. Similarly, pregnant women and their fetuses are at higher risk. In the elderly the immune system is less robust due to age. And literally millions of others are immunocompromised because they are undergoing chemotherapy, are taking steroidal or antimicrobial medication, or have an immune deficiency disease (whether genetically based or acquired, such as AIDS). Foodborne diseases in these vulnerable groups can cause serious complications and even death.

Although dozens of different "bugs" or pathogens are responsible for foodborne illnesses, several characteristics are common. They are carried by food that isn't handled carefully, washed adequately, cooked thoroughly, or stored properly. This simple knowledge and the associated food safety practices go a long way in reducing exposure. In addition, Americans now eat away from home between 30 and 50 percent of the time. This requires additional vigilance and precautions as you make choices about where and what you eat. For example, be observant and select carefully at salad bars, buffets, and those prolonged group picnics or summer reunions.

Restaurants are inspected routinely (or should be) by local health departments to make sure they are clean, have adequate kitchen facilities, and follow established food safety practices. Look at the score from the most recent inspection report (usually posted), and use that score to help guide your choice in where you eat. Some restaurants have specifically trained their staff in principles of food safety. Simple observation of the kitchen staff and servers in their handling of the food and cleaning of tables can reveal whether hygienic practices are being followed.

Whether the "food handler" is the cook at a restaurant or you at home, a few simple precautions can greatly reduce the risk of microbial foodborne diseases. Key recommendations regarding food safety include:

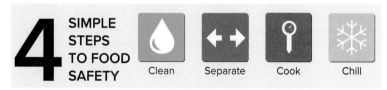

Source: U.S. Department of Health & Human Services.

- *Clean hands, food contact surfaces, and fruits and vegetables.* Wash your hands with soap and water before and after preparing food. Don't be a source of foodborne illness yourself.
- *Separate raw, cooked, and ready-to-eat foods while shopping, preparing, or storing foods.* Avoid cross-contaminating by washing hands, utensils, and cutting boards after they have been in contact with raw meat or poultry and before they touch another food.

- ***Cook*** *foods to a safe temperature to kill microorganisms.* For example, cook ground beef to an internal temperature of 160°Fahrenheit. Eggs should be cooked until the yolk is firm.
- ***Chill*** *(refrigerate) perishable food promptly and defrost foods properly.* Bacteria can grow quickly at room temperature, so refrigerate leftovers within two hours.

In addition to these four steps, remember to avoid raw (unpasteurized) milk or any products made from unpasteurized milk, raw or partially cooked eggs, raw or undercooked meat and poultry, unpasteurized juices, and raw sprouts.

Remember to watch over the most vulnerable (e.g., infants and young children, residents in nursing homes or chronic care facilities, cancer patients) as they must depend on others to ensure their food is wholesome and safe. In short, for most Americans the overall risk of food poisoning is high—about one out of four per year—but the consequences are relatively low—acute gastrointestinal distress for 6–48 hours—except for those in vulnerable groups. Yet even the healthiest among us should be smart about prevention. No one wants to be sick as a dog, not even for one night.

For additional information, see the gateway site on foodborne illness and food safety provided at **www.foodsafety.gov.** A companion site is operated by the CDC at **www.cdc.gov/foodsafety.**

DIETARY SUPPLEMENTS

As the name indicates, **dietary supplements** are intended to augment the diet. Most contain vitamins, minerals, or plant-based substances (botanicals). Dietary supplements are intended to be taken as a pill, capsule, or liquid. The topic of dietary supplements is one of the most controversial and at times contentious in all of nutrition—an inevitable result when private enterprise, science, quackery, public health, politics, and the mass media get tangled together. From blatantly fraudulent to alluringly sophisticated, advertisements for dietary supplements are ubiquitous—on the Internet, social media, TV, radio, and in magazines and newspapers.

The market for dietary supplements is huge: U.S. sales exceeded $36 billion in 2014. Yes, that's "b" as in billion or 36 thousand million dollars! Over half of all American adults use supplements, with the most common being the standard multivitamin/mineral supplement followed by calcium products, vitamin C, vitamin E, botanicals, and sport nutrition supplements. Literally hundreds of different dietary supplements are marketed. Claims for supplements are across-the-board—from treating the entire spectrum of medical conditions (from acne to cancer) to improving performance (sexual, sports, cognitive), to combating general malaise (low energy, poor appetite, insomnia). And the list goes on. Dietary supplements are available at grocery stores, pharmacies, and health food stores, and are also easily purchased on the Internet.

Contrary to what the general populace believes, the federal government does *not* evaluate supplements before they are marketed. In 1994 the dietary supplement industry successfully lobbied Congress to pass legislation favorable to their products—the Dietary Supplement Health and Education Act. The definition of dietary supplement was broadened to include a wide array of products: vitamins, minerals,

Dietary supplements are food products, added to the total diet, that contain vitamins, minerals, herbs, botanicals, amino acids, metabolites, constituents, extracts, or combinations of these ingredients.

herbs, botanicals, amino acids, and other constituents and extracts of animal and plant origin. Based on this legislation—which is the law of the land—*there is no requirement for premarket review of dietary supplements by FDA.*

Rather, FDA must prove a supplement is unsafe *before* it can restrict consumer use. This can be a long, long battle, as in the case of ephedra, a supplement promoted for weight loss and improved athletic performance. After years of investigation, FDA found ephedra use was responsible for five deaths and many more heart attacks, strokes, and seizures. As ephedra clearly posed an unreasonable risk, FDA banned its sale in 2004. The manufacturer went to court, and the ban was struck down in 2005. The next step was the U.S. Court of Appeals, which in 2006 ruled in favor of FDA and upheld the ban. FDA continues to monitor "the wild west" of supplements to try and protect consumers. Of particular concern are fraudulent, unsafe products with undeclared or mislabeled ingredients marketed for weight loss, sexual enhancement, and bodybuilding.

In truth, federal oversight of dietary supplements is limited. Action will be taken only in the most serious cases when a supplement has been shown to be dangerous. Questions of effectiveness or truth in advertising are not routinely evaluated. Supplement manufacturers are not supposed to make unsubstantiated health claims, but often do with a caveat in small print. In stark contrast to the limited regulation of dietary supplements, FDA has stringent approval guidelines for the development of new prescription drugs. For the pharmaceutical industry to get a new drug to market, the drug must be shown to be safe and effective *prior* to its release.

In summary, dietary supplements encompass hundreds of products. Some may be beneficial, many are not. For example, evidence supports the use of standard multivitamin/minerals and selected vitamins and minerals for some individuals, particularly those not eating a well-balanced diet or with known deficiencies. In general though, it is "buyer beware," since supplements with proven benefits make up only a small fraction of the entire dietary supplement market. Examine all advertising with skepticism. (See the section on complementary and alternative medicine [CAM] in Chapter 12.) Before buying any dietary supplement, do your research. The Office of Dietary Supplements at the National Institutes of Health provides an excellent website: **ods.od.nih.gov/HealthInformation.**

✓ **NEED TO KNOW**

ChooseMyPlate.gov is a web-based, consumer-friendly version of the *Dietary Guidelines.* The website provides practical messages and tools designed to educate and motivate us to improve our eating habits and overall health. Alternative approaches to healthy eating include a Mediterranean-style diet and vegetarian diets. An understanding of the related topics of food labels, food safety, and dietary supplements is also necessary to be a savvy consumer in today's food wonderland.

➤ Weight Control

News stories on obesity appear almost daily. The Centers for Disease Control and Prevention (CDC) report that obesity rates doubled among American adults between 1980 and 2010. The World Health Organization (WHO) documents similar trends in Canada, Britain, Australia, and other developed countries around the world. Based on national data from 2015, one out of three American adults are obese while for children and teenagers the frequency is one out of seven.

How have we arrived at this current crisis with America's ballooning body weight? In large part, it can be understood as an unintended consequence of major technological advances over the past 50 years. Our 21st-century lifestyles require only minimal levels of physical activity, and our food choices are more plentiful and convenient than ever before. Sedentary living, combined with drive-through fast food and huge portions, has become the norm.

Given these conditions, it's not surprising that most Americans struggle with their weight. Moreover, the idealized body image advertisers promote to girls and women is to be thin while the message targeted at boys and men is to be muscular. Although less prevalent than obesity-related behaviors, eating disorders—anorexia and bulimia—have been increasing for decades. Females in particular are vulnerable to the Madison Avenue illusion that equates thinness with beauty, success, and self-control.

The key to understanding weight control is the fundamental principle of energy balance—energy intake versus energy expenditure. The basic science and practical aspects of energy balance will serve as the link between our discussion of nutrition in the first part of this chapter and the material to be presented on physical activity in the next chapter.

In the following section, the primary focus is on understanding healthy weight. We start with the questions, What is it, and how is it measured? We will look at selected medical and scientific issues and key resources on obesity and eating disorders and then discuss energy balance. The aim is to present the basics on developing a weight management program and insights on weight-related health issues. The best approach to reducing prejudice and dispelling myths about those who are obese or have an eating disorder is to become informed.

WHAT IS A HEALTHY WEIGHT?

A *healthy weight* simply refers to a body weight at which you feel good and physically function at a high level of well-being. Similar terms such as *optimal weight, ideal weight,* and *desirable weight* are also often used, but generally with reference to athletes where the focus is on the best body weight for competing in a particular sport. A healthy weight varies widely from one person to the next based on age and gender as well as body size, shape, and composition. We will limit our discussion of healthy weight to physically mature individuals from young adults to those in middle age.

As with most mammals, the male of the species *Homo sapiens* is on average significantly taller, heavier, and leaner than the female. Yet it's important to remember that large variability for height, weight, and leanness exists within each gender as well. Beyond the influence of gender, the basic body shape of a person (stockiness, tallness, roundness) is greatly influenced by heredity. These body characteristics can be assessed by measuring limb and torso dimensions and skinfolds. Individuals with extreme body shapes may be well suited to excel in specific sports—such as horse racing, gymnastics, basketball, football—but may not fare well in a world designed for average-sized people.

Although measurements of body size and shape can be used as indicators of a healthy weight, the aspect of physique that is most highly related to healthy weight is leanness or, more technically, body composition. The term *body composition* is used to describe the relative amounts of fat weight (adipose tissue) and lean weight (predominantly muscle and bone) and is reported as percent body fat (fat weight/body weight). A more popular and simpler approach to estimate healthy weight is to simply use height and weight and calculate body mass index.

Body Mass Index (BMI)

Body mass index, or **BMI,** is a ratio of body weight to height (kg/m^2). Instead of converting units and computing BMI, use Table 2.2 to determine your BMI. Find your height (in inches) in the left column and scan across to your weight, then follow the column up to find your BMI. Interpolate as necessary. For example if you are 65″ (5′5″) tall and weigh 144 lb., your BMI is 24. A BMI between 18.5 and 24.9 is considered healthy.

Population-based (epidemiological) studies have found that an increase in BMI is associated with an increase in early death. The mortality curve, described by a J-shaped curve, represents a continuum. As BMI rises from 25 to 30, relative risk begins to increase slightly. As BMI rises above 30, the relative risk increases more steeply and is cause for concern: 30 to 35 is considered moderate risk and 35 to 40 is high risk. This association is similar for men and women and across racial groups. The chances of dying early increase mainly due to heart disease, cancer, and diabetes. The slight rise in death rate for low BMI (underweight) is associated with smoking and preexisting conditions.

Based on this type of evidence, overweight is operationally defined as a BMI of 25 to 29.9, and obesity as 30 or higher. These are the federal standards used in surveillance studies that report on the prevalence of overweight and obesity among Americans. BMI standards are the same for men and women. For individuals with a BMI of 25 or higher, an additional measurement of waist circumference is recommended to further assess risk level. Risk is lower for women with a waist size less than 35 inches and for men with a waist size less than 40 inches.

Body Composition (Percent Fat)

As mentioned earlier, the preferred approach to estimating healthy weight is based on the concept of **body composition** in which the body is viewed as consisting of different tissue components. The most common body composition model is a simple two-component one where the body is divided into fat weight (adipose tissue) and lean body weight (the remaining weight, primarily muscle and bone). The body composition approach is widely used in clinical and sports/fitness settings.

In individuals of normal weight, the majority of body fat is stored immediately beneath the skin—in the subcutaneous fat layer—with the remainder distributed in smaller quantities throughout other tissues and organs. Among obese individuals, large amounts of the excessive body fat can be found within nearly all tissues of the

Body mass index, or **BMI,** is a ratio of weight to height (kg/m^2) that is widely used as a measure of healthy weight (18.5–25), overweight (25–29.9), obesity (30 and above), and underweight (less than 18.5).

Body composition is the partitioning of body weight into fat (adipose tissue) and lean (primarily muscle and bone) components. Body composition is typically expressed as percent body fat (fat weight/body weight) and used to recommend a healthy weight range.

TABLE 2.2 BODY MASS INDEX (BMI) CHART

BMI	NORMAL							OVERWEIGHT				OBESE					
HT (inches)	19	20	21	22	23	24	25	26	27	28	29	30	32	34	36	38	40
								WT (pounds)									
60	97	102	107	112	118	123	128	133	138	143	148	153	163	174	184	194	204
61	100	106	111	116	122	127	132	137	143	148	153	158	169	180	190	201	211
62	104	109	115	120	126	131	136	142	147	153	158	164	175	186	196	207	218
63	107	113	118	124	130	135	141	146	152	158	163	169	180	191	203	214	225
64	110	116	122	128	134	140	145	151	157	163	169	174	186	197	209	221	232
65	114	120	126	132	138	144	150	156	162	168	174	180	192	204	216	228	240
66	118	124	130	136	142	148	155	161	167	173	179	186	198	210	223	235	247
67	121	127	134	140	146	153	159	166	172	178	185	191	204	217	230	241	255
68	125	131	138	144	151	158	164	171	177	184	190	197	210	223	236	249	262
69	128	135	142	149	155	162	169	176	182	189	196	203	216	230	243	257	270
70	132	139	146	153	160	167	174	181	188	195	202	209	222	236	250	264	278
71	136	143	150	157	165	172	179	186	193	200	208	215	229	243	257	272	286
72	140	147	154	162	169	177	184	191	199	206	213	221	235	250	265	279	294
73	144	151	159	166	174	182	189	197	204	212	219	227	242	257	272	288	302
74	148	155	163	171	179	186	194	202	210	218	225	233	249	264	280	295	311
75	152	160	168	176	184	192	200	208	216	224	232	240	256	272	287	303	319

TABLE 2.3 BODY COMPOSITION: % FAT GUIDELINES*

	TOO LEAN	LEAN	MODERATE	OVERFAT
Men	<4	4–12	13–22	>22
Women	<12	12–20	21–30	>30

*Varies by age and goals.

body. Conversely, having too little fat can also lead to an unhealthy state, because fat is an essential component of many tissues (e.g., cell membranes, nervous system).

It's estimated that the amount of fat essential for normal physiological function (the lower limit) is equal to about 4 percent of body weight. In women, another 7 to 9 percent of body weight is gender-specific fat (located in breasts and hips) and is necessary to maintain reproductive function, pregnancy, and lactation. In addition to the essential fat (and gender-specific fat in women), another 8 to 10 percent of body weight as fat is considered to be within an acceptable range and normal for body functions such as insulation, protection, and energy storage.

Table 2.3 presents a set of body fat guidelines for adults. These body composition values reflect a general consensus from many studies, although there are in fact no universally accepted norms. Note the different standards for men and women due to differences in gender-specific fat. A healthy body composition for young adult women may range from 12 to 30 percent fat and for young adult men from 4 to 22 percent fat, with the majority of people in these large ranges falling within the "moderate" subranges. After the age of 30, the norms can be adjusted upward at one percentage point per decade. For example, a 42-year-old man with a body composition of 24 percent would be at the upper end of the moderate range.

The challenge of the body composition approach is that measurement of percent fat is not straightforward like BMI where only height and weight are needed. Body composition measurements are categorized as either field-based or lab-based. Common field methods include (1) measurement of skinfolds and/or circumferences, and (2) use of various instruments to measure bioelectric impedance. As the name implies, field methods provide only rough estimates of percent fat—errors are large (±3–4 percentage points). For example, if your value is estimated as 20 percent fat, your true value probably lies between 17 and 23 percent.

The laboratory method of choice today is dual-energy X-ray absorptiometry (DXA). Although primarily used to assess bone mineral density to screen for osteoporosis, it's now routinely used to measure percent fat, particularly at universities and sports medicine clinics. DXA measurements are reliable and accurate (+1 percentage point). DXA not only provides a percent fat value but also measures total bone mass. This added information is valuable as changes in eating and exercise patterns can selectively bring about changes in body fat, muscle mass, and bone mass. It's an easy procedure for the subject—the only requirement is to lie quietly on a scanning platform.

Body Fat Distribution

For people with excessive levels of body fat, the pattern of fat distribution is another factor to be considered in determining the degree of risk—high or very high—for obesity-related cardiovascular and metabolic diseases. Researchers have shown upper body fat (abdominal fat) may be more dangerous for long-term health than lower body fat (hips, buttocks). For example, two men—Mr. A and Mr. P—have the same high BMI of 35 (e.g., 70″, 243 lb.), well into the obese category. However, since Mr. A has more of an apple shape (upper body fat), he is at greater risk compared to Mr. P, who has a pear physique (lower body fat). This is the basis for the recommendation to measure waist circumference for those with a BMI of 25 or higher. Although men tend to be "apples" and women "pears," both forms of body fat distribution occur within each gender.

Limitations and Interpretation

Body mass index (BMI) is the standard metric used in public health to track the incidence and prevalence of overweight and obesity in our population. As with most simple measures, though, there are limitations. What do you think are the primary shortcomings of using BMI?

Since BMI is not a direct measure of percent fat or fat distribution, misclassification can result. While percent fat and BMI are highly correlated in the population, the relationship is not always true for every individual. Muscle and bone are more dense than fat, so an athlete or muscular person may have a high BMI but not be overfat. Generally, BMI is a good indicator of overweight, because few adults add muscle and bone after their early 20s. Consequently, nearly all weight gained from about age 25 on is adipose tissue. Not surprisingly, weight gain during adulthood is an important predictor of many medical conditions.

To illustrate the use and interpretation of BMI versus percent fat, let's consider three 30-year-old men—a professional football player, an Amish farmer, and a computer programmer—who have identical heights and weights (72″, 221 lb.). The resulting BMI is 30, which is just into the obese category, a category associated

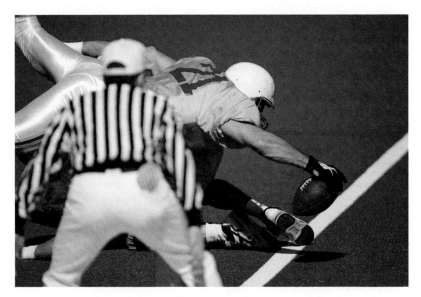

Some athletes may have higher BMIs due to more muscle mass than average, rather than from excess fat.

© Comstock Images

with increased risk for multiple chronic diseases. Waist circumferences are 34, 37, and 41 inches, respectively. And body composition assessments are 14, 20, and 28 percent fat. It's easy to visualize these three physiques.

Although all three men are categorized as obese based solely on their BMI, the football player and Amish farmer are not truly at an increased disease risk as indicated by their normal waist circumferences and percent fat values. They are exceptions. The football player is a muscular, highly trained professional athlete, while the farmer also has a relatively large lean weight and is physically conditioned from the routine manual chores he performs in working a farm. Yet most Americans with a BMI of 30 are probably more like the computer programmer, who leads a sedentary lifestyle, with regular snacking and lots of sitting. His large waist circumference and high percent fat confirm that he is overfat.

Knowing what each man's weight was at age 20 would provide added insight into interpreting or rating their current weights. However, be assured that as BMI rises to 30 and beyond, it's less and less likely that a person is simply a healthy exception with a large muscle mass, a normal waist circumference, and a healthy percent body fat. Are you at a healthy weight? Use the BMI approach as a first screening. If your BMI is higher than desired, check your waist circumference and perhaps also obtain a body composition assessment. And, remember that both BMI and body composition values are presented as recommended *ranges* for a reason. There is no evidence that a BMI of 21 is healthier than 23 or that a body composition of 20 percent fat for a young adult woman is healthier than 22 percent. Any fine-tuning of body weight within recommended ranges depends on individual preferences and circumstances.

THE OBESITY EPIDEMIC

A national poll revealed that 30 percent of overweight people think their weight is fine, 70 percent of obese people feel they are merely overweight, and 39 percent of morbidly obese people think they are overweight but not obese. *Obesity* is a loaded word with many negative connotations. Being referred to as obese or fat is offensive to many people who simply think of themselves as big or large. Judgmental and prejudicial views of the obese by normal-weight individuals are not uncommon. Unless you have firsthand experience coping with excess weight, it's difficult to be sensitive to this issue. In *iHealth,* the term *obesity* is used only in the scientific or medical sense. We encourage you to be tactful when discussing obesity and to dispel unfounded characterizations of those who are obese, while at the same time recognizing the serious health consequences of obesity.

Obesity is the consequence of chronic energy imbalance in which the body stores excess energy in the form of adipose tissue. When a person consistently eats more calories than he or she expends, body fat storage will increase. Genetics also plays a role in the likelihood of developing obesity but is not the primary determinant. Recent evidence also shows the influence (both negative and positive) of shared attitudes about body weight and size among family and friends. As illustrated in

Obesity is the storage of excessive amounts of fat that increases a person's risk for multiple chronic diseases. The accepted definition for obesity is a body mass index (BMI) of 30 or greater.

FIGURE 2.5   KEY FACTORS CONTRIBUTING TO OBESITY

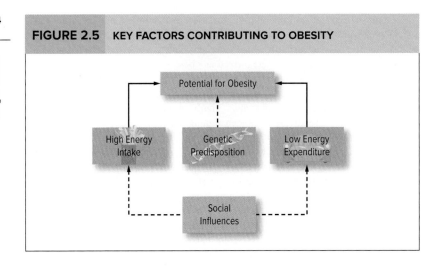

Figure 2.5, a person's potential for obesity is associated with high energy intake, low energy expenditure, genetic predisposition, and social factors that influence eating and activity patterns. Remember, though, regulation of body weight is predominantly determined by our eating and physical activity patterns. The underlying principle of energy balance is discussed more fully in a later section. A key point is that few of us are truly destined to be obese because it's written in our genes.

Public health officials view obesity as a serious epidemic: The most recent data indicate that 34 percent of American adults meet the criteria for obesity (BMI ≥ 30). Perhaps even more dire is the fact that 17 percent of children and adolescents are obese. These percentages have increased twofold over the last 35 years. If the exponential rise in obesity continues, 99 percent of all American adults will be obese by the year 2053! While this statement seems preposterous to consider, it highlights the phenomenal increase in the number of overweight Americans since 1980. This poses a grave health challenge to our society.

Obesity and overweight contribute to the development of many medical conditions and diseases. People who are obese have an increased rate of high blood pressure, lipid abnormalities, and diabetes—all factors that increase risk for cardiovascular disease and stroke. People with obesity are at increased risk for cancers, including colon cancer, breast cancer, gall bladder cancer, and uterine cancer. Obesity is associated with arthritis and mobility problems as well as sleep disturbances and breathing problems. Obesity is also linked to problems with childbearing, premature birth, learning disabilities, and other adverse outcomes for infants. Nationwide, obesity accounts for poorer health-related quality of life and higher health care costs than either smoking or problem drinking.

If we continue down the same path as we've been on for the past three to four decades, researchers believe that the generation in school now will be the first in American history to have a shorter life than its parents. Despite the bleak outlook, the tide can turn. Scientists know that obesity can be prevented with a two-pronged approach: (1) the right combination of individual lifestyle behaviors—namely, healthful eating and regular physical activity—*and* (2) supportive public policies that are accepted by American society. Let's do our part to embrace and promote both aspects for ourselves, our families, and our communities.

With all the attention on the obesity epidemic, we must not overlook the serious health issues that occur at the other end of the body weight continuum. **Eating disorders** are one of the key health issues facing young women and increasingly young men too. The number of Americans with an eating disorder has doubled during the past three decades. Although less widespread than obesity, the rapid rise of these disorders is similar. Professionals estimate that 20 million women and 10 million men suffer from a clinically significant eating disorder at some time in their life.

Extreme dieting to reach a body weight lower and leaner than needed for good health is implicitly promoted by the fashion industry and some sports groups. The National Eating Disorders Association reports that the average female model is 5′11″ and weighs only 117 lb., which is thinner than 98 percent of American women. Is this idealized female image related to why the vast majority of American girls and women are discontent with how they look? Some get caught up in the desire to meet unrealistic expectations to be thin or succumb to pressures from family, coaches, or peers.

Eating disorders are a major concern among female athletes, particularly among elite athletes in appearance sports (e.g., gymnastics, diving, figure skating), endurance sports (e.g., distance running, triathlon), and weight-classification sports (e.g., judo). These disorders are serious disturbances in eating behavior and can include extreme reduction of food intake, severe overeating, and feelings of distress or excessive concern about body image. Eating disorders occur across all socioeconomic, ethnic, and cultural groups. Heredity may play a part in why certain people develop eating disorders, but these disorders afflict many people who have no family history.

The exact causes of eating disorders are not clearly understood. However, their characteristics are well known. Eating disorders are complex psychological conditions that may begin with preoccupations about food and weight. But they are often about much more and serve as a way to focus control in one's life. People with eating disorders tend to be perfectionists who suffer from low self-esteem and are extremely critical of themselves and their bodies. They usually "feel fat" and see themselves as overweight, sometimes even despite life-threatening semi-starvation. An intense fear of gaining weight and of being fat may become all-consuming. In early stages of these disorders, patients often deny that they have a problem. Eating disorders often coexist with other psychological disorders like depression, anxiety, obsessive-compulsive disorder, and alcohol and drug abuse.

The two main types of eating disorders are anorexia nervosa and bulimia nervosa, commonly referred to as anorexia and bulimia. Anorexia is a dangerous condition in which people can literally starve themselves to death. Anorexia afflicts approximately 1 out of every 100 to 200 girls and young women. Patients with anorexia are usually extremely thin (BMI $\leq$ 18.5). They don't maintain a normal weight because they refuse to eat, often exercise obsessively, and sometimes force themselves to vomit or use laxatives to lose weight. Severe physical symptoms accompany starvation.

Eating disorders include a spectrum of clinical disorders involving disturbed eating patterns, with the two main types being anorexia nervosa and bulimia nervosa. These disorders are most common in adolescent girls and young women.

Although less life-threatening, bulimia is more widespread than anorexia, affecting about 1 out of every 30 to 100 girls and young women. Individuals suffering from bulimia follow a routine of secretive, uncontrolled binge eating—ingesting an abnormally large amount of food within a set period of time—followed by behaviors such as vomiting, using a laxative, or fasting to rid the body of food consumed. Persons with bulimia can be slightly underweight, normal weight, or overweight. Because people with bulimia binge and purge in secret and are not excessively thin or heavy, they can hide the disorder for years. Multiple medical complications develop with repeated and chronic purging behaviors. Bulimia disorder may be constant or occasional and often occurs independently of anorexia.

Eating disorders are not due to a personal failure in one's will or behavior. Rather, they are psychological illnesses in which maladaptive patterns of eating take on a life of their own. The good news is that anorexia and bulimia are treatable conditions. Treatment teams generally consist of a psychiatrist or psychologist; a physician, who provides general medical care; and a nutritionist. As with most disorders, the earlier the condition is diagnosed, the more likely treatment will be successful.

If you know of someone who may have an eating disorder, persuade her or him to get professional counseling. Few who suffer with eating disorders seek help on their own, especially in the early stages. And remember that eating disorders can occur in boys and men as well as girls and women. For more information on eating disorders, see Chapter 7 and the website of the National Eating Disorders Association: **www.nationaleatingdisorders.org.**

ENERGY BALANCE

Calories do count. Despite compelling marketing to the contrary, the first law of thermodynamics cannot be broken. Energy is neither created nor destroyed; it only changes forms. Conservation of energy is a law of physics because it always works. As depicted in Figure 2.6, maintaining body weight is fundamentally a balance between energy consumed in the food we eat and energy expended throughout the day based on our body size and level of physical activity. If we eat fewer calories than we expend—known as negative energy balance—then the scale tips and we lose weight. If our energy consumption is consistently higher than our energy expenditure—positive energy balance—then the scale tips the other way and we

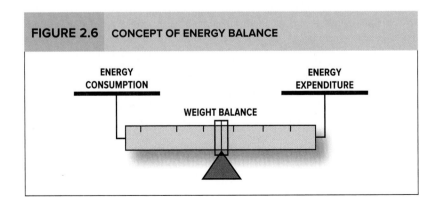

FIGURE 2.6   CONCEPT OF ENERGY BALANCE

ENERGY
CONSUMPTION

ENERGY
EXPENDITURE

WEIGHT BALANCE

gain weight. The goal, of course, is to strike a balance so weight is maintained. **Energy balance** is the essential principle of weight regulation, period.

This is not to say that innate biological variability in energy metabolism (efficiency of deriving energy from food and using it to fuel body processes and activities) does not exist from person to person. Individual differences are present in how we derive and use energy. But in the vast majority of cases, such differences amount to only negligible or very small differences in a person's overall energy balance. Occasionally, medical disorders have been shown to cause obesity; however, these cases are the exception, not the rule.

The principle of energy balance is easy to comprehend but difficult to implement

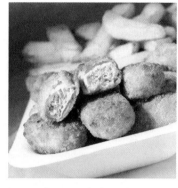

Larger-than-needed meals are popular at restaurants, but add to the problem of energy imbalance and weight gain.

© BananaStock/PunchStock

because contemporary lifestyle encourages consumption of energy and discourages expenditure of energy. Think of the fast-food menus with portions referred to not just as large but as giant, huge, and jumbo or those omnipresent restaurants with the all-you-can-eat buffets. And consider the increase in time spent sitting (at work, at home, and in the car) and the decline in pedestrian-friendly suburbs and cities. Do you walk or bicycle to school or to the store from your home? To achieve and maintain a healthy weight, we must be vigilant and determined. If we choose to remain intellectually and physically passive, the odds are against us. The calories will add up and pounds will accumulate.

On the energy intake side of the equation, control requires a familiarity with the caloric content of the foods and beverages we consume. (Energy expenditure will be discussed in the following chapter on physical activity.) Knowing, for instance, that a medium piece of fruit (banana, apple, orange) is 50–100 Cal, a small soft drink (12-oz. can) 140 Cal, a small order of French fries about 250 Cal, and a standard fast-food burger (e.g., Big Mac, Whopper) 500–700 Cal is important to understanding the "energy currency" of foods and beverages. If the average American woman needs only 2,000 Cal per day to maintain her weight, then one "value-pack" meal (drink, burger, fries) will provide half the energy she needs for the day! Moreover, how often do we opt to get the larger size of this or that because it's only another quarter? Or how many soft drinks or snacks do we consume throughout the day?

If a person consumes only 100 Cal more than needed every day for a year, this will amount to 36,500 surplus Cal that will be stored as body fat (adipose tissue). Since 1 lb. of body fat is equal to about 3,500 Cal, this small imbalance—only 100 Cal per day—will result in a 10-lb. gain! A slight but steady positive energy balance—less than the energy in a single soft drink, candy bar, or pack of snack

Energy balance is the relationship between energy input (caloric intake) and energy output (caloric expenditure). If input and output are matched, then a balance occurs and body weight is maintained.

crackers each day—can result in a significant weight gain in only a few months. And, conversely, cutting back by the same amount can result in a significant weight (fat) loss.

A more gradual increase in body weight of merely 1–2 lb. a year over many years is even easier to comprehend (an excess 10–20 Cal per day). This seemingly trivial energy imbalance results in the slow weight gain that the majority of Americans experience. This process known as creeping obesity is subtle. Several years pass and "suddenly" people notice that they are 5–10 lb. heavier. Continue the process for two to three decades, and the extra poundage becomes substantial.

This is why it's important to periodically consider everything you eat on a typical day and to assess how many calories are contained in those foods and beverages. Refer back and review the individual energy intake results you generated using the Food Tracker analysis tool. Interpret the results and plan accordingly. Make it a habit to read food labels. Knowledge of energy intake is a key to being nutrition savvy and achieving energy balance.

Understand, respect, and follow the principle of energy balance, and you will be able to reach and/or maintain a healthy body weight. Due to individual differences in physiology and eating behaviors, doing so will be more difficult for some and easier for others. Regardless though, basic knowledge, vigilance, and action are the keys to achieving a healthy weight.

NEED TO KNOW

Maintaining a healthy weight in today's society is a challenge. Body mass index (BMI), a ratio of weight to height (kg/m^2), is a widely used method to define healthy weight. Body composition (percent fat) is a more meaningful measurement for evaluating body weight but requires special equipment and expertise. The detrimental health consequences due to obesity are evident. Although less prevalent than obesity, eating disorders are also a significant health concern, particularly for teenage girls and young women. Energy balance is a concept fundamental to achieving a healthy weight and to treating weight-related problems.

➤ Translating Knowledge into Action

Article
2.3

If it were easy to eat well, we all would be doing it. For most of us, the next step is to translate our newfound nutrition knowledge into positive actions—to improve the everyday choices we make about food. This is no small challenge as we live in a society that gobbles up diet books in the search for the "one true diet" that produces results, whether it is losing body fat, gaining muscle, or removing supposed toxins. Of course, no one true diet exists. This is wishful thinking. We need to accept the fact that "dieting" is not an effective long-term solution. The dieting approach— "let's try the new X-week diet by celebrity Z"—promotes a temporary mind-set, which is counter to making lasting changes in lifestyle by developing healthier habits. Moreover, most special diets are restrictive, *not* without risk, and seldom successful, not to mention monotonous and illogical—the rice diet, the grapefruit diet, the detox diets.

We must remember that eating is one of our most basic human behaviors. As we eat multiple times every day, it should come as no surprise that we have developed eating habits highly resistant to change. Awareness and the desire to improve are important for change but often not sufficient. As discussed in Chapter 1, if we wish to change a behavior, the likelihood of success is much better if first we take the time to develop a sound plan.

As you map out a plan, consider these behavior-change strategies from the Mayo Clinic for achieving and maintaining a healthy weight. And be aware that these strategies are useful for those who are normal weight or underweight as well as those who aim to shed a few pounds.

1. **Make a commitment.** Be specific about what you are *willing* to do.
2. **Draw on support from others.** Rely on spouse, family, friends, professionals.
3. **Set a realistic goal.** Use the energy balance principle, monitor, be patient.
4. **Learn to enjoy healthier foods.** Explore healthy foods and dishes.
5. **Get active.** Engage in regular exercise and be active throughout the day—more on this in Chapter 3.

Implementing these strategies will assist you in establishing a healthier lifestyle and move you further along the positive health continuum.

For those who have struggled with their weight over many years, a general perception exists that almost no one succeeds in long-term maintenance of weight loss. This is not true. The National Weight Control Registry (**www.nwcr.ws**) estimates that 20 percent of people who are overweight and obese have been able to achieve lasting success. Established in 1994, the National Weight Control Registry enrolls and tracks individuals who have not only lost weight but, more importantly, maintained weight loss.

Article 2.4

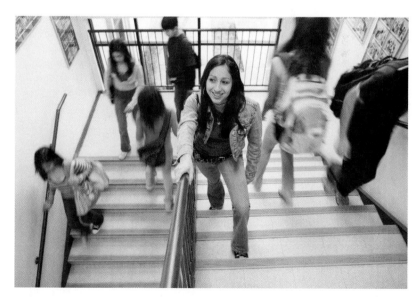

Exercise is important, but any physical activity, such as walking stairs rather than taking the elevator, helps maintain a healthy weight.

© Somos Photography/Veer

In this ongoing monitoring program, long-term maintenance is defined as intentionally losing at least 10 percent of body weight and keeping it off for at least one year. Based on over 10,000 people in the registry, three key characteristics are evident. Successful weight maintainers eat a diet low in saturated fats and *trans* fats, engage in high levels of regular physical activity (about an hour per day), and monitor their food and weight. These findings are real-world evidence that support the *Dietary Guidelines*. If you are overweight or obese, incorporate these practices in your program.

Once you develop a personalized plan, use the following four questions as a final checklist to ensure that your plan meets the essential criteria for healthy eating and weight management. Again, these criteria apply equally to those who are normal weight or underweight as well as those who plan to lose excess weight.

1. **Is it based on wholesome, everyday foods?**
2. **Is it nutritionally balanced?**
3. **Is the energy content appropriate?**
4. **Does it include regular exercise?**

Affirmative answers to these questions fit well with recommendations of the *Dietary Guidelines*. Remember that good results begin with a good plan.

In this chapter we reviewed basic nutrition information and dietary guidelines and provided tools and strategies for choosing a healthy diet. In the final analysis, eating good food is one of the real pleasures in life. And remember that enjoying good food and healthy eating are fully compatible, so nourish your body with only the best. *Bon appétit.*

✓ NEED TO KNOW

Nutrition is about understanding what types and how much food are recommended for good health and reconciling that with our typical eating patterns. Even though our habits are ingrained, we can change. Using ChooseMyPlate tools and the *Dietary Guidelines*, assess your diet, modify as needed, and apply proven strategies to implement change. Design a plan that meets *your* needs and circumstances. No one size fits all.

ARTICLES

2.1 "The More We Learn on Nutrition, the More We Ignore." *New York Times*. Jane Brody explains why it's difficult for us to eat healthier.

2.2 Ancel Keys, Acclaimed Researcher and Promoter of Mediterranean Diet. *iHealth* author Phil Sparling profiles the life of a remarkable scientist.

2.3 "How I Learned to Love Breakfast (Or at Least What to Eat)." *New York Magazine*. A piece that looks into the science behind the idea that breakfast is the most important meal of the day.

2.4 "Six Rules for Eating Wisely." *Time*. Michael Pollan translates the complex guidelines of healthy nutrition into easy-to-remember rules of thumb.

SELF-ASSESSMENTS

2.1 Fruit, Vegetable, and Fiber Screener
2.2 Fat Intake Screener

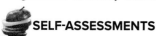

GENERAL

American Academy of Nutrition and Dietetics (professional society)
   www.eatright.org
Center for Science in the Public Interest (watchdog group) **www.cspinet.org**
International Food Information Council Foundation (corporate-funded)
   www.foodinsight.org/
Rudd Center for Food Policy and Obesity (university-based)
   www.uconnruddcenter.org

EAT WELL

Alternative Diets **oldwayspt.org/resources/heritage-pyramids**
ChooseMyPlate **www.choosemyplate.gov**
Dietary Guidelines for Americans **www.health.gov/dietaryguidelines**
Harvard Healthy Eating Plate
   www.hsph.harvard.edu/nutritionsource/healthy-eating-plate
Smart Nutrition 101 gateway **www.nutrition.gov/smart-nutrition-101**
Vitamins & Minerals **ods.od.nih.gov/factsheets/list-VitaminsMinerals**

FOOD LABELS

Labeling & Nutrition, FDA **www.fda.gov/Food/IngredientsPackagingLabeling/LabelingNutrition**

FOOD SAFETY

Centers for Disease Control and Prevention **www.cdc.gov/foodsafety**
Federal Food Safety gateway **www.foodsafety.gov**

DIETARY SUPPLEMENTS

Herbs & Supplements, MedlinePlus, National Library of Medicine
   www.nlm.nih.gov/medlineplus/druginfo/herb_All.html
Office of Dietary Supplements, National Institutes of Health
   https://ods.od.nih.gov

WEIGHT MANAGEMENT

Healthy Weight, CDC **www.cdc.gov/healthyweight**
National Weight Control Registry **www.nwcr.ws**

EATING DISORDERS

National Eating Disorders Association **www.nationaleatingdisorders.org/learn**

Knowing the Language

body composition, 59
body mass index (BMI), 59
Calorie (Cal), 40
carbohydrates, 41
dietary supplements, 56
eating disorders, 65
energy balance, 67
fats, 41

foodborne illness, 54
kilocalorie (kcal), 40
macronutrients, 39
micronutrients, 40
minerals, 44
obesity, 63
protein, 42
vitamins, 44

Understanding the Content

1. What are the six types of nutrients and their roles in the human diet?
2. What is the Choose MyPlate guide, and how can it be used to tailor your diet?
3. What are four basic rules of food handling that minimize risk of illness?
4. What is body mass index, or BMI, and how is it used to define overweight and obesity?
5. What is energy intake, and how would you measure it?

1. Why has the prevalence of overweight Americans increased so much over the past three to four decades?
2. How has the food industry changed its products to provide healthier options to the consumer? Identify three specific examples.
3. Why are so many Americans addicted to trying fad diets? Discuss the possible societal, social, psychological, and behavioral influences.
4. Why are dietary supplements so widely used by Americans? Discuss the pros and cons of dietary supplements.

Selected References

American Academy of Nutrition and Dietetics. Position paper: Promoting and supporting breastfeeding. *Journal of the Academy of Nutrition and Dietetics* 115: 444–449, 2015.

American Academy of Nutrition and Dietetics. Position paper: Total diet approach to healthy eating. *Journal of the Academy of Nutrition and Dietetics* 113: 307–317, 2013.

Bailey RL, Gahche JJ, Lentino CV, et al. Dietary supplement use in the United States, 2003–2006. *Journal of Nutrition* 141: 261–266, 2011.

Bray GA. *Contemporary Diagnosis and Management of Obesity and the Metabolic Syndrome* (3rd ed.). Newtown, PA: Handbooks in Health Care, 2003.

Centers for Disease Control and Prevention. Overweight and Obesity. **www.cdc.gov/obesity/**

Donnelly JE, Blair SN, Jakicic JM, et al. Appropriate physical activity intervention strategies for weight loss and prevention of weight regain for adults: ACSM position stand. *Medicine and Science in Sports and Exercise* 41: 459–471, 2009.

Finucane MM, Stevens GA, Cowan MJ, et al. National, regional, and global trends in body-mass index since 1980: Systematic analysis of health examination surveys and epidemiological studies with 960 country-years and 9.1 million participants. *Lancet* 377: 557–567, 2011.

Harmon K. How obesity spreads in social networks. *Scientific American,* May 2011.

Harris Interactive Poll. Overweight? Obese? Or Normal Weight? Americans Have Hard Time Gauging Their Weight. September 2, 2010.

Heymsfield SB, Lohman TG, Wang Z, Going SB (eds.). *Human Body Composition* (2nd ed.). Champaign, IL: Human Kinetics, 2005.

Hill JO, Wyatt HR, Peters JC. Energy balance and obesity. *Circulation* 126: 126–132, 2012.

Katzen M, Willett W. *Eat, Drink, and Weigh Less.* New York: Hyperion, 2007.

Kenney WL. Dietary water and sodium requirements for active adults. *Sports Science Exchange* 92, 2004.

Kushi LH, Doyle C, McCullough M, et al. American Cancer Society guidelines on nutrition and physical activity for cancer prevention. *CA: Cancer Journal for Clinicians* 62: 30–67, 2012.

Kushner RF. Clinical assessment and management of adult obesity. *Circulation* 126: 2870–2877, 2012.

Mayo Clinic. Weight Loss: 6 Strategies for Success. **www.mayoclinic.com/health/ weight-loss/HQ01625**

National Institutes of Health. *Managing Overweight and Obesity in Adults: Systematic Evidence Review, 2013.* **www.nhlbi.nih.gov/sites/www.nhlbi.nih.gov/ files/obesity-evidence-review.pdf**

Olshansky SJ, Passaro DJ, Hershow RC, et al. A potential decline in life expectancy in the United States in the 21st century. *New England Journal of Medicine* 352: 1138–1145, 2005.

Pollan M. *Food Rules: An Eater's Manual.* New York: Penguin, 2009.

Popkin BM, Armstrong LE, Bray GM, et al. A new proposed guidance system for beverage consumption in the United States. *American Journal of Clinical Nutrition* 83: 529–542, 2006.

Sparling PB. Obesity on campus. *Preventing Chronic Disease,* July 2007.

World Health Organization. Obesity. **www.who.int/topics/obesity**

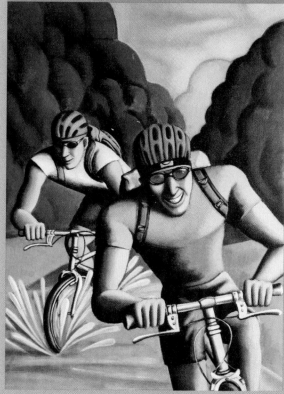

Exercise will make you feel better, function better, look better, and live longer.

— Steven N. Blair,

Senior Scientific Editor,

Physical Activity and Health:

A Report of the Surgeon General

Chapter 3

DEVELOP A FITNESS PROGRAM

The main topics in this chapter are health-related physical fitness, responses and adaptations to exercise, and exercise guidelines including national physical activity recommendations to improve health and prevent disease. Strategies are provided to assist you in developing an individualized plan that is enjoyable and sustainable.

THE HUMAN SPECIES was designed for movement. Until the mid-19th century, humans lived as gatherers, toolmakers, hunters, farmers, and artisans. For 99 percent of human history, physical tasks and manual labor were as much a part of daily life as eating and sleeping. Walking great distances, lifting and carrying loads, working with tools—muscular efforts of all types—were simply part of the everyday world. Our species not only survived but also flourished for several thousand generations prior to the advent of the automobile, television, and Internet. Then abruptly— within only a few generations—the physical activity demands of work and domestic chores decreased so dramatically as to be nearly nonexistent in present-day urbanized societies. Most of our waking hours are spent sitting.

Without question, the nearly universal adoption of labor-saving technology has brought marvelous advances to nearly all facets of human living. Yet, it's become evident that many of the chronic diseases we face today are associated with the resulting sedentary lifestyle. Physical *inactivity* is a risk factor for heart disease, diabetes, osteoporosis, and colorectal cancer, to name a few. These "diseases of inactivity" begin to emerge as early as the second and third decades of life. Moreover, the roots of obesity are at least as much in physical inactivity as in overeating.

From an evolutionary viewpoint, Dr. Thomas Rowland makes the case that habitual physical activity has a biological basis with a central neural control, not unlike hunger. In young children (and the young of most mammals), movement, which is central to growth and development, is often playful and spontaneous. The joy of movement in children is undeniable. Although the nature of this enjoyment— such as the discovery and mastery aspects—changes from childhood to adulthood, the enjoyment itself need not stop. If this natural drive to be active is severely limited, normal physiological function may be hampered. In modern America, the design of our living spaces restricts activity. Most of our leisure pursuits are in fact sedentary. Consider how our physical environments and social norms subdue our innate biological drive to be physically active.

Article
3.1

To be clear, this is not a plea to return to the physical toil that our ancestors endured. Rather, it's a frank reminder that the pendulum has swung too far to the other side. Our bodies were designed and wired for movement, yet we live in an environment where activity is no longer needed and in many ways discouraged (e.g., fewer sidewalks, more drive-throughs).

Based on extensive evidence, public health researchers have identified physical activity as one of the key health behaviors that must be promoted. This is no small challenge. Across the country, rates of participation in fitness and exercise activities decline steadily during the teenage and young adult years—throughout high school, throughout college, and then even more steeply in the years immediately following college.

This widespread decline in physical activity is understandable. In the college setting, considerable time is spent sitting (in classes, studying, computer use). And, in nearly all cases, you are being educated for sedentary occupations. These patterns of inactivity are likely to persist through adult life unless *you* decide otherwise. On the positive side, colleges provide multiple exercise and fitness resources (i.e., extensive facilities, intramurals, sports clubs, credit and noncredit exercise classes) and often a pedestrian- and bicycle-friendly campus. Most students have flexible schedules, making it easier to accommodate fitness and sports activities compared to what lies ahead with full-time jobs following graduation.

To optimize our well-being, we need to be physically active on a regular basis as well as reduce prolonged sitting throughout the day. Colleges provide a wide range of exercise and fitness opportunities just waiting to be explored. It's important to note that in addition to the enjoyment and challenge of regular physical activity, exercise can relieve stress, alleviate anxiety and depression, and boost higher-level thinking. These are valuable benefits indeed, especially for college students. The key to reaping the benefits lies with your decision to take a proactive approach.

➤ Physical Activity, Exercise, and Physical Fitness

The terms *exercise* and *physical fitness* are probably spoken in every home in America. Although these and related terms have specific meanings, the way in which they are used in everyday conversations varies widely among individuals and across groups. Let's eliminate any possible confusion by setting operational definitions for key terms at the onset.

PHYSICAL ACTIVITY AND EXERCISE

Let's begin by defining two core terms: *physical activity* and *exercise*. They have similar but distinct meanings. Then we'll define *intensity* because it is a common descriptor used to characterize physical activity or exercise.

Physical Activity

Physical activity is bodily movement produced by muscle contraction that increases energy expenditure above a resting level. Simply put, *physical activity* refers to moving around using our own muscle power. Physical activity includes all movement whether getting out of bed in the morning, getting dressed, preparing a meal, or walking to class. Research shows that consistently incorporating more physical activity into one's lifestyle (e.g., increasing incidental walking, commuting by foot or bike) can yield significant health benefits, particularly for those who have been sedentary. This active lifestyle approach may be more viable and appealing for many who are not interested in playing sports or training in a gym.

Exercise

Exercise is a subcategory or type of physical activity. Exercise is physical activity that is planned and structured with the primary purpose of improving or maintaining one or more aspects of our physical capacity, commonly known as physical fitness (defined in the next section). Thus, *exercise* refers to virtually all physical training and sports activities. Sports camps, physical education classes, and basic training in the military are all examples of exercise. Exercising regularly—whether it's training on a sports team or working out at the fitness center—improves health as well as physical capacity and performance.

Physical activity is muscular movement of the body that results in significant energy expenditure above the resting metabolism.

Exercise is structured physical activity that focuses on improving or maintaining physical capacity.

TABLE 3.1 PHYSICAL FITNESS: HEALTH-RELATED COMPONENTS

Cardiorespiratory (or aerobic) fitness
Musculoskeletal (or muscular) fitness
   Muscular strength
   Muscular endurance
   Flexibility
Body composition

Intensity

Intensity is arguably the most important element of physical activity or exercise, yet the concept remains fuzzy to many. *Intensity* refers to the physiological or perceptual effort given during a physical activity. Intensity is assessed with objective measurements (e.g., heart rate, energy expenditure) or subjective ratings (e.g., light, moderate, vigorous, all-out). Although intensity may be measured somewhat differently from setting to setting (e.g., health club, sports performance center, medical clinic), heart rate and perceived exertion are two widely used methods. Both are reviewed in the section "Recommendations for Healthy Adults."

PHYSICAL FITNESS

Physical fitness is a multifaceted concept whose definition has evolved over the past several decades. A generally accepted and enduring definition of physical fitness is "the ability to carry out daily tasks with vigor and alertness, without undue fatigue, and with ample energy to enjoy leisure time pursuits and meet unforeseen emergencies" (Clarke, 1971; *Physical Activity Guidelines*, 2008). A succinct definition from the *Surgeon General's Report on Physical Activity and Health* (1996) is "a set of attributes that people have or achieve that relates to the ability to perform physical activity." Three aspects of physical fitness are particularly noteworthy. First, improved fitness means an enhanced capacity to perform physical tasks of daily living as well as work-related and leisure-time physical activities. Second, as fitness improves so does physiological well-being, providing protection against numerous inactivity-related diseases. And third, physical fitness is divided into two types—health-related fitness and skill-related fitness—and each type has several components.

Health-Related Physical Fitness

Health-related physical fitness includes three fundamental components—cardiorespiratory or aerobic fitness, musculoskeletal or muscular fitness, and body composition (Table 3.1). The second, musculoskeletal fitness, is in turn composed of three subcomponents—strength, muscular endurance, and flexibility. These

Intensity is the effort associated with physical activity and is typically measured using heart rate or subjective ratings.

Physical fitness is a developed physical capacity that enables people to perform routine physical tasks with vigor, participate in a variety of physical activities, and reduce their risk for multiple, inactivity-related chronic diseases.

terms will be defined and discussed in detail in subsequent sections. Cardiorespiratory fitness, musculoskeletal fitness, and body composition are probably familiar concepts because they have long been included in school health and physical education classes.

As the name implies, developing health-related physical fitness is health-protective. Cardiorespiratory fitness lowers risk of disability and early death, especially from heart disease and stroke. Musculoskeletal fitness increases bone density, muscle mass, and joint health and thereby lowers the risk of osteoporosis, low back pain, and degenerative joint diseases. Maintenance of a healthy weight (body composition) through physical activity and good nutrition protects against obesity, diabetes, and related diseases including heart disease, arthritis, and some cancers. How many of these diseases have you witnessed among family members and friends? As we experience these events firsthand, the connection between physical activity and health becomes more real and less abstract.

Body composition, which partitions body weight into lean tissue (muscle and bone) and fat tissue, prescribes a healthy weight from one's level of relative body fatness (% body fat). This health-related fitness component is plainly dependent on *both* eating patterns and physical activity, more so than either cardiorespiratory or musculoskeletal fitness. As body composition answers to two masters, it is sometimes presented as a topic under diet and nutrition and sometimes under exercise and physical fitness. Everyone must eat, but physical activity is largely optional. For that reason, we provide our main discussion of body composition and the importance of healthy weight in Chapter 2; see the section on weight control.

When considering fitness components, it's natural to think of high-level sports performance. For elite endurance athletes such as Tour de France cyclists or Olympic marathoners, or elite strength athletes such as world-ranked power lifters or Olympic weight lifters, the focus is necessarily narrow and specialized—to be faster or stronger and have the best performance. The sole aim of the champion endurance or strength athlete is to train relentlessly to improve performance in a single fitness component. Other fitness components are important only if proficiency means an additional competitive edge. Such is the nature of national and international sports competition.

Most elite athletes compete at the highest level for only a few years. Upon retiring from competition, they dramatically reduce training levels and (hopefully) transition toward general health and fitness goals. For most of us, training and competing in sports and physically challenging activities are enjoyable leisure-time pastimes, not our livelihood or full-time pursuit. Thus, we are free to take a more balanced approach to our fitness programs. Regardless of our athletic abilities or sports interests, each of us can develop an exercise program that includes the three components of health-related fitness—cardiorespiratory fitness, musculoskeletal fitness, and body composition—in a measured and meaningful way.

Skill-Related Physical Fitness

The second type of fitness is skill-related physical fitness. While there are many skill-related components of physical fitness, the best known are agility, speed, coordination, and balance. Skill-related components are associated primarily with sport and motor skill performance and only secondarily with improved health. Among young adults, a finely tuned or specialized physical skill can translate into success in a variety of individual and team sports, from golf and

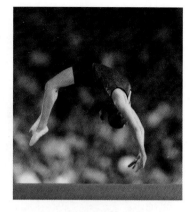

tennis to baseball and basketball. Among older adults, fitness classes to improve balance are increasing popular, as loss of balance is the major cause of falls among elderly individuals.

As many of us know from personal experience, components from both skill-related and health-related fitness intertwine in many sports. Soccer players must develop high levels of cardiorespiratory fitness in combination with soccer-specific skills, and gymnasts require high levels of musculoskeletal fitness to execute their skillful performances. Consider your favorite sports for other examples. As recreational athletes, many of us share a common goal—to develop the right combination of fitness components, both health-related and skill-related, to improve performance in our preferred sport(s).

Well-developed skill-related components of fitness, such as speed and agility, are essential to many sports.

© 2009 Jupiterimages Corporation

✓ NEED TO KNOW

Physical activity refers to movement due to muscle contraction, which results in an increase in energy expenditure. Exercise is one type of physical activity; it involves planned, structured activity with a focus on physical fitness. *Physical fitness* is a multidimensional concept that relates to a person's ability to perform physical activity. Physical fitness includes both health-related and skill-related components. To counter the development of chronic diseases and to enhance overall quality of life, personal fitness programs should emphasize the health-related components: cardiorespiratory fitness, musculoskeletal fitness, and body composition.

➤ How the Body Responds to Exercise

In miraculous fashion, the human body transforms the food we eat into our cells and tissues—blood, bone, muscle—and also uses food as fuel to supply the body's many energy needs. To understand how exercise can improve health and fitness, it's necessary to review the basic concept of energy metabolism, or how energy is produced for different types of physical activity.

ENERGY PRODUCTION FOR MUSCLE CONTRACTION

Energy for physical activity is produced in the muscle cells through a complex series of reactions that converts chemical energy into mechanical energy, resulting in muscle contraction. The most immediate source of energy comes from the high-energy chemical bonds of adenosine triphosphate (ATP). However, ATP—the energy currency of cells—is stored in the muscle in very small

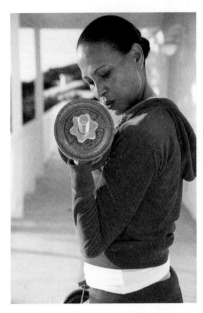

Weight lifting relies primarily on the anaerobic pathway.

© Corbis/Jupiterimages

amounts and can supply energy for only a few seconds. Only momentary movements such as turning your head or opening a door can be accomplished using stored ATP.

As movement is continued, ATP must be replenished from available macronutrients—primarily carbohydrate (glycogen) and fat. This is when the real work of energy production for muscular activity begins. Energy can be generated to replenish ATP via anaerobic or aerobic pathways. **Anaerobic metabolism** is the production of energy without oxygen present. This pathway of energy production is also relatively short-lived. It can provide a very high energy output but only for about 30 seconds. Anaerobic metabolism is the predominant pathway for short-term, high-intensity activities such as weight lifting and sprinting. Lactic acid is a byproduct (see the "Breaking It Down" discussion on lactic acid).

Energy production in the presence of oxygen is called **aerobic metabolism.** This pathway can provide moderate energy output for many hours. Prolonged activities such as distance running, cycling, swimming, and other endurance sports rely on aerobic metabolism for continued energy production. Aerobic metabolism depends on the cardiorespiratory system to transport oxygen from the air we breathe to the working muscles, where energy for muscle contraction is released during the oxidation of carbohydrates and fats. Carbon dioxide is a byproduct. The oxygen transport and uptake processes are complex yet efficient.

Only a few types of exercise are purely anaerobic or aerobic. For example, performance in short-duration events such as a bench press, high jump, or 40-yard sprint is essentially completely dependent on the anaerobic pathway. In contrast, performance in events lasting several hours such as running a marathon (26.2 miles) or cycling 50 miles is almost totally dependent on the aerobic pathway, which in turn reflects the capacity of the cardiorespiratory system to transport oxygen to the active muscles.

For sports competitions or other physically demanding tasks that are intermediate in duration, such as events lasting 1–10 minutes, both aerobic and anaerobic pathways contribute proportionately, with the relative significance of each

Anaerobic (which means "without oxygen") **metabolism** refers to biochemical pathways that do not require oxygen to produce energy for muscle contraction.

Aerobic (which means "with oxygen") **metabolism** pertains to biochemical pathways that use oxygen to produce energy for muscle contraction.

Among athletes and coaches, it's commonly thought that the buildup of lactic acid in the muscles leads to muscle pain, fatigue, and soreness. Scientists, though, have known for years that lactic acid does not cause muscle soreness. In fact, many of the side effects ascribed to lactic acid are simply not true. Let's take a quick look at how the lactic acid story arose.

In the early 1900s, prominent British researchers W. M. Fletcher and F. G. Hopkins found that isolated muscle fibers (from a frog) accumulated large amounts of lactic acid as they fatigued (when stimulated electrically). Following exercise, as the lactic acid dissipated, the muscle fibers recovered and were soon ready to contract again. This finding supported the hypothesis that a buildup of lactic acid causes muscle acidosis, which diminishes force production and in turn leads to fatigue. Good scientists always consider the most obvious or simplest explanation first. Follow-up studies appeared to support the hypothesis, so the finding was published and within years become part of common coaching knowledge.

With better techniques and high-tech tools, our understanding of exercise physiology and energy production advanced enormously, particularly from the 1970s forward. George Brooks, a professor at the University of California, Berkeley, led the way in unraveling the complexities of lactic acid. For example, his findings show that the body can efficiently use lactic acid as a source of fuel on par with carbohydrates stored in muscle (glycogen) and sugar in blood (glucose). In fact, it appears that lactic acid plays a role in linking the two metabolic cycles—the oxygen-based aerobic pathway and the oxygen-free anaerobic pathway—previously thought to be distinct.

So what is the bottom line on lactic acid? First, lactic acid can serve as an important fuel during exercise, and plays an important role in physiological adaptations (the training effect). Second, although lactic acid may be responsible for some of the discomfort of intense exercise, its role in muscle fatigue remains unclear. The evidence is mixed; some shows lactic acid may prevent fatigue, and some indicates just the opposite. Third, and still surprising to many, lactic acid does not cause muscle soreness. The likely explanation—with substantial evidence to support it—is that the muscle soreness we experience a few days following exercise is due to cellular-level disruption to muscle fibers and surrounding tissue.

Interestingly, these scientific revelations about lactic acid have little practical impact on how coaches train athletes. Through trial and error, coaches have learned what works, and to a large degree, this coaching knowledge is independent of understanding the details of human physiology. Since these scientific insights don't directly affect day-to-day training of athletes, it's easy for misconceptions to persist.

As with many aspects of human physiology and performance, the conventional wisdom is often a simplified version of early research and once established in popular thinking becomes difficult to revise or update. Now you know the real story about lactic acid, so spread the word and illuminate your friends. Lactic acid is not the cause of muscle soreness and it is more than just a byproduct of intense exercise.

| TABLE 3.2 | CONTRIBUTIONS OF AEROBIC AND ANAEROBIC METABOLISM TO ENERGY OUTPUT DURING EVENTS OF DIFFERENT DURATIONS | |

DURATION	% ANAEROBIC	% AEROBIC
10 seconds	95	5
30 seconds	85	15
1 minute	70	30
2 minutes	50	50
4 minutes	40	60
8 minutes	30	70
12 minutes	15	85
30 minutes	5	95

Source: Adapted from Astrand PO, Rodahl K. *Textbook of Work Physiology*. New York: McGraw-Hill, 1977.

depending on the duration of the effort. Table 3.2 presents the relative contributions of energy from aerobic and anaerobic pathways to perform maximally in events of different durations.

Many physical activities and sports are "stop and go," or intermittent in nature. Tennis is a good example. For these activities, both aerobic and anaerobic systems are called on to varying degrees throughout the game. Other factors being similar, the more continuous the activity, the greater the dependence on aerobic metabolism and thus the cardiovascular system. For instance, soccer and basketball, although not pure aerobic activities, are relatively more aerobic than baseball or volleyball.

CARDIORESPIRATORY FUNCTION AND OXYGEN UPTAKE

Cardiorespiratory function refers to the integration of the heart, lungs, and blood vessels to transport oxygen in the blood to muscles and other tissues and to remove carbon dioxide, a byproduct of oxidation. Oxygen delivery to the working muscles is paramount to sustain physical activities.

To understand the circulation of blood through the body, remember that arteries are vessels carrying blood away from the heart, and veins are vessels carrying blood to the heart (refer to Figure 3.1). As blood circulates through the lungs, hemoglobin in the red blood cells binds oxygen. This freshly oxygenated blood (red) returns to the heart via the pulmonary veins, flows through the left side of the heart, and is then pumped through the aorta, the main artery from the heart, to the major parts of the body (systemic circulation).

Arteries distribute the oxygen-rich blood to the working muscles, where oxygen is removed (or taken up, thus the term *oxygen uptake*) and used for aerobic metabolism. Carbon dioxide is produced, and the veins return the oxygen-poor, carbon dioxide–rich blood (blue) back to the heart and then to the lungs, where carbon dioxide is released in exhaled air and exchanged for oxygen. And the cycle repeats with hemoglobin binding oxygen.

The heart is a special type of muscle (cardiac muscle), and like skeletal muscle, it must have an adequate oxygen supply to continue its work. Delivering oxygen and nutrients to the heart muscle is the role of the coronary arteries, which branch off the aorta back onto the heart's surface. If these vessels become narrowed with

FIGURE 3.1 FLOW OF BLOOD THROUGH THE CIRCULATORY SYSTEM

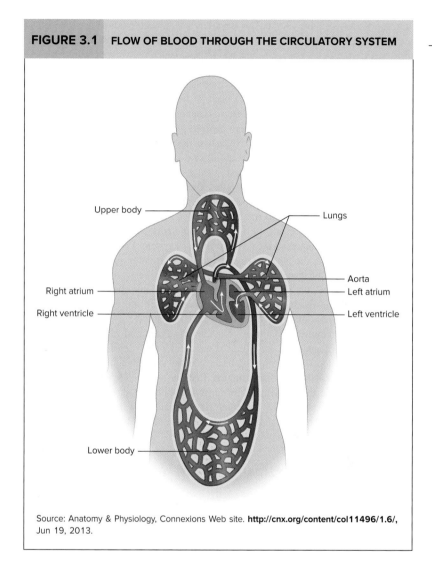

Source: Anatomy & Physiology, Connexions Web site. **http://cnx.org/content/col11496/1.6/**, Jun 19, 2013.

fatty deposits (atherosclerosis), blood flow can become restricted. This can lead to chest pain and heart attack.

Each beat of the heart can be felt as a pulse wherever an artery is close to the surface of the body, such as at the wrist or neck. Heart rate is expressed as beats per minute. The amount of blood ejected with each contraction (beat) of the heart is known as the stroke volume and is measured in milliliters per beat. The product of heart rate and stroke volume is cardiac output, which is the rate of blood flow in liters per minute. Cardiac output is directly proportional to oxygen transport: the greater the rate at which blood is being circulated, the greater the delivery of oxygen to the working muscles.

For most physical activities, the body responds in specific, predictable ways. As exercise begins—for example, going from sitting at your desk to walking across campus—the leg muscles need additional oxygen, so heart rate and stroke volume ramp up to deliver more blood. The elevation in heart rate is directly proportional to the demand for oxygen. Perhaps you are late for a class, so you walk quickly or jog. Again, your heart rate will increase proportionately as your exercise intensity increases. This is why heart rate is a widely used measure of exercise intensity.

Whether training or competing, if the exercise is demanding and prolonged, heart rate will continue to increase until the person's **aerobic capacity,** or maximal oxygen uptake, is reached. This is the case for runners, cyclists, and triathletes during the final stages of their races. Aerobic capacity refers to one's maximal ability to produce energy aerobically during exhaustive exercise. It can be measured in the lab via a graded exercise test on a treadmill or a stationary bike (cycle ergometer), or it can be estimated from a field test such as a 2-mile run. Aerobic capacity is the single best measure of cardiorespiratory fitness and is the main determinant of endurance performance. This concept plays a central role in individualizing exercise programs and will be discussed in more detail later in this chapter.

For exercise that is focused on musculoskeletal fitness, such as weight training or calisthenics, the demand on the cardiorespiratory system is much less pronounced. As mentioned earlier, the physiological demands of different types of exercise vary widely. At one end of the continuum is cross-country skiing—a total-body form of exercise that requires the simultaneous use of the large muscles in the legs, trunk, and arms to sustain the high energy output necessary to move one's body weight over a long distance. This type of exercise is clearly aerobic.

At the other end of the continuum is a one-arm bicep curl in which a relatively small muscle is producing force over a distance of only a few feet per repetition. The energy demand on the single muscle can be very high, but it is localized. Multiple repetitions take less than a minute. Relative to the energy required to move the entire body, the energy demand to move a dumbbell a short distance is small and short-lived. Consequently, muscular fitness training relies primarily on the anaerobic pathway. The contribution and interaction of aerobic and anaerobic systems vary depending on the duration, continuousness, and type of exercise.

ADAPTATIONS TO PHYSICAL TRAINING

The physiological and performance changes that occur with regular training are collectively termed the **training effect.** A primary adaptation to aerobic exercise is improved oxygen delivery to the muscles. At the level of the lungs, training enhances the exchange of oxygen and carbon dioxide at higher rates. Concurrently, as the heart strengthens, it can eject more blood with each beat. This increase in stroke volume results in the decrease in resting heart rate commonly observed after a few weeks of training. These cumulative pulmonary and cardiovascular changes account for the improved delivery of oxygen to the muscles.

Another fundamental adaptation that improves oxygen uptake and thus energy production takes place within the muscle cells themselves. Most of the cellular

---

Aerobic capacity, or maximal oxygen uptake, is the highest amount of oxygen the body can consume during exhaustive exercise. It is considered the single best measure of cardiorespiratory fitness.

The **training effect** is the physiological changes (adaptations) and improved fitness resulting from regular physical training.

changes occur in the cell structure known as the mitochondrion. This is the actual site of aerobic metabolism, where food is converted to usable energy in the presence of oxygen. Training causes the mitochondria to increase in size and number. The aerobic enzymes, catalysts in the aerobic pathway of energy production, also increase in quantity. Moreover, endurance is further improved by the enhanced ability of the muscles to use fats as fuel, sparing muscle carbohydrate stores (glycogen).

Resistance or weight training to improve musculoskeletal fitness can bring about significant increases in muscle size (hypertrophy), strength, muscular endurance, and flexibility. Improvements in muscle tone and force production are induced in several ways. A program of resistance training coupled with flexibility exercises improves blood flow to and neural control of muscle fibers, allowing for more efficient energy production, fiber recruitment, and muscle recovery. Over the same period, concentrations of anaerobic and/or aerobic enzymes are increased in the muscle cells, depending on the energy pathways being challenged. Resistance/flexibility training maintains healthy joints and connective tissues such as tendons, ligaments, and cartilage, and is protective against musculoskeletal injury.

A balanced exercise program develops or maintains both cardiorespiratory and musculoskeletal fitness. Such a program improves performance whether in specific fitness tests, sports competitions, or challenging physical tasks in daily life. A balanced exercise program also yields direct health benefits modulated through the body's multiple biological systems. Primary health benefits include

- Improved metabolism (namely, normalized blood lipids and glucose) and lower risk for heart disease and diabetes
- Improved body composition and weight control and lower risk for obesity
- Maintenance of healthy bones, muscles, and joints and lower risk for osteoporosis, joint diseases, and low back pain
- Improved psychological health and reduced risk for anxiety and depression

A dose-response relationship is evident for both cardiorespiratory and musculoskeletal exercise. That is, the more you exercise, the greater the improvements in health and fitness. If a pill could bring about this impressive combination of benefits, it would be hailed as a wonder drug. Moreover, regular physical activity has few unwanted side effects, and costs are easily minimized. As top researcher Steven N. Blair succinctly affirms, exercise will make you feel better, function better, look better, and live longer. A final point to remember about the training effect: Improved fitness and associated health benefits are reversible and diminish with inactivity. We can't store up fitness. The key is to establish exercise as a habit.

✓ NEED TO KNOW

Energy for most physical activity is provided via aerobic metabolism, which is dependent on the cardiorespiratory system to transport oxygen to the working muscles. Aerobic capacity (maximal oxygen uptake) is the single best measure of cardiorespiratory fitness. The *training effect* refers to both the physiological adaptations and performance improvements that occur as a consequence of regular training. A balanced physical activity program to promote health and fitness includes both cardiorespiratory and musculoskeletal training.

➤ Recommendations for Healthy Adults

The physical activity recommendations presented in this section focus on the amounts and type of exercise known to improve health. These recommendations are based on the *Physical Activity Guidelines for Americans,* and position statements from leading scientific and public health organizations including the American College of Sports Medicine, Centers for Disease Control and Prevention, World Health Organization, American Heart Association, and American Cancer Society.

For those who lead a sedentary lifestyle, these guidelines provide a reasonable goal. For those who are fit and engage in more advanced training programs, these guidelines serve as a benchmark for comparison. You can glean tips to adjust your current program and insights on how to assist a friend in starting or maintaining a program.

First, we'll review the basic principles of exercise training as a prelude to presenting the physical activity recommendations for cardiorespiratory fitness followed by those for musculoskeletal fitness. Then we'll present the concept of the physical activity continuum to illustrate where the recommendations fall within the broad spectrum of activity levels.

PRINCIPLES OF EXERCISE TRAINING

Exercise training is based on four principles: overload, reversibility, specificity, and individual differences. Consider each principle when planning an exercise program.

Principle of Overload

To improve a physiological system, it must be challenged, stressed, or taxed—in other words, exposed to a stimulus greater than it is normally accustomed to, such as a faster pace or a heavier weight. This is the fundamental principle on which all exercise training is based. Repeated exposure over time to progressively greater loads (amounts of exercise) results in responsive changes by the lungs, heart, muscle, and connective tissue—structural and functional adaptations from the molecular to the system level. This translates into enhanced capacities and efficiencies in cardiorespiratory and musculoskeletal functions and, thus, improved fitness.

Principle of Reversibility

This principle is simply the converse of the principle of overload. When one stops exercising and the training overload is removed, the previously developed physiological systems will over time return to pretraining levels. To maintain fitness, one must continue to exercise. Fitness cannot be stored.

Principle of Specificity

Many training effects are specific to the type of exercise, the particular muscles involved, and the intensity. For example, if the goal is to run a 5-kilometer (5K) race at a 7-minute-per-mile pace, then the principle of specificity suggests that the person should focus on *running* and include training sessions *at the goal pace.* If all training is done at an 8- to 9-minute-per-mile pace, it will be difficult to shift gears on race day because the body has not been exposed to the specific demands of running at the faster pace. Moreover, swimming and cycling, although excellent aerobic exercise, will do little to improve running performance because the muscles are used in different ways for each activity. Training specificity is critical for reaching performance goals.

Principle of Individual Differences

There is tremendous variability from one person to the next in both natural fitness level and in the rate of improvement that occurs with exercise training. Due to different genetic endowments, each of us begins at a different point on the fitness continuum. This is no different from variability among individuals in height or hair color. What is not as apparent, though, is the variability among individuals in their responses to a similar training program. A standard exercise dose may be just right for many people but too hard for others and not enough for some. For best results, customize your exercise program as you learn how your body responds. The exercise guidelines that follow are just that, a *guide*, a place to start, a point of reference. The fine-tuning is left to each individual.

CARDIORESPIRATORY FITNESS

Cardiorespiratory fitness, also known as aerobic fitness or cardiorespiratory endurance, is the ability of the respiratory and circulatory systems to supply oxygen to the working muscles during sustained physical activity. For most people, being fit means having good cardiorespiratory fitness. Due to the multiple benefits that come with cardiorespiratory fitness, most scientists and clinicians believe this fitness component to be the most important.

The FITT Acronym

Four factors constitute an exercise plan: frequency, intensity, time (duration), and type. Conveniently, the first letters of these four factors form the acronym FITT, which is an easy way to remember them. The details for each factor are presented below:

Frequency: How Often?

The recommended exercise frequency is at least three and up to seven days per week. One should consider frequency relative to both intensity and duration. For example, those who enjoy vigorous exercise should consider training every other day, while those who prefer moderate intensity activity could probably exercise most days of the week (e.g., hard running three to four days per week vs. brisk walking five to six days per week).

Intensity: How Hard Do I Have to Push Myself?

Exercise intensity should be within 50–85 percent of aerobic capacity, with **moderate intensity** defined as 50–59 percent and **vigorous intensity** as 60–85 percent. For most

---

Cardiorespiratory fitness is a health-related component of physical fitness that relates to the ability of the circulatory and respiratory systems to supply oxygen to the working muscles during sustained physical activity.

Moderate-intensity physical activity is brisk walking or similar activities that require 50–59 percent of one's aerobic capacity (equivalent to 50–59 percent of one's heart rate training range using the heart rate reserve method).

Vigorous-intensity physical activity is running and similar sweat-producing activities that require 60–85 percent of one's aerobic capacity (equivalent to 60–85 percent of one's heart rate training range using the heart rate reserve method).

young adults, a moderate-intensity activity is similar to brisk walking (about 4 miles per hour), and a vigorous-intensity activity is like jogging/running. A lower threshold of 40 percent of aerobic capacity may be appropriate for people who are older or chronically sedentary.

Heart Rate (HR) as a Measure of Intensity Since oxygen uptake and heart rate are highly correlated, heart rate can be used to gauge intensity. There are several approaches to using heart rate to calculate training zones (ranges). Although it is common to take a straight percentage of a person's estimated maximal heart rate, we prefer the heart rate reserve method because it takes into account resting heart rate and is directly proportional to increases in oxygen uptake (energy expenditure). The heart rate reserve is simply the difference between the resting heart rate (HR_{rest}) and the maximal heart rate (HR_{max}). Maximal heart rate is estimated by subtracting age from 220. To calculate the training heart rate range, determine the lower and upper limits as follows:

$$HR \text{ at } 50\% \text{ intensity} = [(HR_{max} - HR_{rest}) \times 0.50] + HR_{rest}$$
$$HR \text{ at } 85\% \text{ intensity} = [(HR_{max} - HR_{rest}) \times 0.85] + HR_{rest}$$

For example, using these equations, the heart rate training range (from 50 to 85 percent intensity) for a 20-year-old with a resting heart rate of 70 would be 135–181 beats per minute. As this is a large range, the next step would be to decide whether to train in the moderate or vigorous part of the range. The training heart rate zone for different ages is plotted in Figure 3.2.

How to Measure Heart Rate Measuring heart rate is easy to learn. Take your pulse on the inside of the wrist (at the radial artery) by placing the tips of your first

FIGURE 3.2 TRAINING HEART RATE ZONE BY AGE, USING THE HEART RATE RESERVE METHOD

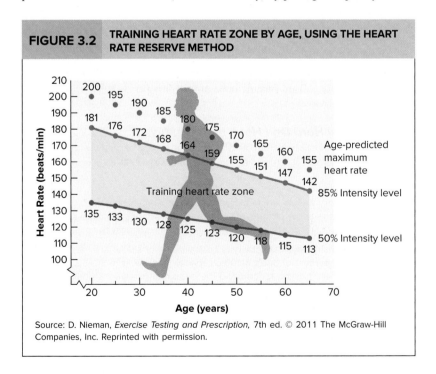

Source: D. Nieman, *Exercise Testing and Prescription,* 7th ed. © 2011 The McGraw-Hill Companies, Inc. Reprinted with permission.

two fingers about an inch below the base of the thumb. When you feel the pulse, count the beats for 10 seconds and then multiply the 10-second count by six to determine your heart rate in beats per minute. To measure resting heart rate, check your pulse after sitting quietly for at least 10 minutes or upon waking in the morning. To estimate exercise heart rate, count your pulse immediately after exercise. Take time to practice so you can reliably measure the higher heart rates. An option is to use a heart rate monitor that displays heart rate continuously. Light-weight heart rate monitors that consist of a chest strap (transmitter) and watch (receiver) are reliable, durable, and relatively inexpensive.

Perceived Exertion as a Measure of Intensity Another approach for monitoring intensity is to use the **rating of perceived exertion (RPE).** Developed by Professor Gunnar Borg, this scale links a person's subjective rating of physical exertion to a number between 6 and 20 using verbal descriptors (Table 3.3). For example, if the exercise effort feels "very light," the rating would be a 9; "somewhat hard" would be a 13; and "extremely hard" a 19. The RPE scale correlates well with heart rate and is routinely used during exercise testing and in exercise classes. The scale is useful in teaching people how *hard* or *easy* to work to achieve an appropriate intensity. For most young adults, ratings from 12 to 14 correspond to about 50–60 percent of the heart rate training range (HR reserve method), and ratings from 15 to 18 correspond to 60–85 percent.

Exercise intensity is arguably the most important factor in determining the rate of improvement. For the highly motivated, it's tempting to work out very hard (at high intensities) from the onset of an exercise program with the aim of improving quickly. Yet, exercising too hard without appropriate transition time to build up is generally counterproductive. High-intensity "starter" programs often lead to prolonged fatigue, extreme soreness, and an increased risk of injury. Forget the crash programs and limit the intensity the first few weeks of a new program.

Time: How Long?

Consensus guidelines recommend engaging in a minimum of 150 minutes a week of moderate-intensity, or 75 minutes a week of vigorous-intensity, aerobic activity, or an equivalent combination. Intensity and duration generally balance each other— the higher the intensity, the shorter the duration, and vice versa. For moderate-intensity aerobic activities like brisk walking, the guideline is at least 30 minutes per day, five days per week. Durations as short as 10 minutes can be accumulated throughout the day. Because of the dose-response relationship between physical activity and health, more is better: 45–60 minutes per day is preferable, and 60–90 minutes may be necessary for weight control (refer to Chapter 2).

Type: Which Activities?

The type or mode of activity should stress the cardiorespiratory, or aerobic, system. Such activities have the following characteristics: require use of major muscle groups, are rhythmic or repetitive, and can be done continuously. The most common

> **Rating of perceived exertion (RPE)** is a subjective measure of the strenuousness of a physical activity, based on one's overall perception of effort; it is widely used as a measure of exercise intensity. The RPE scale ranges from 6 to 20 with accompanying verbal descriptors (e.g., light, hard).

Recommendations for Healthy Adults

TABLE 3.3 RATING OF PERCEIVED EXERTION: BORG RPE SCALE®

6	No exertion at all
7	
8	Extremely light
9	Very light
10	
11	Light
12	
13	Somewhat hard
14	
15	Hard (heavy)
16	
17	Very hard
18	
19	Extremely hard
20	Maximal exertion

Source: © Gunnar Borg, 1970, 1985, 1994, 1998. Reprinted with permission of Gunnar Borg.

Instructions to the Borg RPE Scale®

While exercising, we want you to use this scale to rate your perception of exertion. How heavy and strenuous does the exercise feel to you, combining all sensations and feelings of physical stress, effort, and fatigue? Do not concern yourself with any one factor, such as leg pain or shortness of breath, but try to focus on the total feeling of exertion.

6 "No exertion at all," means you don't feel any exertion whatsoever—no muscle fatigue, no breathlessness or difficulty breathing.

9 "Very light" exertion, such as taking a short walk at your own pace.

13 "Somewhat hard" work, but it still feels OK to continue.

15 "Hard" and tiring, but continuing isn't terribly difficult.

17 "Very hard" means very strenuous work. You can still go on, but you really have to push yourself and you are very tired.

19 "Extremely hard" is for most people the strongest exertion they have ever experienced.

Try to appraise your feeling of exertion as honestly as possible, without thinking about what the actual physical load is. Try not to underestimate and not to overestimate your exertion. It's your own feeling of effort and exertion that is important, not how it compares with other people's. Look at the scale and the expressions and then give a number.

Sources: © Gunnar Borg, 1985, 1994, 1998, 2006. Reprinted with permission of Gunnar Borg.

aerobic activities are walking, running, cycling, and swimming, but many other activities meet the criteria as well. The key is to select an activity that you like. If the activity is not enjoyable, it's unlikely you will continue. A word of caution for beginning exercisers or older people: avoid high-impact activities like running and aerobic dance as initial choices because of their higher injury rates.

MUSCULOSKELETAL FITNESS

Musculoskeletal fitness, or muscular fitness, is composed of three intertwined elements: muscular strength, muscular endurance, and flexibility. **Muscular strength** is a muscle or muscle group's maximal capacity to exert force against an external resistance—that is, the most weight you can lift one time (e.g., one-repetition maximum, 1RM), such as with the arm curl for the biceps muscle or the leg extension for the quadriceps. **Muscular endurance** is slightly different. It refers to the muscle's ability to sustain a submaximal force or to persist at some relative level—for example, the number of repetitions you can complete at a resistance equal to 50 percent of 1RM. **Flexibility** is the functional range of motion in a joint or group of joints. Flexibility varies from joint to joint and depends on the muscles, tendons, and ligaments at the involved joint(s).

Musculoskeletal fitness is demonstrated in nearly all sports. To varying degrees during a competition, muscles are called on to exert peak force, resist fatigue, and perform well through multiple ranges of motion. Musculoskeletal fitness is certainly related to our health status, too. It enables us to perform demanding physical tasks—both routine and unplanned—that arise in everyday situations as well as helping to combat osteoporosis, low back pain, joint disease, loss of mobility, and frailty.

To develop musculoskeletal fitness, we must engage in some form of **resistance training.** Although it is better known as strength training or weight training, *resistance training* is the preferred term for several reasons. First, strength *and* muscular endurance are usually developed in combination. Second, "resistance" can be applied to the muscles using traditional iron weights (dumbbells, barbells, weight stacks), but it can also be accomplished using muscle- and movement-specific equipment with pneumatic, hydraulic, and computer-controlled resistance, as well as simply body weight (e.g., calisthenics—sit-ups, push-ups, pull-ups). Resistance training coupled with appropriate attention to flexibility exercises is the basis for improving musculoskeletal fitness.

Musculoskeletal fitness, a health-related component of physical fitness, refers to the combination of muscular strength, muscular endurance, and flexibility.

Muscular strength is the maximal force that a muscle (or muscle group) can exert against a resistance.

Muscular endurance is the ability of a muscle (or muscle group) to apply a submaximal force repeatedly or to sustain a muscular contraction over an extended period.

Flexibility is the range of motion available in a joint (or group of joints).

Resistance training, commonly known as weight training or strength training, is exercise that develops strength and muscular endurance using free weights, machine weights, body weight (calisthenics), or some combination.

Hundreds of scientific studies have been conducted to determine what constitutes a sufficient (health-promoting) exercise dose for developing strength and muscular endurance. The evidence base for recommending flexibility exercises is much sparser. Although stretching exercises have proven effectiveness in regaining range of motion during rehabilitation from musculoskeletal injury or surgery, there is little quality research on the health benefits of flexibility for people with no physical limitations. Among the many official statements on physical activity recommendations from scientific organizations, only the American College of Sports Medicine provides specific commentary and suggestions on flexibility. Although of less overall importance than either aerobic or resistance training, flexibility training is certainly important as a complementary component and should be included as part of a balanced program of physical activity.

Using the FITT acronym's categories, we present recommendations for achieving a healthy level of musculoskeletal fitness.

Frequency: How Often?

The recommended training frequency for resistance training is two or more nonconsecutive days per week. Training three days per week will result in greater benefits. The standard practice is to allow two days of rest between resistance training sessions to give muscles time to recover and adapt (e.g., work out Monday, Wednesday, Friday or Tuesday, Thursday, Saturday).

Intensity: How Hard Do I Have to Work?

Intensity is a function of the resistance (e.g., amount of weight lifted). The recommendation is to complete at least one set of 8–12 repetitions of 8–10 exercises that condition the major muscle groups. Through trial and error, you will learn to select the proper resistance for each exercise—that is, a weight that results in substantial muscle fatigue during the final 1–2 repetitions of the set. The RPE scale can also be used to gauge intensity. In Table 3.4, we provide a sample program of 10 exercises.

TABLE 3.4	**STANDARD RESISTANCE EXERCISES AND ASSOCIATED MUSCLE GROUPS**
EXERCISE*	**MUSCLE GROUP**
1. Bench press	Chest (pectoralis, triceps)
2. Leg press	Legs, buttocks (quadriceps, gluteals)
3. Shoulder press	Shoulders (deltoids, triceps)
4. Leg extension	Front of thigh (quadriceps)
5. Pull down	Back (latissimus dorsi)
6. Leg curl	Back of thigh (hamstrings)
7. Triceps extension	Back of arm (triceps)
8. Heel raise	Calves (gastrocnemius)
9. Arm curl	Front of arm (biceps)
10. Curl-ups	Abdomen (abdominals)

*These or very similar exercises can be done with free weights or on exercise machines. Also, note that all the major muscle groups can be developed with calisthenics (e.g., push-ups, pull-ups, bar-dips, curl-ups, heel raises, bench stepping with added weight).

Time: How Long?

As a practical matter, the time or duration is the length of the entire workout session. This includes the actual time exercising (e.g., lifting weights) and the recovery time between exercises, which should be kept to 1–2 minutes. A duration of 20–30 minutes is a reasonable estimate for the total time needed to complete one set of 8–10 exercises.

Type: Which Activities?

In contrast to training for cardiorespiratory fitness, the options for improving or maintaining muscular fitness are more limited. Such training must involve resistance exercise whether it is traditional weight training, calisthenics, or newer variations of resistance-based exercise. Regardless of the type of equipment or specific program, the overall goal is the same: to condition all the major muscles, not just a couple specific muscles. End-of-chapter Website Resources provide detailed information on resistance exercises and programs for different levels (novice, intermediate, advanced).

To maintain range of motion, flexibility exercises should be included as part of a musculoskeletal training program. Although flexibility training per se is not included in the physical activity position statements of all organizations, it is an accepted component for individual exercise plans. Stretching should focus on muscle/tendon groups at major joints (e.g., ankle, knee, hips, back, neck, shoulder, elbow, wrist). Stretches should be slow and steady (static), maintained at a position of mild discomfort for about 30 seconds, and repeated two or three times. Refer to end-of-chapter Website Resources for descriptions and illustrations of flexibility exercises.

PHYSICAL ACTIVITY CONTINUUM

It's convenient to categorize everyone into two groups: exercisers and nonexercisers. This oversimplification neglects a fundamental fact: Physical activity levels vary tremendously across a broad continuum, from no physical activity beyond the routine activities of daily living to enormous amounts of training required for high-level sports competition. In Figure 3.3, the physical activity (PA) continuum is depicted as three overlapping spheres representing low, moderate, and high activity. Within each sphere, multiple levels exist. During various periods in our lives, we shift among levels within a sphere and from one sphere to another. Additionally, our "background activity level" continues to shrink—sitting has become the predominant feature of our waking hours.

Many college students may find themselves in the low-activity sphere in which the sedentary lifestyle rules. They engage in few if any physical activities other than those required to get through the day and are plainly falling short of recommended activity levels. Some may be taking small steps toward incorporating more activity into daily routines, such as frequent standing/walking to break up prolonged sitting or walking across campus instead of taking the bus. These actions are additive and in the right direction. The goal is to move into the next sphere in the continuum.

Those who are achieving recommended levels of physical activity for both cardiorespiratory and muscular fitness are in the middle sphere of the continuum. The recommendations allow wide latitude in developing programs to meet individual needs and preferences. For example, some people prefer vigorous aerobic exercise, while others find moderate-intensity physical activity more to their liking. Similar options exist for meeting recommendations for muscular fitness. Lifting weights and

Article 3.2

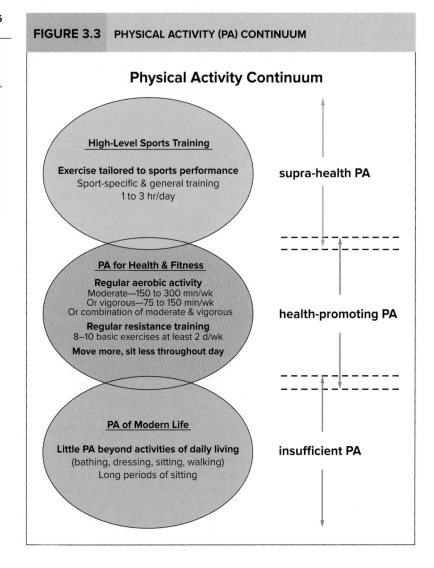

FIGURE 3.3 PHYSICAL ACTIVITY (PA) CONTINUUM

Physical Activity Continuum

High-Level Sports Training

Exercise tailored to sports performance
Sport-specific & general training
1 to 3 hr/day

supra-health PA

PA for Health & Fitness

Regular aerobic activity
Moderate—150 to 300 min/wk
Or vigorous—75 to 150 min/wk
Or combination of moderate & vigorous
Regular resistance training
8–10 basic exercises at least 2 d/wk
Move more, sit less throughout day

health-promoting PA

PA of Modern Life

Little PA beyond activities of daily living
(bathing, dressing, sitting, walking)
Long periods of sitting

insufficient PA

stretching at a fitness center is a popular choice, but others may prefer a home-based program of calisthenics and flexibility exercises.

This sphere is expansive and includes those expending 800–1,000 Cal per week (e.g., briskly walking 2 miles per session five days per week) up through those expending twice that amount through a variety of activities (e.g., a combination of running, swimming, basketball, and soccer). Approaches are variable: Some choose a lifestyle approach such as accumulating 10-minute walks throughout the day, while others opt for structured exercise classes. Within this middle sphere, regardless of the approach, the greater the total physical activity, the greater will be the health benefits.

The top sphere of the continuum is the realm of high-level exercise and sports training. Many of you have been in this sphere, perhaps as an age group or high school athlete. And some of you are in this sphere now, enjoying the challenge of advanced training on a sports team or for personal fitness. Competing at a high level requires a commitment to training, often several hours a day most days of the week. The goals at this level are focused on performance, not on health. In fact, few additional health benefits are derived from training at this level beyond those achieved from training in the middle sphere. Remember, though, successful training at this level depends on a solid fitness base and robust health developed in the middle sphere.

Throughout this section, physical activity recommendations have been presented as ranges for frequency, intensity, time, and type of activity. The public health standard—equivalent to 30 minutes of brisk walking at least five days per week—imparts significant health benefits for those who have been sedentary. If the entire population could achieve this standard, it would significantly improve the nation's health. However, this level of physical activity is the minimal, *not* the optimal—it's the lowest level within the middle sphere. Let's be clear on this point. Greater amounts of physical activity result in greater health benefits. Individuals who can maintain an exercise program that is of longer duration and/or more vigorous (a high level within the middle sphere) will be both more fit and healthier.

✓ **NEED TO KNOW**

The physical activity "dose" needed to impart significant health benefits is known. Exercise is prescribed in terms of frequency, intensity, time, and type (FITT) for both aerobic and musculoskeletal conditioning. The basic training principles of overload (and reversibility), specificity, and individual differences can guide you in applying exercise recommendations. The physical activity (PA) continuum has three spheres: physical activity of modern life (insufficient PA), physical activity for health and fitness (health-promoting PA), and training for high-level performance (supra-health PA).

➤ Personalizing an Exercise Program

Developing a fitness program involves linking consensus recommendations to individual goals. And goals vary widely—increase stamina, gain strength, improve muscle tone, lose body fat, add muscle mass, control weight, relieve stress, improve sports performance—and the list goes on. What are your goals? Since many exercise goals are related to losing body fat or gaining muscle mass, the energy expenditure side of the energy balance equation will be reviewed in the first part of this section.

From time to time, each of us are drawn to try a new sport or special event —perhaps a local 10K road race or an active, adventure vacation centered on downhill skiing, ocean kayaking, mountain biking, or scuba diving. The challenge then becomes to devise a fitness plan to prepare accordingly. The more fit you are, the more enjoyable the experience—and the more you'll be able to do! List your main short-term goals and a few long-term goals too. In the latter part of this section, key practical points are shared to help you develop an exercise program that works.

ENERGY BALANCE: ENERGY EXPENDITURE

One of the primary reasons people exercise is for weight control—that is, to help keep a balance between energy intake and energy expenditure. In Chapter 2, the *energy intake* or food consumption side of the energy balance equation was discussed. Now let's take a closer look at the *energy expenditure* side. Understanding how physical activity contributes to energy expenditure is critical to preventing unwanted weight gain and to successful long-term weight management.

Estimating Daily Energy Expenditure

Three factors determine a person's daily energy expenditure: (1) resting metabolic rate, (2) the thermic effect of food, and (3) the amount of physical activity. Resting (or basal) metabolic rate is a function of body size and accounts for the majority of one's daily energy expenditure (about 60–75 percent). Plainly, the larger your mass (the more you weigh), the more energy you need to keep all physiological functions operating at the resting level (e.g., sleeping or sitting quietly).

The *thermic effect of food* refers to the energy required for digestion. This is associated with that slight but noticeable warm-up one feels an hour or two after a large meal. This energy expenditure component is small (5–10 percent) and generally included as part of the resting metabolic rate.

The third factor is the amount of physical activity. This is the only factor that we control. Physical activity is highly variable among people and within an individual. It may account for as little as 25 percent of daily energy expenditure in sedentary folks whose only physical activity is that required by daily living—such as dressing, bathing, and necessary walking. Or physical activity can account for as much as 40 percent or more among highly active people who get an hour or more of exercise every day.

Daily energy expenditures for a moderately active 121-lb. woman and a moderately active 154-lb. man would be about 2,000 and 2,500 Cal, respectively. Your energy expenditure will vary accordingly based on your weight and activity level.

Self
Assessment
3.1

Additional Caloric Expenditure through Physical Activity

Average calories burned for different types of moderate and vigorous physical activities are shown in Table 3.5. Note that the energy expended during resistance training is quite a bit lower than what is expended for aerobic activities. This should be clear from the earlier discussion on energy pathways and the different energy demands of aerobic training versus resistance training.

A second point to highlight is the trade-off between intensity and duration among aerobic activities. If your primary aim is to expend calories, you have a choice between exercising at a higher intensity for a shorter duration or longer at a lower intensity. The total energy required to move a mass—in this case, a person's body weight—over a given distance is not substantially affected by the speed at which it occurs. The energy expended by running 2 miles in 15 minutes (about 200 Cal) is only about 10 percent more than is expended by walking the same distance in 30 minutes (about 180 Cal). For a beginning exerciser or a person with a high-BMI, the preferable option is to extend duration and go at a moderate pace.

When considering healthful levels of physical activity, the target range for energy expenditure is 150–400 Cal per day. This is in addition to the energy expenditure from activities of daily living. The lower end of the range represents a minimal level of about 1,000 Cal per week, which equates to the public health physical activity recommendation of 30 minutes of brisk walking five days per week. Based on the positive dose-response relationship between physical activity and health, gradually moving toward the 300–400 Cal per day level is encouraged. Intentional energy expenditure at 2,000 Cal per week and higher (60–90 minutes per day) has been shown to be successful for both initial weight loss and weight maintenance.

TABLE 3.5	ENERGY EXPENDITURE FOR INTERMITTENT AND CONTINUOUS ACTIVITIES

INTERMITTENT ACTIVITIES	CAL EXPENDED IN 30 MINUTES
Resistance training—light	100
Volleyball	100
Golf—walking	150
Resistance training—vigorous	150
Aerobic dance	215
Basketball	220

CONTINUOUS ACTIVITIES	CAL EXPENDED IN 30 MINUTES
Walking at 4 miles/hour	200
Bicycling	245
Swimming	255
Stair climbing	300
Jogging at 6 miles/hour	310
Running at 8 miles/hour	440

These are estimates of total energy expended in 30 minutes for a 154-lb. person. Those who weigh more will expend more, and those who weigh less will expend less. These values are approximations that allow for relative comparison among different activities. Actual calories expended can vary depending on the intensity and continuousness of the activity.

Source: Compendium of physical activities. **https://sites.google.com/site/ compendiumofphysicalactivities/.**

DEVELOPING AN EXERCISE PLAN

It's time to translate the cardiorespiratory and musculoskeletal guidelines into a specific exercise prescription based on your goals. Alternatively, if you are already a regular exerciser, take the time to assess your program in light of the current recommendations. To help with the translation process, consider the following points.

Physical Activity or Exercise?

Most people in their 20s still have moderate to high functional capacities due to their youth. Relying solely on moderate-intensity physical activity, such as brisk walking, may not be sufficiently challenging unless you have been very sedentary—in that case, moderate-intensity activity *is* the appropriate choice. The majority of college students report they *prefer* exercise that is more vigorous whether it's recreational sports, basic fitness training, or a combination.

Many colleges have excellent fitness centers and programs. This provides a special opportunity to explore all types of classes. The variety of physical education and campus recreation classes taught by high-caliber instructors is impressive. High school offerings pale in comparison. Moreover, after college, your choices will likely be much more restrictive—fewer choices, higher costs, less convenient—and you'll have less time. So, make the most of your campus resources. Develop an exercise program based on activities and sports you enjoy, and, at least once a year, take the plunge and try a new exercise/activity class for a semester.

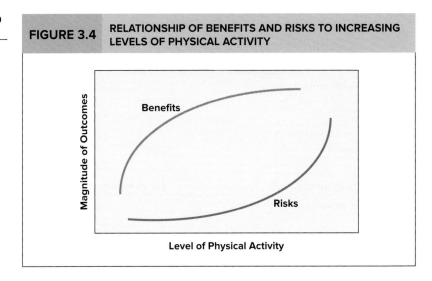

FIGURE 3.4 RELATIONSHIP OF BENEFITS AND RISKS TO INCREASING LEVELS OF PHYSICAL ACTIVITY

Initial Screening and Risks of Exercise

For nearly all apparently healthy young adults, it is safe to begin or intensify an exercise program. In fact, some experts contend that you put yourself *at greater risk for medical problems if you remain physically inactive.* However, as a precaution to identify individuals who may need medical clearance, take the seven-question Physical Activity Readiness Questionnaire available online: **PAR-Q.**

Every year a few sudden deaths occur among high school and college athletes during training or competition. There is always immediate speculation as to the cause of death because the official explanation is typically not known for several weeks pending medical tests. At that point, the official cause of death receives only back-page coverage. Nearly all confirmed causes of sudden deaths in young athletes are attributable to inherited cardiac abnormalities, heat stress, drug or supplement use, or a combination of these factors.

A sensible program of exercise is very safe, especially for young people. The greatest risk for college students is simply overdoing it—too much, too fast. As shown in Figure 3.4, low-to-moderate levels of training impart many health and fitness benefits with minimal risks. In contrast, as training levels continue to increase, the benefits level off while the risks increase.

This rise in risk is most often due to overtraining—exercising too hard, too long, and/or too often. This cumulative overload exceeds the body's capacity to adapt. Overtraining commonly results in musculoskeletal injuries or respiratory infections (e.g., common cold, flu). These "breakdowns" are highly treatable with rest, medical management, and common sense.

Initial Fitness Level

One's initial fitness level is the foundation on which an individualized plan or exercise prescription (frequency, intensity, time, type) is built. If you don't already know your fitness level, consider using standard fitness tests to see where you stand; for example, time yourself in a 1-mile walk or a 1.5-mile run to assess cardiorespiratory fitness and use push-up, sit-up, and trunk-flexion tests to assess muscular fitness. A variety of fitness tests with instructions and scoring are available online: **adultfitnesstest.org.**

How you score will be of interest; however, the true value of assessment is in using the results as a baseline for tailoring an exercise plan. Be honest in self-appraisal and carefully set the initial training level to your current condition. One of the main reasons the exercise recommendations are presented as ranges is to accommodate the variability in initial fitness levels. Once started, the question becomes: How fast to increase the exercise overload? Progression depends on the principle of individual differences. Simply put, you learn your dose-response curve through trial and error.

Envision an exercise program as having three stages: an initial conditioning stage, which lasts two to three weeks; an improvement stage, which can be highly variable in length; and a maintenance stage, which goes on indefinitely. A systematic increase in overload is applied during the second stage. Small, steady increments in the exercise dose (5–15 percent) every one to two weeks is a reasonable rate of progression. Ramping up too quickly is often counterproductive.

Anatomy of the Exercise Session

The format for an exercise session or workout is a warm-up period, the main conditioning phase that involves aerobic and/or resistance training, and a cool-down period. In Figure 3.5, this format is illustrated for a 30-minute aerobic workout in which heart rate is plotted against time. Warm-up facilitates the transition from rest to exercise, and cool-down allows gradual recovery and transition back to the resting level.

When feasible, aerobic training and resistance training should be performed on alternate days, although both activities can be combined into the same workout. If combined, the training you wish to emphasize (aerobic or resistance) should be done first. Stretching is typically done during the cool-down, as stretching is more effective when the muscles are warm. However, flexibility exercises are also often included as part of a warm-up and are sometimes done at a separate time altogether.

FIGURE 3.5   **FORMAT OF AN AEROBIC TRAINING SESSION WITH WARM-UP, CONDITIONING PHASE, AND COOL-DOWN**

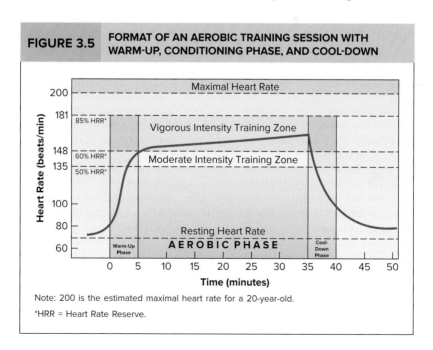

Note: 200 is the estimated maximal heart rate for a 20-year-old.

*HRR = Heart Rate Reserve.

Aerobic, resistance, and flexibility training are the components of a complete fitness program. There is wide latitude in how you choose to mix or blend these activities. For example, participation in sports such as basketball, soccer, and tennis can be a core element of your fitness program or simply be included for competitive and social pleasures. Yet, regardless of the specific sport or fitness activity, it's wise to follow the exercise session format and include a warm-up and a cool-down.

CONSUMER ISSUES

Many consumer issues can arise when developing an exercise program or moving from one setting to another (e.g., new school, new job, new living arrangement). Three topics of wide interest are fitness centers, personal trainers, and home exercise equipment.

Fitness Centers

Most colleges have very good sports/exercise facilities for their students. Having a state-of-the-art fitness center is increasingly viewed as not just important but necessary. A modern, well-equipped facility provides an edge with student recruitment. These fitness centers are usually well staffed, open long hours, and conveniently located. Generally, no monthly fee is assessed as operational costs are underwritten from student fees paid with tuition.

You may also want to investigate what's available at community health clubs as an alternative to using a campus facility. Fitness programs can be categorized as for-profit health clubs (e.g., 24 Hour Fitness, Gold's Gym, LA Fitness), not-for-profit centers (e.g., YMCAs, YWCAs, Jewish Community Centers), and hospital-affiliated fitness centers.

Off-campus fitness clubs vary widely by size of facility, type of equipment, breadth and quality of programs and services, and costs. Carefully consider your options before joining one. High-pressure sales pitches are still the norm for many of the for-profit clubs. To help make a wise decision, use guidelines available from trusted sources such as the American College of Sports Medicine: "Selecting and Effectively Using a Health/Fitness Facility."

Personal Trainers/Expert Instructors

Article
3.3

Campus fitness centers usually offer a number of classes and individualized training sessions at reasonable rates by well-qualified instructors and personal trainers. Depending on your particular exercise plan, it may be smart—and fun—to use these services. For example, if you are ready to start a resistance-training program, consider getting a personal trainer to work with you for the first few sessions to familiarize you with the proper lifting technique and use of equipment. Exercise equipment—both resistance and aerobic—can vary widely from one center to another.

A personal trainer provides expert instruction, immediate feedback, and motivation. This individualized coaching is especially helpful for novices, but also for those who have been away from exercise for an extended period or who simply want reassurance and guidance in getting started.

Before hiring a personal trainer, be sure to check the trainer's qualifications and experience—having a good body is *not* enough! For example, does the trainer have a college degree in the field (e.g., exercise science, kinesiology, physical education)? Or is he or she certified as a personal trainer by a nationally recognized, nonprofit organization such as the American College of Sports Medicine, National Strength and Conditioning Association, or the American Council on Exercise?

For most college students, home exercise equipment is not a pressing issue. Yet, for those considering such a purchase, begin by asking key questions:

- Will the equipment help me reach my goals?
- Will I really use the equipment regularly?
- Is the equipment well made?
- Do I have room for the equipment?
- Can I afford a quality piece of equipment?

Remember that health-related fitness can be developed without any special equipment. Moreover, high-quality equipment for cardiorespiratory training (e.g., treadmills, stationary bicycles, elliptical trainers) or resistance training is expensive. Just as in selecting a health club, do your research first and take your time before making a purchase. Be realistic. Basements and attics are full of hardly used exercise equipment.

✓ **NEED TO KNOW**

Developing an individualized exercise plan involves tailoring the physical activity recommendations to meet your goals, with due consideration of initial fitness level, rate of progression, and available campus resources (i.e., facilities, programs, personal trainers). Selected websites listed at the end of the chapter provide additional guidance, expertise, and detail on specific types of exercise training.

➤ Establishing the Exercise Habit

Article 3.4

Motivated to lose weight and get in shape, a friend joined a health club several months ago. I asked him how it was going and he said, "Paid my 300 bucks but haven't lost a pound. Guess you actually have to go and work out!" His comeback quip was a humorous way to describe an unsuccessful effort to begin an exercise program. He is not alone.

During the last two decades, the year-by-year growth in the number of health clubs mirrored the increase in obesity in the United States with a near perfect correlation (>0.9). While the growth in health clubs is obviously not causing America's obesity epidemic, it is intriguing that the increase in fitness facilities appears to have no impact on helping Americans reach or maintain a healthy weight. This ironic finding shows that for many, many people, facilities alone are not sufficient to make the transition from couch potato to regular exerciser.

When it comes to changing a behavior, we often have good intentions but poor results. This is especially true regarding exercise because it's voluntary, is time-consuming, and requires effort. Let's examine a few factors that influence change in physical activity and consider strategies that may enable you to successfully implement and maintain an exercise program.

IDENTIFYING BARRIERS AND INCENTIVES TO EXERCISE

The large majority of college students report they enjoy exercise and sports activities, and over 80 percent indicate they know how to set up a fitness program

Health & the Media A Sport for Every Body

Can you identify these sports legends nattily attired in white tuxedos? This photo by portrait photographer Annie Leibovitz is from a 1987 American Express print ad. Basketball star Wilt Chamberlain towers above champion jockey Willie Shoemaker. Chamberlain—who once scored 100 points in a game—was 7′1″ and weighed over 300 lb., while Shoemaker—winner of over 9,000 races—was 4′11″ and weighed less than 100 lb. The contrast in body size and dimensions is striking and wondrous. This image should remind us that there is no single ideal form when it comes to sport. Every person can find a sport that matches his or her physique. Clearly, body size does not have to interfere with the innate enjoyment of exercise and one's quest to become physically fit.

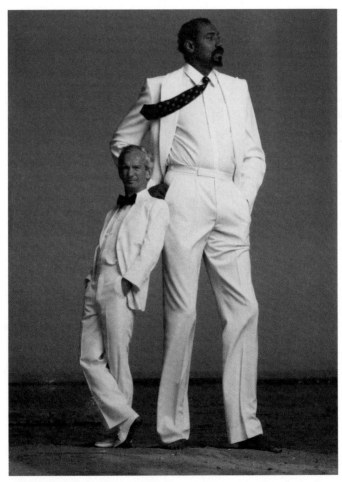

© Annie Leibovitz/Contact Press Images

Yet, according to the Centers for Disease Control and **105**
Prevention, only about one in three engages in recommended levels of exercise.
Why does this large gap exist?

Assessing self-motivation can be useful in determining likelihood of exercise
adherence. Take the assessment and calculate your "dropout" score. Do the results
agree with your past exercise experiences?

A BMI of 30 or higher is also associated with discontinuing exercise. If your
self-motivation score or your BMI indicates you are likely to drop out, view this as
a challenge to remain active. Remember, these are simple predictors about groups
of people and not necessarily true for every individual within a group. If you qualify as a dropout, how might you shift your approach—from this point forward—to
improve consistency with your exercise routine?

Readiness to change as described in the stages of change model (see Chapter 1)
provides another baseline measure that is useful in putting an exercise plan into
action. Most students find themselves in one of the three middle stages—contemplation,
preparation, or action. Ten to 15 percent are already in maintenance, and a smaller
percentage are in precontemplation.

To determine your current stage, select the statement in the following list that
best reflects your recent physical activity pattern. Note that *exercise* refers to jogging
or similar vigorous activities lasting at least 20 minutes at a time, and *walk* refers
to brisk walking or similar moderate activities lasting at least 30 minutes at a time.

Self
Assessment
3.2

1. I don't exercise or walk regularly and don't intend to start.
2. I don't exercise or walk regularly, but I have been thinking of starting.
3. I'm trying to begin exercising or walking.
4. I exercise or walk but not on a regular basis (vigorous less than three days per
   week or moderate exercise less than five days per week).
5. I have been exercising or walking regularly for the last few months (vigorous
   three or more days per week or moderate exercise five or more days per week).
6. I have been exercising or walking regularly for more than six months.

If you chose 1, you're in the precontemplation stage; 2 is contemplation; 3 is preparation; 4 is action; 5 is maintenance; and 6 is when exercise has become an established behavior. For example, perhaps you are stuck in the preparation stage (#3);
you play soccer or run a couple times per week but can't seem to get beyond that.
Identifying your current stage can help you see what you need to do to reach the
next stage—in this case, to add a third session per week.

There are many barriers to adopting or maintaining an exercise program.
Americans often report lack of time and limited access to facilities and equipment. Yet, for most college students these are not significant barriers. In fact,
just the opposite—a flexible schedule, fewer family responsibilities, and an accessible campus fitness center provide opportunities. So let's focus on other variables that are more likely to influence exercise adherence. Each can be viewed
as a negative or a positive. Consider the following list in relation to your current
or planned exercise routine:

- Boring versus enjoyable.
- Disapproval versus encouragement by close friends, family.
- Injuries, physical limitations versus injury free, no limitations.
- Haphazard schedule versus regular routine.
- Inadequate instruction versus expert instruction.
- Previous experience versus complete novice.

The combination of negative factors often outweighs that of positive factors. Consequently, it's important to take stock of key variables and work at turning each negative into a positive whenever possible. Also, despite a sound plan and your best efforts, know that interruptions can occur at all stages. If you have to discontinue exercise for a short time, don't let that stop you from starting again. Relapses are a natural part of the long-term process of establishing a new behavior.

STRATEGIES FOR INCREASING EXERCISE ADHERENCE

The aim is to leverage every feasible strategy to establish exercise as a permanent habit. If we don't, then exercise will frequently lose out to the many other interests that compete for our time. Consider the following practical strategies to tip the scale—the balance between the pros and cons—in the right direction.

- Make exercise fun.
- Schedule your exercise.
- Set specific long-term and short-term goals.
- Keep a log and include periodic testing to monitor your progress.
- Reward yourself for consistency and milestones.
- Minimize injuries by starting out with a moderate program.
- Try something new from time to time.
- Be patient but consistent—remember, the tortoise beat the hare.
- Exercise to feel better.

Apply as many of these suggestions as possible, especially if you are in the contemplation, preparation, or action stage. Another useful strategy is to exercise with a friend. Although some people prefer to exercise by themselves as a break away from everything and everybody, most of us enjoy the camaraderie of exercising with others. Why should all social time with family and friends revolve around eating and other sedentary activities? Physical activity—whether merely a long walk or sports and fitness activities—provides excellent opportunities to share time together.

The aim of applying behavioral strategies is to make it difficult to *not* exercise. A sensible, individualized program of exercise can directly improve quality of life. Only by engaging in a long-term exercise routine can we experience this health enhancement. The natural consequence is that the value of exercise is elevated, and the behavior becomes more ingrained. Eventually, a behavior repeated over months and years becomes a lifelong habit. Follow your individualized plan, apply the most helpful strategies, and with time and commitment you will establish the exercise habit.

NATIONAL PHYSICAL ACTIVITY PLAN

Establishing the exercise habit is not just an individual goal, it's a societal goal. The vision of the National Physical Activity Plan—a large-scale, private–public collaboration—is that one day, all Americans will be physically active and will live, work, and play in environments that facilitate regular physical activity.

Launched in 2010, the National Physical Activity Plan provides a comprehensive set of initiatives and policies to increase physical activity across America, from large cities to small towns. Recommendations are organized by key sectors including education, business, health care, recreation/sports, transportation/land use, and public health. For example, with respect to transportation/land use, city planners are encouraged to prioritize and integrate infrastructure (sidewalks, bikeways) and green space for active commuting within larger highway projects.

Look for and support the National Physical Activity Plan initiatives in your communities. The ultimate aim is to create a national culture that supports physically active lifestyles, and in turn improve health, prevent disease, and enhance quality of life: **www.physicalactivityplan.org.**

✓ **NEED TO KNOW**

Integrating a fitness program into your lifestyle is not just a matter of choice. Becoming a regular exerciser requires a plan and perseverance. By identifying barriers and incentives and applying strategies that fit your situation, you stack the odds in your favor. Exercise empowers living. And it's a metaphor for life. You get out of it what you put into it. Enjoy the good feelings and positive health that come with fitness.

connect Resources

ARTICLES

3.1 "The Play of the Year." *Sports Illustrated*. The benefits from engaging in sports aren't just in the records set. This story captures a special moment that reflects the goodness in people and transcends a single event in a single game.

3.2 "Should Athletes Stretch Before Exercise?" Gatorade Sports Science Institute. Surprisingly little scientific evidence supports the idea that stretching before exercise prevents injuries and improves performance. The article reviews the science and summarizes unanswered questions.

3.3 "Body Image: Are You Imagining the Wrong Image?" *ACSM's Health and Fitness Journal*. An article written for personal trainers and group exercise leaders that examines how to help a client improve his or her body image.

3.4 *The Courage to Start: A Guide to Running for Your Life*. Fireside Press. The author shares how he went from an out-of-shape klutz to a marathon runner—albeit a slow one. He shows us that the fun of running is not limited to the swift.

SELF-ASSESSMENTS

3.1 Assessment of Daily Energy Expenditure
3.2 Self-Motivation Assessment for Exercise

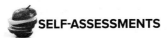 Website Resources

PHYSICAL ACTIVITY RECOMMENDATIONS

National Physical Activity Plan **www.physicalactivityplan.org**
U.S. Physical Activity Guidelines **www.health.gov/paguidelines**
WHO Physical Activity Recommendations **www.who.int/dietphysicalactivity/factsheet_recommendations/en/**

EXAMPLES OF EXERCISE RESOURCES

Adult Fitness Tests **www.adultfitnesstest.org/**
Resistance Exercises **www.exrx.net/Lists/Directory.html**
Resistance Training for Health and Fitness **www.acsm.org/docs/brochures/resistance-training.pdf**
Selecting a Health/Fitness Club **www.acsm.org/docs/brochures/selecting-and-effectively-using-a-health-fitness-facility.pdf**
Stretching Exercises **www.mayoclinic.com/health/stretching/SM00043&slide=1**

GENERAL

American College of Sports Medicine **www.acsm.org**
Centers for Disease Control and Prevention: Physical Activity **www.cdc.gov/physicalactivity**
National Strength and Conditioning Association **www.nsca.com**
Sport & Exercise Medicine: BJSM multimedia portal **bjsm.bmj.com**

Understanding the Content

1. Contrast and define the following terms: *physical activity, exercise,* and *physical fitness.*
2. What are the three primary components of health-related physical fitness? How are they related to our health?
3. What are the minimum levels of aerobic activity and resistance training recommended to improve and maintain health for adults?
4. An exercise session has three phases. Name and describe them and illustrate with an example.

Exploring Ideas

1. Physical activity and health have a dose–response relationship. Explain this concept and comment on the advantages and limitations of prescribing exercise as a medicine.
2. Approximately how many calories should one burn in intentional physical activity (per day or week) to improve and maintain health? Where does this level of energy expenditure fall within the physical activity continuum? Explain.
3. How do the basic principles of exercise training—overload, specificity, and individual differences—relate to tailoring an individual exercise plan? Explain with examples.
4. Most of us enjoy exercise and know it's beneficial. Yet, only a small percentage of Americans exercise regularly. Explain this quandary and suggest strategies to enable folks to become more active.

Selected References

Academy of Nutrition and Dietetics. Position of the Academy of Nutrition and Dietetics, Dietitians of Canada, and American College of Sports Medicine: Nutrition and athletic performance. *Journal of the Academy of Nutrition and Dietetics* 116: 501–528, 2016.

Ainsworth BE, Haskell WL, Herrmann SD, et al. 2011. Compendium of Physical Activities: A second update of codes and MET values. *Medicine and Science in Sports and Exercise* 43: 1575–1581, 2011.

American College of Sports Medicine. *ACSM's Guidelines for Exercise Testing and Prescription* (9th ed.). Baltimore: Lippincott Williams & Wilkins, 2013.

American College of Sports Medicine. Progression models in resistance training for healthy adults. *Medicine and Science in Sports and Exercise* 41: 687–708, 2009.

American College of Sports Medicine. Quantity and quality of exercise for developing and maintaining cardiorespiratory, musculoskeletal, and neuromotor fitness in apparently healthy adults. *Medicine and Science in Sports and Exercise* 43: 1334–1359, 2011.

American College of Sports Medicine and American Heart Association. Physical activity and public health: Updated recommendation for adults from the American College of Sports Medicine and the American Heart Association. *Circulation* 116: 1081–1093, 2007.

American Heart Association. Exercise standards for testing and training. *Circulation* 128: 873–934, 2013.

American Heart Association. Interventions to promote physical activity and dietary lifestyle changes for cardiovascular risk factor reduction in adults. *Circulation* 122: 406–441, 2010.

American Heart Association. The National Physical Activity Plan: A call to action. *Circulation* 131: 1932–1940, 2015.

Anderson B. *Stretching*. Bolinas, CA: Shelter Publications, 2010.

Borg G. *Borg's Perceived Exertion and Pain Scales*. Champaign, IL: Human Kinetics, 1998.

Bouchard C, Blair SN, Haskell WL. *Physical Activity and Health* (2nd ed.). Champaign, IL: Human Kinetics, 2012.

Clarke HH (ed.). Basic understanding of physical fitness. *Physical Fitness Research Digest*. Washington, DC: Presidents Council on Physical Fitness and Sport, July 1971.

Gladden, LB. Personal communication with PB Sparling on the lactic acid–muscle performance relationship. May 2011.

Hertzog C, Kramer AF, Wilson RS, et al. Fit body, fit mind? Your workout makes you smarter. *Scientific American,* July 2009.

Kolata G. Lactic acid is not muscles' foe, it's fuel. *New York Times,* May 16, 2006.

Marcus BH, Forsyth L. *Motivating People to Be Physically Active,* 2nd ed. Champaign, IL: Human Kinetics, 2009.

McArdle WD, Katch FI, Katch VL. *Exercise Physiology: Energy, Nutrition, and Human Performance* (8th ed). Baltimore: Lippincott Williams & Wilkins, 2014.

Owen N, Sparling PB, Healy GN, et al. Sedentary behavior: Emerging evidence for a new health risk. *Mayo Clinic Proceedings* 85 (12): 1138–1141, 2010.

Powell KE, Paluch AE, Blair SN. Physical activity for health: What kind? How much? How intense? On top of what? *Annual Review of Public Health* 32: 349–365, 2011.

Powers SK, Howley ET. *Exercise Physiology: Theory and Application to Fitness and Performance* (9th ed.). New York: McGraw-Hill, 2014.

Ratey JJ. *Spark: The Revolutionary New Science of Exercise and the Brain*. New York: Little, Brown, 2008.

Rowland TW. The biological basis of physical activity. *Medicine and Science in Sports and Exercise* 30 (3): 392–399, 1998.

Sparling PB. College physical education: An unrecognized agent of change in combating inactivity-related diseases. *Perspectives in Biology and Medicine* 46: 579–587, 2003.

Sparling PB, Snow TK. Physical activity patterns in recent college alumni. *Research Quarterly for Exercise and Sport* 73: 200–205, 2002.

U.S. Department of Health and Human Services. *Physical Activity and Health: A Report of the Surgeon General.* **www.cdc.gov/nccdphp/sgr/sgr.htm**

U.S. Department of Health and Human Services. *Physical Activity Guidelines for Americans, 2008.* **www.health.gov/paguidelines**

Voss MW, Nagamatsu LS, Liu-Ambrose T, et al. Exercise, brain, and cognition across the lifespan. *Journal of Applied Physiology* 111: 1505–1513, 2011.

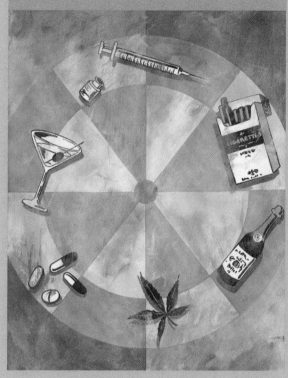

© Lisa Zado/Photodisc/Getty

There are people who strictly deprive themselves of each and every eatable, drinkable, and smokable pleasure which has in any way acquired a shady reputation. They pay this price for health. And health is all they get for it.

—Mark Twain

Chapter 4

AVOID DRUG ABUSE

In Chapter 4 we provide a foundation for an understanding of the principles regarding drug use, misuse, and abuse. The chapter begins with an overview of the scope of drugs in society today and then explains key language and terminology. The chapter moves on to explain various categories of drugs and ends with a discussion of drug testing and drug abuse treatment options. The goal is to provide a grounding in the concepts integral to understanding the risks associated with drugs.

DRUG USE, misuse, and abuse not only alter an individual's body chemistry and perception of reality, but drugs have widespread economic and social costs. Murder, child abuse, drowning, rape, assault, suicide, spousal abuse, and traffic fatalities all too often have improper use of controlled substances as a contributing factor. And substance abuse among young adults is especially common. According to the National Center on Addiction and Substance Abuse at Columbia University (CASA, 2007), college students have higher rates of drug dependence than the general public, with almost 23 percent of them classified as substance dependent. Alcohol abuse is especially common and costly in this age group, with about 30 percent of students meeting the criteria of alcohol abusers. Other alcohol-related problems each year include:

- 1,800 deaths from accidents.
- Approximately 600,000 injuries.
- Over 646,000 physical assaults.
- Over 110,000 occasions when students were unsure if they consented to sex.
- Over 97,000 sexual assaults.
- 400,000 instances of unprotected sex.

Instances of drug misuse and abuse among other groups in the United States are also quite high. The United States consumes a whopping 60 percent of the world's supply of illicit drugs.

According to *Monitoring the Future* (Johnston et al., 2014), in 2013 among college students in the United States in their lifetime and in the past 30 days:

- 51 percent had ever used any illicit drugs and 22.5 percent in the previous 30 days.
- 26.7 percent had ever used any illicit drugs other than marijuana and 8.2 percent in the previous 30 days.
- 50.5 percent had ever used any illicit drugs including inhalants and 22.5 percent in the previous 30 days.
- 47.7 percent had ever used marijuana/hashish and 20.6 percent in the previous 30 days.
- 4.3 percent had ever used inhalants and 0.1 percent in the previous 30 days.
- 7.8 percent had ever used hallucinogens and 1.0 percent in the previous 30 days.
- 4.4 percent had ever used LSD and 0.4 percent in the previous 30 days.
- 8.1 percent had ever used Ecstasy (MDMA) and 0.8 percent in the previous 30 days.
- 5.1 percent had ever used cocaine and 0.9 percent in the previous 30 days.
- 0.7 percent had ever used crack and 0.3 percent in the previous 30 days.
- 5.2 percent had ever used other cocaine and 0.9 percent in the previous 30 days.
- 0.4 percent had ever used heroin and 0.2 percent in the previous 30 days.
- 0.1 percent had ever used heroin with a needle and 0.1 percent in the previous 30 days.
- 0.8 percent had ever used heroin without a needle and 0.3 percent in the previous 30 days.
- 15.3 percent had ever used amphetamines and 5.3 percent in the previous 30 days.
- 0.9 percent had ever used methamphetamine and 0.0 percent in the previous 30 days.

- 5.4 percent had ever used sedatives (barbiturates) and 0.9 percent in the previous 30 days.
- 7.8 percent had ever used tranquilizers and 1.2 percent in the previous 30 days.
- 78 percent had ever had alcohol and 63.1 percent in the previous 30 days.
- 66.5 percent had ever been drunk and 40.2 percent in the previous 30 days.
- 67.5 percent had ever had flavored alcoholic beverages and 29.1 percent in the previous 30 days.
- 14 percent had used cigarettes in the previous 30 days.
- 0.8 percent had ever used steroids and 0.0 percent in the previous 30 days.

The frequency of drug use among college students is alarming. According to the SIUC/Core Institute (2014), 32.2 percent of college students reported being involved in public misconduct (trouble with police, fighting, arguing, DUI/DWI, vandalism) at least once during the past year as a result of drinking or drug use. Also, 21.8 percent reported experiencing some personal problem(s) such as suicide ideation, sexual assault, or injury at least once in the past year as a result of drinking or drug use. The National Institute on Alcohol Abuse and Alcoholism (2015) reports that 25 percent of college students report academic consequences from drinking including missing class, falling behind in class, and doing poorly in class. The Center on Young Adult Health and Development (Arria et al., 2013) reports that *substance use has an insidious way of interfering with a student's ability to take advantage of all that college has to offer.*

It is clear that drug use behavior does not begin in college. *Monitoring the Future* (Johnston et al., 2014) results show that alcohol continues to be the drug of choice among high school students (40 percent of 12th-graders reporting using alcohol in the past 30 days). The most recent data released show that among high school students, alcohol use has decreased and marijuana and illicit drug use has increased.

Article
4.1

➤ Drug Administration and Terminology

Drug administration and absorption are key issues that influence safety in drug doses. For any drug to have an effect, it must enter the blood, where it can potentially affect any cell in the body within minutes. There are six types of drug administration:

1. **Oral administration** is when the drug, normally in pill or liquid form, is swallowed and absorbed through the stomach and intestines. This is the most common way to administer drugs, but it is also the least efficient because of differences in rates of digestion between people.
2. **Parenteral administration** is the injection of a drug with a needle. Types of injection include intravenous (into the vein), intramuscular (into muscle), and subcutaneous (under the skin). The effects of parenteral administration are quick since the drug is absorbed into the bloodstream almost immediately.

Oral administration is the taking of a drug by mouth in pill or liquid form.

Parenteral administration refers to injected drugs.

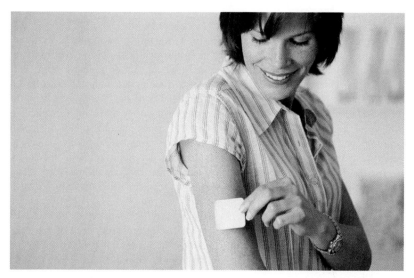

A nicotine patch, used to help smokers deal with cigarette withdrawal symptoms while quitting, is an example of a drug that uses transdermal administration.
© Stockdisc/PunchStock

3. **Inhalation administration** is when a drug is inhaled into the lungs as a gas or snorted into the nose as a powder. Again, there is an almost immediate effect because blood vessels in the lungs and nose aid quick absorption. Vaping, as in the use of electronic cigarettes, is a form of inhalation administration.

4. **Rectal administration** is the insertion of suppositories into the rectum. As the suppository melts, the drug enters the many blood vessels that support the lower digestive system.

5. **Transdermal administration** takes place when a drug is contained in an adhesive patch that is affixed to the skin. The drug diffuses into the bloodstream via the skin.

6. **Vaping administration** is inhaling the vapor from the device called an "electronic cigarette." Other drugs besides nicotine can be put into the device, vaporized, and inhaled. Once inhaled the drug immediately enters the blood. Vaping could be included under inhalation administration but because vaping is becoming more popular, it begs to be identified as its own method of administration.

Inhalation administration is breathing in a drug as a gas or vapor.

Rectal administration is used for drugs in suppositories that are absorbed through rectal membranes.

Transdermal administration refers to drugs given through adhesive patches put on the skin.

Vaping administration is inhaling the vapor from the device called an "electronic cigarette."

It is important to understand some basic drug terminology. **Drug use** refers to taking a drug for its intended purpose, such as swallowing an antihistamine capsule to treat symptoms of allergy. **Drug misuse** is the taking of a drug for a reason other than that for which it was intended—for example, taking an antihistamine to feel a "buzz." **Drug abuse** is the chronic, long-term, and consistent taking of a drug for a reason other than the intended use. If someone regularly takes antihistamines to achieve a high, that is considered abuse. These terms can also be applied to alcohol consumption: having a drink to relax is considered drug use, drinking enough to get drunk is misuse, and getting drunk regularly, by definition, is considered abuse.

There are also factors beyond the frequency of use that can influence the effect of drugs. **Set** is a powerful variable that refers to a person's expectations regarding how a drug will be experienced. If people believe a drug has a certain effect before they take it—for example, that it causes hallucinations—then there is a good chance that they will experience what they expect while under the influence of the drug. The placebo effect is an example of a set variable. In this case, people take a placebo (sugar pill) rather than a real drug but still display the effect of the drug they thought they took.

The **setting,** or environment in which a drug is taken, also influences the effect. For example, alcohol is a depressant and should induce drowsiness when consumed. If someone drinks in a quiet environment, then the most likely result is sleepiness. But if the same amount of alcohol is consumed in an environment where there is a festive atmosphere and social interaction, chances are that the user will feel stimulated.

Dependence is another important concept related to drug use. **Physical dependence** is when the body learns to require a certain drug in order to function normally. When the drug is removed from the dependent person's body, he or she will have withdrawal symptoms, or physical reactions that can range from a headache to seizures, depending on the type of drug and the extent of dependence. Withdrawal symptoms eventually subside over time if the drug remains out of the person's system, but they will also subside if the person immediately consumes more of the drug. To become physically dependent, a person usually needs to take a drug for a long period of time. However, drugs such as methamphetamines are capable of reinforcing a craving very quickly, so physical dependence on them can develop in a short period of time.

Drug use is using a drug for its intended purpose.

Drug misuse is using a drug for a reason other than the intended use.

Drug abuse is chronically using a drug for a reason other than the intended use.

Set is the mental expectation regarding the effects of a drug.

The **setting** is the environment in which a drug is consumed, which can influence its effect.

Physical dependence occurs when the body requires a drug, and withdrawal symptoms occur if the drug is not administered and absorbed.

Psychological dependence is an emotional attachment to a drug that develops in the person taking it. If the user does not take the drug at regular intervals, then withdrawal symptoms such as anxiety or irritability result. In this case, the drug fulfills an underlying emotional need in the user. Many drugs result in both physical and psychological dependency. For example, a person who usually smokes a cigarette after dinner each night may feel irritable and anxious if he or she is prevented from doing so, even when wearing a patch that prevents nicotine levels from dropping to the point where physical cravings are triggered. Drugs that cause both physical and psychological dependence tend to be the hardest for users to stop taking.

Last, there are a few concepts relating to the amount of drugs taken. An **effective dose** of a drug is the amount of the substance it takes to achieve the therapeutic or desired effect. A **lethal dose** is the amount of drug that will overwhelm the body's systems and result in death.

Normally, effective doses and lethal doses are expressed with respect to the percentage of people experiencing the effect at that dose. For example, if we say the effective dose for 50 percent of people (ED50) for a certain drug is 10 mg, that means that 50 percent of people will experience the desired therapeutic effect after taking 10 mg. But it also indicates that the other 50 percent of people will need more or less of the drug to achieve the intended effect. The same concept holds true for the lethal dose—the amount of a drug that may cause one person to die may even be an effective dose for another person.

The effect of different doses varies depending on body mass and underlying health, as well as tolerance. **Tolerance** is a condition that occurs when a drug is taken repeatedly over time, and the effects at the original dose diminish. To get the same original effect, the user must take increasingly larger doses. A person who has established a tolerance has probably taken the drug over an extended period of time, and the body has adapted to certain levels of the drug in the blood.

NEED TO KNOW

Drugs can be administered orally, transdermally, rectally, and parenterally; through inhalation; and through vaping. Taking a drug for its intended purpose is called *drug use*. *Drug misuse* is the taking of a drug for a reason other than the one for which it was intended; and *drug abuse* is the chronic, long-term, and consistent taking of a drug for a reason other than the intended use. Set and setting are perhaps as important in determining a drug's effect as the actual physical action of the drug itself because mental expectations and environment influence a person's behavior.

Psychological dependence is an emotional attachment to a drug.

Effective dose is the dose necessary to produce a desired effect.

Lethal dose is the dose capable of causing the user's death.

Tolerance is a condition in which a person needs an increased amount of a drug to achieve the desired effect.

In the United States, the Drug Enforcement Administration (DEA) is in charge of regulation and classification of controlled substances. It "schedules" drugs according to five categories (I, II, III, IV, and V) that describe effects, legal availability, and potential for abuse (Figure 4.1). The drug schedule weighs the negative risks and effects of various drugs against their possible beneficial uses and then assigns penalties and use parameters accordingly. Drugs with the fewest accepted medical uses and the most negative or dangerous effects are often banned outright and carry the highest penalties for improper trafficking and distribution. Drugs that are dangerous under most circumstances but still have therapeutic medical uses are made available only under strict controls and with high penalties for misuse or improper possession. At the other end of the scheduling spectrum are drugs deemed as having little chance for misuse, abuse, and dependency. These drugs are more readily available, and the penalties for abuse tend to be lower.

FIGURE 4.1   DRUG SCHEDULES AND LEGAL PENALTIES

A new class of substances was created by the Anti-Drug Abuse Act of 1986. Controlled substance analogues are substances that are not controlled substances but may be found in the illicit traffic. They are structurally or pharmacologically similar to Schedule I or II controlled substances and have no legitimate medical use. A substance that meets the definition of a controlled substance analogue and is intended for human consumption is treated under the Controlled Substances Act (CSA) as if it were a controlled substance in Schedule I. [21 U.S.C. 802(32), 21 U.S.C. 813]

SCHEDULE I

- The drug or other substance has a high potential for abuse.
- The drug or other substance has no currently accepted medical use in treatment in the United States.
- There is a lack of accepted safety for use of the drug or other substance under medical supervision.
- Examples of Schedule I substances include heroin, lysergic acid diethylamide (LSD), marijuana, and methaqualone.

SCHEDULE II

- The drug or other substance has a high potential for abuse.
- The drug or other substance has a currently accepted medical use in treatment in the United States or a currently accepted medical use with severe restrictions.

FIGURE 4.1 DRUG SCHEDULES AND LEGAL PENALTIES (*concluded*)

◆ Abuse of the drug or other substance may lead to severe psychological or physical dependence.

◆ Examples of Schedule II substances include morphine, phencyclidine (PCP), cocaine, methadone, and methamphetamine.

SCHEDULE III

◆ The drug or other substance has less potential for abuse than the drugs or other substances in Schedules I and II.

◆ The drug or other substance has a currently accepted medical use in treatment in the United States.

◆ Abuse of the drug or other substance may lead to moderate or low physical dependence or high psychological dependence.

◆ Anabolic steroids, codeine and hydrocodone with aspirin or Tylenol®, and some barbiturates are examples of Schedule III substances.

SCHEDULE IV

◆ The drug or other substance has a low potential for abuse relative to the drugs or other substances in Schedule III.

◆ The drug or other substance has a currently accepted medical use in treatment in the United States.

◆ Abuse of the drug or other substance may lead to limited physical dependence or psychological dependence relative to the drugs or other substances in Schedule III.

◆ Examples of drugs included in Schedule IV are Darvon®, Talwin®, Equanil®, Valium®, and Xanax®.

SCHEDULE V

◆ The drug or other substance has a low potential for abuse relative to the drugs or other substances in Schedule IV.

◆ The drug or other substance has a currently accepted medical use in treatment in the United States.

◆ Abuse of the drug or other substances may lead to limited physical dependence or psychological dependence relative to the drugs or other substances in Schedule IV.

◆ Cough medicines with codeine are examples of Schedule V drugs.

Source: Drug Enforcement Administration, *Drugs of Abuse,* 2015 (**www.usdoj.gov/dea/pubs/scheduling.html**).

According to the DEA, Schedule I drugs are the ones with the highest potential for abuse and dependency and are not currently acceptable for medical use. Examples of Schedule I drugs include heroin, marijuana, and LSD. Possessing or taking these drugs is banned outright in the United States. The government also considers Schedule II drugs highly addictive, but these drugs have widely accepted medical uses. Examples of Schedule II substances include morphine, cocaine, and methamphetamines.

Schedule III drugs have common uses in medical treatment, and they include anabolic steroids, most barbiturates, and the antinausea drug Marinol. Like Schedules I and II drugs, these drugs are addictive, and they may cause moderate physical or high psychological dependence.

Finally, Schedules IV and V drugs have medical uses but low potential for abuse and the risk of only limited physical or psychological dependence. The anti-anxiety drug Xanax and the sedative barbital are examples of Schedule IV drugs. Mixtures having small amounts of codeine, such as a prescription cough syrup, are examples of Schedule V drugs.

Now we will turn to the second way drugs are classified—by their effect—and discuss some of the major types of drugs that medical professionals and regulators are concerned with today.

NEED TO KNOW

There are two types of drug dependence: physical and psychological. Effective and lethal doses of drugs can vary according to many factors, including body mass and tolerance. Tolerance of a drug can develop over time, requiring larger doses to achieve the desired effect. The government regulates the selling and taking of all drugs and classifies use and penalties under a system of "schedules." Penalties regarding unlawful use and trafficking of controlled substances are severe and aggressively prosecuted by state and federal governments.

➤ Depressants

Depressants are drugs that decrease or slow down body processes. These drugs include opioids, sedative-hypnotics, and the number one drug of use, misuse, and abuse in the United States—alcohol.

ALCOHOL

The major forms of alcoholic beverages are beer, wine, and distilled liquor. Generally beer has a 3–6 percent concentration of ethyl alcohol, wines have 10–14 percent, and distilled liquors such as whisky and bourbon have 35–40 percent. The term *proof* is used to designate the amount of alcohol in a beverage. One-half of the proof number equals the percentage of alcohol. For example, a 90-proof beverage contains 45 percent alcohol. In terms of standard serving sizes, a can or bottle of beer is usually 12 oz., a glass of wine is 5 oz., and a mixed drink contains one shot (1–1.5 oz., depending on the proof of the liquor). It is interesting to note that although the concentration of alcohol in each type of beverage is different, the standard size adjusts total volume so that in the end, one serving of beer, wine, or liquor each contains 0.5 oz. of ethyl alcohol. This guide can be a handy measure for monitoring your alcohol consumption. Just be aware that certain mixed drinks such as margaritas and Long Island iced teas contain more than one shot of alcohol, so they count as more than one serving.

Because alcohol is a liquid, it quickly absorbs into the bloodstream, where it moves on to affect the nervous, circulatory, endocrine, and digestive systems. The higher the dose, the greater the effect. In the central nervous system, alcohol's depressant effect is most noticeable in the cerebrum, cerebellum, and medulla areas of the brain. Alcohol affects memory, awareness, and reasoning—collectively, these are what we call *judgment*—and it diminishes balance and coordination. Heart rate and breathing are also slowed. With smaller doses of alcohol, such as 1–2 drinks in an hour, the main effect felt is relaxation—hence alcohol's reputation as the social lubricant. With high doses, such as 7–8 drinks in one hour, the user would have impaired judgment, movement, and balance, and decreased heart rate and breathing. With extremely high doses of alcohol, say 15–20 drinks in one hour, loss of consciousness and death can result because in addition to the continuing depression of the cerebrum and cerebellum, the medulla is being depressed to a point where it no longer instructs the heart to beat or the lungs to breathe (Figure 4.2).

Alcohol causes blood vessels to expand, so the drinker feels very warm and sweats. The more alcohol in the system, the longer the vessels will dilate, and the longer one will feel uncomfortably warm or hot. Alcohol also increases urination, so it is easy to become dehydrated while drinking too much alcohol.

The digestive system is affected in two ways. First, alcohol is a gastric irritant that causes food to move through the system quicker, so there is poor absorption of nutrients, and constipation, diarrhea, or both can result. People who have digestive problems such as ulcers or gastric reflux should abstain or significantly limit drinking and never drink on an empty stomach. Second, alcohol also affects the liver, which is chiefly responsible for breaking down alcohol in the body in a process called *oxidation*, in which alcohol, as it cycles through the liver, is eventually broken down into water and carbon dioxide. The liver oxidizes the amount of alcohol in a standard size drink (half an ounce) in about one hour. Oxidizing alcohol is hard on the liver, and prolonged excessive drinking will damage it. But most experts agree that 1–2 drinks per day won't cause a negative impact on the liver of an otherwise healthy person.

Blood Alcohol Level

The effects of alcohol are directly related to the amount of alcohol in the blood, referred to as *blood alcohol level (BAL)* or *blood alcohol concentration (BAC)*. Figure 4.2 shows the effects of alcohol at selected blood alcohol concentrations.

The higher the level of alcohol in the blood, the greater the effect: from relaxation (0.01) to death (0.40). Four variables influence blood alcohol concentration: (1) the amount of alcohol consumed in a given time period, (2) the weight of the drinker, (3) the gender of the drinker, and (4) the amount of food in the stomach. Figures 4.3 and 4.4 bring together the first three variables. Here we can see that blood alcohol levels are influenced by the amount consumed as well as the weight and gender of the drinker. When they consume the same number of drinks, a person who weighs less will have a higher BAL than a person who weighs more. In addition, if a man and a woman consume the same number of drinks and they also weigh the same, the woman will still have a higher blood alcohol level than the

FIGURE 4.2 — BLOOD ALCOHOL CONCENTRATIONS AND BEHAVIORAL EFFECTS

0.01–0.03 BAC

- slight euphoria, loss of shyness
- depressant effects are not apparent
- mildly relaxed and maybe a little light-headed

0.04–0.06 BAC

- euphoria
- feeling of well-being, relaxation, lower inhibitions, sensation of warmth
- minor impairment of reasoning and memory
- lowering of caution
- exaggerated behavior
- intensified emotions

0.07–0.09 BAC

- 0.08 is legally impaired, and it is illegal to drive at this level
- slight impairment of balance, speech, vision, reaction time, and hearing
- euphoria
- reduced judgment and self-control
- impaired caution, reason, and memory
- belief that they are functioning better than they really are

0.10–0.125 BAC

- significant impairment of motor coordination
- loss of good judgment
- speech may be slurred
- impaired balance, vision, reaction time, and hearing
- euphoria

0.13–0.15 BAC

- gross motor impairment and lack of physical control
- blurred vision
- major loss of balance
- severely impaired judgment and perception

Health & the Media Alcohol Advertising and Behavior

It has been reported that by age 18 the typical American youth has seen or heard over 100,000 alcohol advertisements on television, in print, and on the radio. Billions of dollars are spent each year on alcohol advertising. In a 2006 *Archives of Pediatrics and Adolescent Medicine* study, researchers reported that underage youth viewed, on average, 23 alcohol ads per month. The study also found that such advertising contributes to an increase in drinking among underage youth, and that for each additional dollar per capita spent on alcohol advertising in a local advertising market, young people drank 3 percent more. Does alcohol advertising work? The short answer is yes.

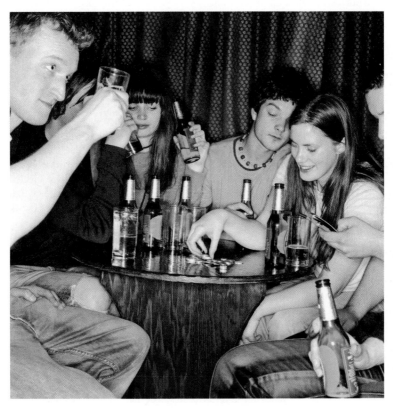

© Punchstock/Image Source

the fact that women tend to process alcohol in their system more slowly than men. A more precise, individualized measure can be obtained with a breathalyzer, a machine that analyzes alcohol content when a person exhales into it. The concentration of alcohol in the breath is an excellent indication of the concentration of alcohol in the blood, and it is legally defensible, as in the case of a Driving Under the Influence (DUI) or Driving While Intoxicated (DWI) legal charge.

Alcohol-Related Problems

Alcohol is a caustic substance that over time can lead to debilitating conditions such as deterioration of the heart muscle and cirrhosis of the liver. But perhaps the most common alcohol-related problem is the headache, nausea, dehydration, and light-headedness collectively referred to as a *hangover*. A number of factors come into play with a hangover. The expansion of cerebral blood vessels can cause the headache. Furthermore, the first step in the liver's breaking down of alcohol produces a toxic chemical that, in abundance, can also cause nausea and headache. Finally, the dehydration that comes with excessive drinking can also cause symptoms such as headache, nausea, and light-headedness.

Hangovers are for the most part self-limiting—their symptoms pass after the body oxidizes the alcohol, and systems have cycled back to normal. There is no cure for a hangover except time. Hangover symptoms can be treated, but one must be careful because certain common over-the-counter medications, such as acetaminophen (Tylenol) and ibuprofen (Advil), can interact with alcohol and damage the liver. People who take too much pain reliever medication after a hangover can experience profound liver problems, including liver failure.

Another alcohol-related problem is drinking and driving. Driving Under the Influence **(DUI)** or Driving While Intoxicated **(DWI)** are the most common legal terms describing one who is driving after having consumed alcohol. "Under the influence" and "while intoxicated" are defined as driving while having a 0.08 BAL or above. If you recall (see Figures 4.3 and 4.4), it doesn't take a huge amount of alcohol to reach a 0.08 level, and people with a high tolerance may even appear to have been drinking but have a 0.08 BAL. Tolerance is individual and subjective, but the laws governing drinking are fairly universal and black and white. A 0.08 BAL can impair judgment and driving reflexes in most people, so it is now the main criterion for a DUI or DWI conviction in almost all states.

Article
4.2

In most states conviction of a DUI or DWI is a Class I misdemeanor, which means that the person will have a criminal record forever. Conviction can also mean that the person will not be eligible for certain occupations, especially those that require a security clearance, since these organizations will not hire someone with a criminal record. Also, car insurance premiums can increase 200–400 percent (assuming that the driving record other than the DUI or DWI is good) for two to three years. Finally, legal representation, fines, and court costs can total thousands of dollars. Thomas von Hermet of the Thomas Jefferson Area (Virginia) Community Criminal Justice Board estimated that the financial costs of a DUI could be as high as $20,000. A DUI/DWI is a serious offense with lifelong implications.

Another alcohol-related problem is drinking while under the legal age of consumption, which is 21 years old in all 50 states. The fake ID is a popular way for underage people to misrepresent their age and be allowed to purchase alcohol and attend nightclubs or parties where alcohol is served. Possessing a fake ID is legally considered fraud, and depending on the context of use, it can result in a Class I

DUI stands for "driving under the influence."

DWI stands for "driving while intoxicated."

misdemeanor conviction and criminal record for life. To compound matters, a fake ID Class I misdemeanor can be considered a "crime of moral turpitude," which means that the person convicted is a dishonest person who committed fraud. Many employers, organizations, and segments of the general population view this as a character flaw with far-reaching implications. So the legal and societal penalties related to fake ID convictions can be surprisingly harsh.

High-Risk Drinking

In recent years much attention has been directed at what is termed **binge drinking,** which is defined as four or more drinks for a female and five or more drinks for a male in one setting. There is no time limit inherent in binge drinking, although some researchers attach a two-hour period for consumption of these drinks. Binge drinking is a concern on college campuses, but what is of more concern is consumption of even higher amounts of alcohol in a short period of time, which is referred to as "high-risk drinking."

Much high-risk drinking is done in a game context, such as the "power hour"— 21 shots in an hour during a 21st birthday celebration. As blood alcohol levels rise, judgment gets more impaired, personal safety can be compromised, and blood alcohol content can rise to lethal levels. High-risk drinking is certainly a problem; it can range from being episodic (for festive events) to something done by an inexperienced underage drinker with limited access to alcohol.

Problem drinking, in a clinical context, usually refers to alcohol abuse and alcohol dependence. *Alcoholism*, although a commonly used term, is not typically used in clinical contexts. **Alcohol abuse** is defined as "continued drinking despite recurring social, interpersonal, and legal problems." **Alcohol dependence** is predicated on the presence or absence of tolerance and withdrawal symptoms. How would one know if he or she is a normal drinker or a problem drinker heading toward alcohol abuse, alcohol dependence, or both?

Self
Assessment
4.1

Help for Problem Drinkers

A typical model for assisting a problem drinker involves three steps: detoxification, counseling, and support groups. Detoxification is a medically supervised effort that removes the alcohol from a person's system and helps reduce the related cravings. It is important that the detoxification be medically supervised because of potentially serious withdrawal symptoms, including tremors, rapid heart beat, confusion, nausea, anxiety, and convulsions. Medications can be used to help limit the severity of symptoms.

Once detoxification is over, people should undergo counseling to deal with the issues that drove them to use alcohol in the first place. Counseling can be individual, family, or group. The counseling effort also focuses on coping skills other than the use of alcohol. In addition, emotional support is also important to help people stay clean and sober. Without this, it is more likely that the user will relapse.

Article
4.3

Binge drinking is having four or more drinks in one occasion for a woman and five or more drinks for a man.

Alcohol abuse is continued drinking despite recurring social, interpersonal, and legal problems.

Alcohol dependence is predicated on the presence of withdrawal symptoms.

Support groups are made up of people who are also trying to stay clean and sober. In every community there are numerous support groups that meet daily, and in these groups people hold one another accountable in the effort to stay clean and sober. Perhaps the best example of a support group is Alcoholics Anonymous (AA).

✓ NEED TO KNOW

The amount of alcohol in a standard-size drink is the same in a glass of wine, a shot of liquor, or a glass of beer. Nothing can be done to speed up the oxidation of alcohol by the liver. Women digest alcohol slower than men, so even if they weigh the same, women will have a higher blood alcohol level than men after the same number of drinks. It takes women longer than men to rid their body of alcohol due to differences in levels of certain digestive enzymes between men and women. Taking too many pain relievers (such as Tylenol or Advil) after drinking heavily can lead to liver damage. Excessive alcohol consumption is a high-risk behavior that can have disastrous consequences. DUI and fake ID convictions are economically costly and have lifelong implications in regard to security clearances for certain jobs. Finally, help for problem drinkers usually involves three steps: medically supervised detoxification, counseling, and support groups.

OPIOIDS

Another class of depressant drugs is called *opioids*. This name refers to natural products of crude opium, semisynthetic products containing some natural crude opium, and synthetic opiates, which react in the body in the same manner as opiates but are made without natural products. Collectively, opioids are a very important class of drugs due to their effectiveness at treating pain. But they also have a high potential for dependence and abuse, and their use is highly regulated. The range of effects includes euphoria, including a dreamlike state of significant relaxation; drowsiness; respiratory depression; nausea; and constipation.

Crude opium is a product of a poppy that grows wild in Asia and other parts of the world. For centuries opium was used to treat pain, diarrhea, and coughs. It was also used recreationally to induce euphoria or a sense of well-being. In the early 1800s, morphine, the active ingredient in crude opium, was isolated, and later that century heroin, a semisynthetic drug, was also created. Codeine, another active ingredient in crude opium, was isolated in the 1930s. All of these opiates were used medically for decades. There were originally no laws regarding their sale or use, and it was not until the Civil War, when thousands became morphine addicts after receiving drugs for treatment of war injuries, that the downsides to opiates became widely known in the United States. In the early 1900s the government passed the first legislation to control distribution and use of opium, morphine, heroin, and other drugs referred to as *narcotics*.

Heroin is a Schedule I narcotic, meaning it is illegal and considered to have no medical use. It continues to be widely abused, causing many personal and societal problems. Most heroin addicts do not live long because the habit is expensive, and they often have to turn to crime to pay for drugs. Further, heroin addicts often share needles and eventually expose themselves to bloodborne infections such as HIV and hepatitis.

Many other semisynthetic opioids have medical uses, so they are listed as Schedule II narcotics. These include Demerol, Dilaudid, and Darvon. In recent years two other opioids, methadone and Oxycontin, have received much publicity.

Methadone is primarily used in heroin rehabilitation. So-called methadone maintenance is designed to determine the stabilization dose of methadone necessary to eliminate the craving for heroin. Once that dosage is reached, the heroin addict can undergo both personal and vocational counseling in order to reintegrate back into society as a productive member. Methadone maintenance is controversial, mostly because one drug (methadone) is substituted for another (heroin). There is conflict between the view that drug addiction is a poor life choice (a "disorder of the will") and that it is a disease. However, the two views do intersect. At first, the person is making a choice to modify his or her mood (an act of the will), but after time, if tolerance, physical dependence, and psychological dependence are established, the user has little control, and stopping the drug will lead to withdrawal symptoms requiring medical intervention. There is no easy answer to this conflict, as both views of addiction have merit.

A more recent controversy involves the drug **Oxycontin,** a time-released opioid normally prescribed to people in significant pain, such as cancer patients. It is a powerful opioid, and like many powerful drugs, has become a popular illicit drug because of the euphoria it can produce. Patients taking Oxycontin must be monitored closely because of the potential problems of drug interactions, tolerance, and dependence and the possibility of dosages reaching a lethal level. Recreational abuse of Oxycontin has particularly been a problem in Appalachia (southwest Virginia and eastern Kentucky), where it has been referred to as *hillbilly* heroin. Other opioids that are prescribed and popularly abused include Vicodin, Lortab, and Tussionex.

Vicodin and Lortab are prescription drugs used to treat pain and coughs. The generic name is hydrocodone, and it is an effective pain reliever. Because the drug produces a euphoric effect, it is an attractive recreational drug. Side effects of Vicodin and Lortab include upset stomach, nausea, and dizziness.

Dextromethorphan or DMX is an over-the-counter cough suppressant drug. DMX works on the cough center in the brain, and when the recommended dose is taken, it produces little or no euphoria. When taken in higher-than-recommended doses, a heightened euphoria results. Since it is readily available and a "cheap high," DMX is abused. Long-term effects of abuse are similar to most other depressants: sensory changes, agitation, paranoia, and in some cases hallucinations.

SEDATIVE-HYPNOTICS

Sedative-hypnotic drugs are a category of depressants normally used to induce sedation and sleep (hypnotic). These drugs are medically prescribed and include barbiturates, which are classified as ultra-short, intermediate, and long-acting. Ultra-short barbiturates such as thiopental are used to induce anesthesia; intermediate ones such as Seconal are used to induce sleep; and long-acting ones such as butalbital and phenobarbital are used to treat headaches and prevent seizures, respectively. Of the three types of barbiturates, the intermediate drugs have been the most

Oxycontin is a time-released opioid similar to morphine and extremely potent.

Sedative-hypnotic drugs are capable of producing sedation and sleep.

problematic, since at one point they were popularly used to treat insomnia. Seconal dependence can occur fairly rapidly, and Seconal combined with alcohol can be toxic and result in death. Further, withdrawal from barbiturates can cause serious problems and even be life-threatening.

Nonbarbiturate sedative hypnotics also exist. Meprobamate (Miltown) has the same effect as an intermediate barbiturate, but the risk of dependence is not as serious. With the introduction of minor tranquilizers in the 1960s, there has been less need for barbiturates and nonbarbiturates as sedative-hypnotics.

INHALANTS

Inhalants are solvents and solutions that are used in hair spray, gasoline, paint, glue, and other commonly used items. *Huffing* is the term used to describe use of inhalants. The effects from huffing include euphoria, light-headedness, and lack of coordination. The chemicals in the solvents can interfere with the amount of oxygen reaching the brain and other tissues, resulting in a condition called *hypoxia,* a dangerously low level of oxygen. Inhalant use can introduce toxic levels of the solvent into the system, and brain damage can result.

Nitrous oxide, or "laughing gas," is a popular inhalant. Nitrous oxide is used medically as an anesthetic. Inhaling nitrous oxide results in relaxation and a loosening of inhibitions often resulting in uncontrolled laughter. The amount of nitrous oxide administered for medical purposes must be closely monitored. Recreational users find items such as CO_2 cartridges containing nitrous oxide used in baking and inhale the nitrous oxide right from the cartridge. This is extremely dangerous because of the freezing temperature in the cartridge. Frostbite of the nose and lung damage from freezing can result.

VAPING

The introduction of e-cigarettes has ushered in a new term, vaping, which is defined earlier in the chapter. Technically, the nicotine in the e-cigarette could be replaced with a different drug, vaporized, and inhaled. Since e-cigarettes are unregulated it is difficult to stop the practice of vaporizing different drugs. Vaping does present a danger not only in terms of health risks associated with the drug being vaporized but also with a chemical byproduct of vaping called diacetyl. Diacetyl is a natural substance found in some foods and is safe to eat but not necessarily safe to inhale.

✓ NEED TO KNOW

Other depressants include opioids, sedative-hypnotics, and inhalants. Drugs in the opioid category include morphine, codeine, Vicodin, and Oxycontin. These drugs are powerful and have a high potential for abuse. Sedative-hypnotics is a broad category of depressants with a wide variety of uses ranging from anesthesia to prevention of seizures. Inhalants also have medical uses, but like other depressants, they can be abused, especially by adolescents who have easy access to glue, household chemicals, and other common substances that when inhaled can deprive the brain of oxygen and induce a euphoric effect. Using an e-cigarette device to vaporize nicotine and other drugs can present health risks.

➤ Stimulants

Stimulants are a large category that includes powerful drugs such as cocaine, crack, and amphetamines and milder cerebral stimulants such as nicotine and caffeine. *Speed* is a term used to describe stimulants, particularly amphetamines. All stimulants have the capability to increase functional activity of the nervous system. This can have a significant effect on thought processes to the point where thinking becomes so scrambled that it is difficult for people to focus their thoughts. Sometimes this can serve as a catalyst for creativity, such as in stand-up comedy, but it can also lead to a split from reality involving the personality called a *psychosis*.

COCAINE AND CRACK

Cocaine is a drug found in the leaves of the coca bush, which grows wild in parts of Bolivia, Colombia, and Peru. Ancient civilizations such as the Incas integrated cocaine into their culture through chewing coca leaves for the stimulant effect. Cocaine also has local anesthetic properties. What the common pick-me-ups caffeine and nicotine are to current society, cocaine was to the ancient Incas.

Cocaine has an interesting history that includes Sigmund Freud, who at first espoused the use of cocaine to treat morphine addiction, then renounced it as a scourge when he became addicted himself. The fictional detective Sherlock Holmes is known for his "7 percent solution," the special formula he used in preparing his cocaine. Inventor John Pemberton used cocaine in his original formula for Coca-Cola. In low doses cocaine can increase heart rate and blood pressure, decrease fatigue, and increase mental alertness and sociability. But in high doses it can cause dizziness, blurred vision, and tremors, as well as repress heart enzymes and cause convulsions and death. The cocaine experience is short-lived. After snorting it, users experience a euphoric high for 15–30 minutes. After that they "crash," becoming light-headed and nauseated. The only ways for users to resolve the experience are to wait out the crash or to snort more cocaine to alleviate it. Snorting more cocaine will reinforce the craving—this is why cocaine is considered so addictive.

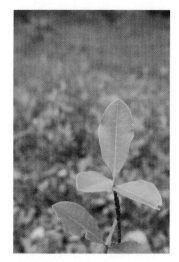

Recreational use of cocaine ebbs and flows in popularity. When it was extremely popular to abuse in the 1980s, a new, purer form called *crack* was created. Crack is about 10 times more powerful than regular cocaine, in terms of both its euphoric high and the painful crash afterward. As such, it is even more addictive than cocaine.

Interestingly, cocaine is not a Schedule I drug. The DEA placed it in Schedule II because it is a powerful local anesthetic used to numb the eyes or nasal passages for surgery.

Cocaine, a stimulant drug derived from the leaves of the coca plant, has been used by humans for at least a thousand years.

© Sayarikuna/iStock/Getty Images

Amphetamines are powerful prescription stimulants used to treat narcolepsy, low blood pressure, and attention-deficit/hyperactivity disorder (ADHD). Amphetamines are similar to cocaine in experience, but their effect lasts much longer, up to 10 or more hours. The crash from amphetamine use is also more prolonged. Because amphetamines have such a long duration, they are popularly taken to help people stay awake for long periods of time. Some students use them to stay awake all night to cram for an exam, and some truck drivers use them to drive for longer periods of time. Unfortunately, the effects of the amphetamines can be scary and even life-threatening. Extreme restlessness, anxiety, confusion, paranoia, high blood pressure, convulsions, and cardiac arrest can result from excessive doses or extended use.

In a medically supervised context, amphetamines improve quality of life. ADHD is a case in point. The stimulant Ritalin is prescribed for children, but adults who are diagnosed with the disorder can also be prescribed the drug. A person with ADHD has a short attention span, has difficulty concentrating, and is easily distracted. Learning is compromised. How Ritalin works is not entirely clear, and it does seem like a paradox that a hyperactive person would find relief from a prescription stimulant, but true ADHD patients receive tremendous benefit from Ritalin. They can take the drug without experiencing euphoria. People who take Ritalin who do not have ADHD will experience an amphetamine high, though. For that reason, Ritalin has become a drug of abuse in non-ADHD populations.

In recent years a form of amphetamine called *methamphetamine* has become a serious problem, especially in communities where the rave culture is prominent. Methamphetamine use has increased in popularity and with that popularity has come an increase in emergency room visits due to methamphetamine-related emergencies. In its oral form, the drug is often called *speed* or *meth*, and in smokable form, *ice* or *crystal*. Both forms are normally made in illegal laboratories from ingredients in common over-the-counter drug products such as appetite suppressants, decongestants, and allergy products. There were over 10,000 methamphetamine lab incidents in 2010. Methamphetamines generally have a much more intense effect on the nervous system than prescription amphetamines, and the addictive potential is more profound.

Methamphetamines are extremely dangerous, and increased use can result in delusions and hallucinations, as well as heart problems. Smoking methamphetamine allows the administration and absorption to be quicker than taking it in tablet form, and the effects are more intense because the drug is getting to the brain quicker. The long-term effects of methamphetamine use include aggressive and violent behavior, weight loss, and psychosis. In addition to these effects, people who smoke methamphetamines can develop "meth mouth" when the teeth become destroyed and look like they are rotting away.

NICOTINE

Nicotine is another naturally occurring stimulant. Found in tobacco, nicotine is highly addictive. Once absorbed into the blood, it exerts a cerebral stimulant effect that is both pleasurable and short-lived. The smoker must inhale again and again to obtain more of the pleasurable feeling, and over time that produces cravings and addiction. Unfortunately, in addition to the nicotine, a smoker inhales tars and carbon monoxide, which starve tissue of oxygen. This is why smokers are at higher risk of both cancer and heart disease. The health hazards associated with any form of tobacco use are documented and well known. And for the approximately

29 percent of the population who smokes, tobacco use is an expensive habit. A pack-a-day cigarette habit will cost most smokers well over $1,000 each year.

The e-cigarette is becoming a popular way to administer nicotine. The device is an electronic unit that vaporizes nicotine and is marketed as being safer than cigarettes, though there is no evidence to this claim. Further, since e-cigarettes are unregulated, it is difficult to implement a public health response.

In addition to the health hazards associated with smoking, those who are exposed to cigarette smoke are also at risk for health problems. Secondhand smoke (the smoke that people around a smoker inhale) contains carbon monoxide and carcinogens and can cause heart disease or even cancer in nonsmokers who spend large amounts of time in the company of smokers.

Getting dependent on nicotine is easy. Quitting tobacco use is hard. The withdrawal symptoms of nicotine include headache, nervousness, fatigue, poor concentration, and sleep disturbances. But users who have a desire to quit have numerous options. First, there is the classic "cold turkey" withdrawal, whereby the user quits tobacco, overcomes the withdrawal symptoms, and stays tobacco free. Second, there are gums that contain nicotine. They provide enough of the drug to reduce the craving for tobacco gradually. Third, there are nicotine patches, which release the drug into the blood at a steady rate through the skin and reduce the craving for nicotine. Finally, there are prescription medications, such as the antidepressant Zyban, which reduce the craving for nicotine and can be effective in helping people quit.

In the continuing effort to educate people on the health effects of cigarette smoking, the FDA sponsored the development of new cigarette warning labels that are very graphic and depict the health effects of smoking. Cigarette companies are required to place the labels on cigarette packs, cartons, and advertisements. Only time will tell how effective this new approach will be in reducing cigarette smoking.

CAFFEINE

Caffeine is the most common cerebral stimulant. It is found in coffee, chocolate, tea, soft drinks, and many over-the-counter drugs from analgesics to weight-loss products. The highest amounts of caffeine are found in coffee, where the dose can range from 75 mg per cup for instant coffee to 150 mg per cup for drip coffee. In soft drinks the caffeine can range from 37.5 mg in a 12-oz. can of Pepsi to 70 mg in extra-caffeinated drinks like Jolt Cola. Other energy drinks contain 120 mg or more. Table 4.1 shows the caffeine content in popular beverages.

Ingesting caffeine results in a higher level of alertness and mild euphoria. A dose of caffeine can exert this effect for about an hour and then it gradually wears off. People can become dependent on caffeine, and this can lead to a craving. The most common withdrawal effect is a headache.

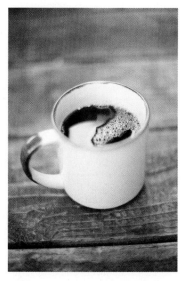

Caffeine is a popular, legal stimulant most commonly found in coffee, sodas, and teas.

© Ingram Publishing/SuperStock

TABLE 4.1   OVERCAFFEINATED: EXAMINING CAFFEINE AND ITS EFFECTS

	8 oz.	12-oz. can	Per oz.
Caffeine in Coke Products			
Coke Classic	23 mg	34.5 mg	2.875 mg
Coke Zero	23 mg	34.5 mg	2.875 mg
Vanilla Coke	23 mg	34.5 mg	2.875 mg
Diet Coke	31 mg	46.5 mg	3.875 mg
Diet Vanilla Coke	31 mg	46.5 mg	3.875 mg
Barq's Root Beer	15 mg	22.5 mg	1.875 mg
Tab	31 mg	46.5 mg	3.875 mg
Pibb Xtra	27 mg	40.5 mg	3.375 mg
Caffeine in Pepsi Products			
Pepsi	25 mg	37.5 mg	3.125 mg
Diet Pepsi	24 mg	36 mg	3 mg
Pepsi One	36 mg	54 mg	4.5 mg
Caffeine in Mountain Dew			
Mountain Dew	36 mg	54 mg	4.5 mg
Diet Mountain Dew	36 mg	54 mg	4.5 mg
Code Red	36 mg	54 mg	4.5 mg
Misc. Sodas			
Surge	53 mg	70.5 mg	6.625 mg
Jolt	47 mg	70.5 mg	5.875 mg
Mello Yellow	35 mg	52.5 mg	4.375 mg
Sunkist	27 mg	40.5 mg	3.375 mg
Dr. Pepper	27 mg	40.5 mg	3.375 mg
	CAFFEINE IN ENERGY DRINKS		
	8 oz.	12-oz. can	Per oz.
Caffeine in Energy Drinks			
MDX	47 mg	70.5 mg	5.875 mg
Diet MDX	50 mg	75 mg	6.25 mg
Amp Energy Drink	71 mg	106.5 mg	8.875 mg

Sometimes caffeine users overcaffeinate themselves and induce a state of **caffeinism.** The symptoms include tremors, restlessness, agitation, confusion, light-headedness, and anxiety. Abstaining from coffee for a few hours will cause the symptoms to subside. Although it is not pleasant, caffeinism is not generally harmful or dangerous. However, people should be aware that caffeine is rather caustic and can aggravate ulcers and acid reflux disease, so those who have digestive problems should not use it. Individuals with anxiety disorders and women who are pregnant should also avoid excessive caffeine in their diets.

Caffeinism is an outcome of an excessive dose of caffeine.

| TABLE 4.1 | OVERCAFFEINATED: EXAMINING CAFFEINE AND ITS EFFECTS *(concluded)* |

	8 oz.	12-oz. can	Per oz.
No Fear	83 mg	124.5 mg	10.375 mg
SoBe Adrenaline Rush	75 mg	112.5 mg	9.375 mg
Adrenaline Sport	35 mg	52.5 mg	4.375 mg
Red Bull	80 mg	—	10 mg
Atomic Rush	100 mg (7 oz.)	—	14.29 mg
Bawls Guarana	67 mg (10 oz.)	—	6.7 mg

CAFFEINE IN COFFEE AND OTHER HOT DRINKS

	8 oz.	12-oz. can	Per oz.
Coffee, Espresso, and Tea			
Espresso	100 mg*	—	50 mg
Coffee, Instant	75 mg	112.5 mg	9.375 mg
Coffee, Decaffeinated	3 mg	4.5 mg	0.375 mg
Coffee, Brewed	135 mg	202.5 mg	16.876 mg
Tea, Green	15 mg	22.5 mg	1.875 mg
Tea, Leaf or Bag	50 mg	75 mg	6.25 mg

CAFFEINE IN FOODS

	Mg	Serving size	Mg per oz.
Chocolate			
Hershey's Special Dark Chocolate	31 mg	1 bar (1.5 oz.)	
Hershey's Milk Chocolate	10 mg	1 bar (1.5 oz.)	
Chocolate Milk	5 mg	7.5 mg	0.625 mg

TABLET

	Mg	Serving size	Mg per oz.
Tablets			
Caffeine Tablet (Vivarin)	200 mg	1 tablet	—
Caffeine Tablet (NoDoz)	200 mg	1 tablet	—
Excedrin Tablet	65 mg	1 tablet	—

*2 oz.

Source: Data from **OverCaffeinated.org.**

✓ NEED TO KNOW

Stimulants make people feel energetic or euphoric, and they may have numbing or pain-relief qualities. Medical uses include anesthesia and treatment of ADHD (hyperactivity). Stimulants are widely abused and can induce dependence quickly, due to both the high and the unpleasant low that comes as the drug leaves the body. Whether it is caffeine, nicotine, cocaine, or amphetamines, all stimulants produce an up-and-down cycle, but their effects differ in degree and intensity.

➤ Hallucinogens

Hallucinogens are a category of drugs capable of inducing a hallucination, which is a perception of sights, sounds, physical senses (touch), or taste with no basis in reality. Similar to a hallucination is a delusion—a misinterpretation of something real. For example, a person who looks at a car and sees a dog instead of the vehicle is having a delusion, while a person seeing a car when nothing is there is having a hallucination.

LSD

LSD was accidentally discovered in the late 1930s when a Swiss chemist was working with ergot, a fungus that grows on rye, in an attempt to find a cure for migraine headaches. LSD proved not to have any headache-relief properties despite numerous experiments to find a medical use for the drug. In the 1960s LSD became popular as a part of the counterculture movement. It is a colorless, odorless, and tasteless drug. A small dose, called a *microdot*, can induce an 8- to 12-hour psychoactive experience that includes hallucinations. This experience can be framed by anxiety, and the beginning, several hours of hallucinations, can be followed by several hours of depression. Like any other drug, the intensity of these effects varies.

There has been no documentation of physiological damage among LSD users. However, some users have experienced a post-hallucinogenic sensory disorder and have hallucinations years after using LSD. Also, during the hallucinogenic phase of the LSD experience, safety can be compromised if the false perception involves a potentially dangerous situation. For example, a person could be unaware of his or her surroundings and walk in front of oncoming traffic or fall out a window. Like cocaine, LSD popularity ebbs and flows. Much of the current LSD use is tied to rave culture.

PSILOCYBIN

Psilocybin is a hallucinogenic drug found in *teonanacatl,* a type of mushroom native to the United States and Mexico. The term *shrooms* is sometimes used for these psilocybin-containing mushrooms. Shrooms are usually eaten, and the effects can last from three to eight hours. Small doses of psilocybin induce a tranquil euphoric state, and higher dosages can induce hallucinations. The shroom experience is similar to LSD, but normally not nearly as intense or potent.

MESCALINE

Mescaline is a hallucinogenic drug found in peyote, a growth or "button" found on a small cactus that grows in Mexico and the southwestern United States. Mescaline produces a total psychoactive experience for about 10 hours, with hallucinations lasting about 2 hours. Although not a very powerful hallucinogen, mescaline can still pack a punch depending on the size and frequency of doses. Unlike many other hallucinogens, mescaline has medical uses; it is prescribed as a respiratory stimulant and as a treatment for heart problems.

Phencyclidine (PCP) was originally developed as a dissociative anesthetic (one capable of keeping patients awake but pain free during surgery and other procedures). The early trials of PCP as an anesthetic found it to be effective, but the patients experienced mood swings and hallucinations, and displayed violent behavior, all symptoms that indicated a narrow margin of safety, so the FDA never approved PCP for human use. However, it was approved for use as a veterinary anesthetic and tranquilizer. Consequently, it was easy to divert to human populations.

The effects of PCP are very unpredictable, causing some experts to characterize PCP as the most dangerous illicit drug. It can induce profound mood swings, delusions, violent primal behavior, and hallucinations. This experience can last for hours, and users may endanger themselves and others while under the influence. To complicate matters, when users are hurt, they do not feel the pain because of PCP's anesthetic properties. So users can continue violent and destructive behavior for much longer than would be possible for anyone who is not under the influence of PCP.

Like PCP, ketamine is a dissociative anesthetic and is used in veterinary medicine. Not as powerful as PCP, ketamine is also used as an anesthetic for humans. It can induce a PCP-like experience, and when used illicitly, it is sometimes called Special K. Often ketamine is marketed as PCP.

KHAT AND SALVIA

Khat is a naturally occurring stimulant that comes from a shrub common to Africa and the Middle East. Cathinone is the active ingredient in khat, and while khat is not scheduled by the DEA, cathinone is, and it is a Schedule I drug. Similar to amphetamines, khat can be effective in eliciting a euphoric effect and increased alertness for about one to three hours, after which the user experiences depression, anorexia, and difficulty in sleeping. Long-term use of khat can result in periodontal disease, gastrointestinal problems, and cardiovascular problems. A synthetic cathinone commonly referred to as bath salts can produce an effect more powerful that khat. In addition, emergency room visits for severe reactions to bath salt use have increased in recent years.

Salvia is an herb commonly found in Mexico and throughout Central and South America. Salvinorin A is the active ingredient in salvia. The salvia leaves are usually chewed, smoked, or consumed in liquid form. The effects of salvia begin within 1 minute after it enters the blood and last for about 30 minutes. Effects include hallucinations and mood swings. Since salvia is an herb, it is not scheduled by the DEA and is readily available in the United States. The legality of salvia will vary from state to state.

✓ NEED TO KNOW

Hallucinogens are powerful drugs with unpredictable effects. PCP and ketamine are particularly dangerous due to the unpredictable, sometimes violent behavior they can cause users to exhibit. Khat and salvia are two newly popular hallucinogens derived from plants and herbs. Khat produces similar effects to amphetamines, and salvia produces hallucinations and mood swings.

➤ Marijuana

Marijuana is the name for products from the cannabis plant that are dried and prepared for smoking. Cannabis has been referred to as a weed because it does grow wild in many areas of the world. A resin called tetrahydrocannabinol (THC) is the chief agent responsible for the physical and psychological effects associated with marijuana.

FORMS AND EFFECTS OF MARIJUANA

How cannabis impacts someone relates to the concentration of THC in the final product. Ganja, the tops and leaves of the cannabis plant, generally contains 3–5 percent concentration THC. Sinsemilla, or "without seeds," refers to a form of marijuana with an 8–10 percent concentration of THC. Hashish is a more concentrated form that is usually smoked in small, square blocks and contains a 14–16 percent THC concentration. Finally, the most potent form is hash oil, which can contain up to 60 percent THC. Hash oil will induce an LSD-like experience. The other forms of marijuana are less potent and can induce significant sedation and possibly delusions but not hallucinations.

Because smoking is the chief method of administration, the effects are felt almost immediately. The psychological effects of THC include relaxation, relief from anxiety, euphoria, laughter, and, if the concentration of THC is high enough, impaired judgment and short-term memory. Physical effects of marijuana include dry mouth, increased appetite, bloodshot eyes, coughing, and decreased muscle coordination. Often the effects of marijuana are compared to alcohol, particularly by those who want to see marijuana legalized. Long-term effects of marijuana use include the development of amotivational syndrome, impaired immunity, respiratory problems, and increased cancer risk.

Physical dependence and tolerance to marijuana have not been shown. Psychological dependence can be related to anything, so it is safe to say that users can become psychologically dependent on marijuana.

Article
4.4

Of note is a recent study in *Clinical Psychological Science* (2016) that reported people who smoked cannabis four or more days a week over many years experienced downward socioeconomic mobility as well as more financial difficulties, workplace problems, and relationship conflict than occasional users of marijuana. As marijuana is subjected to more scientific scrutiny, more will be understood about its benefits and drawbacks.

MARIJUANA'S SAFETY AND THE QUESTION OF LEGALIZATION

Due to its common illicit use since the 1960s, some people feel that using marijuana in moderation is as safe as alcohol or cigarettes and ought to be legalized. Just how safe is marijuana use?

Self
Assessment
4.2

Although THC and alcohol may both be used for relaxation, alcohol is not smoked, so the method of administration is not comparable. Smoking marijuana puts one at risk of the same kinds of conditions that cigarette smokers are at risk for, including heart disease and cancer. **Cannabinoids** are tars in cannabis, many

Cannabinoids are tars in cannabis and marijuana, some of which are carcinogenic.

of which are cancer causing. Further, marijuana smoke, like cigarette smoke, contains high levels of carbon monoxide. Thus tissues become oxygen starved when marijuana is used. The dangers that may come with marijuana smoke have not been studied as closely as the dangers of cigarette smoke, so the long-term impact of marijuana use is not as well understood. See "Breaking It Down" for more information on the legalization controversy.

Breaking It Down   Should More Drugs Be Legalized?

The United States spends billions of dollars on drug regulations, prohibitions, and enforcement. High-profile people such as former secretary of state George Shultz and the late Nobel laureate Milton Friedman have stated that making drugs illegal leads by default to the involvement of organized crime. If drugs were legal, the argument goes, the government could control sales and tax the products. This would generate large amounts of revenue now lost to the government because it cannot currently track illegal sales. Further, if drugs were legal, organized crime might be reduced because people seeking drugs could do so legally. Without the involvement of organized crime in drug trafficking, there might be fewer homicides and other types of violent crime surrounding drug use and sales. There would also be fewer incarcerations and possibly fewer health problems such as overdoses, because if the government enforced quality control of drugs, people would be able to ascertain the exact substance they had and know the safer dose levels. Finally, most of those who favor legalizing some or all drugs feel that drug use is a personal choice and should not be subject to government interference.

In contrast, opponents of legalizing some or all drugs, such as Lee P. Brown, director and spokesperson of the Office of National Drug Control Policy and Drug Enforcement, argue that legalization of drugs is immoral. People who are against legalizing drugs also tend to believe that the stiff penalties for drug use deter many from trying drugs in the first place, and that saves lives. Opponents feel legalization would only increase social problems like addiction and the violent crimes that are committed by people under the influence.

Although the idea of legalizing heroin or cocaine is not widely accepted in the United States, a growing number of Americans seem to feel that the classification of marijuana as a Schedule I drug should be changed. They point out that Marinol, an antinausea drug used by cancer patients, is derived from marijuana, so the government's claim that marijuana is a Schedule I drug without any accepted medical uses is inconsistent and incorrect. Washington, Colorado, and Oregon have legalized recreational use of marijuana. Other states—including Alaska, California, Hawaii, Maine, Montana, Nevada, New Mexico, Rhode Island, and Vermont—have passed laws in the last decade that remove state-level penalties for possessing or growing marijuana if it is intended to be used as a treatment for depression, for chronic pain from illnesses such as cancer, or for the treatment of glaucoma. Furthermore, another 10 states (plus the District of Columbia) have statutes that symbolically support the idea of medical marijuana use.

Opponents of legalization claim that the pro-legalization camp is disingenuous about its motives and simply wants to relax the bans and make the recreational use

(continued)

of marijuana easier for everyone. Opponents point out that although the psychological effects of THC are similar to alcohol, the long-term effects of chronic use of marijuana are more similar to smoking cigarettes. Marijuana smoke has high levels of carbon monoxide and carcinogenic tars. Collectively these substances can starve the tissues of oxygen, leading to cardiovascular disease as well as cancer. So significant health risks are associated with marijuana. Further, marijuana dependence does occur in some people, and marijuana can impair driving performance.

There seems to be more support for the total legalization of marijuana because opinions on its general safety vary, and there may be wisdom in restricting recreational use. But continuing the ban on medical use of marijuana is much more up in the air. The prosecution of medical marijuana cases, both at the federal and the state level, appears to be an issue in flux. Examining what happens in Washington, Colorado, and Oregon will help clarify the issues associated with legalization of marijuana.

SPICE AND K2

Spice and K2 are together a mixture of herbs with psychoactive properties that has been successfully marketed as an incense substitute for marijuana. Since it is an incense, it is commonly available through numerous outlets—health food stores, head shops, convenience stores, and the Internet. Spice and K2 is usually smoked but can be prepared in liquid form and consumed. In addition to the mostly marijuana-like effects, users can also experience rapid heart rate, vomiting, agitation, confusion, and hallucinations. Because of the immediate dangers associated with Spice and K2 use, the DEA was able to effect emergency scheduling, making Spice and K2 a Schedule I drug and essentially banning it.

✓ NEED TO KNOW

Marijuana is a popular recreational drug. The concentration of THC in the marijuana induces the psychoactive effect. The higher the concentration of THC, the more intense the effect. Street-grade marijuana today is much more powerful than it was in the 1960s and 1970s. Use of marijuana carries health risks that are similar to the health risks associated with smoking. The common comparison to alcohol holds true only for THC ingested in some way other than smoking. Spice and K2 are herbs that have been promoted as substitutes for marijuana, and as a result the DEA has banned both.

➤ Psychotherapeutic Drugs

Psychotherapeutic drugs treat mental and emotional problems that range from anxiety to depression. For many, this category of drugs represents a medical miracle—these substances can enable users to continue with their life in a healthful way and be free from symptoms of mental illness. Further, the effectiveness of these drugs confirms the biological basis of anxiety and depression, which previously had been subject to debate. The most common psychotherapeutic drugs include antidepressants, minor tranquilizers, and major tranquilizers.

ANTIDEPRESSANTS

Clinical depression has a biological basis. Abnormalities in the level of neurotransmitters, specifically serotonin, can result in depression. Antidepressants as a category of drugs have improved the lives of millions of people because they "adjust" the neurotransmitters to a point where depression is prevented. Common antidepressants today are selective serotonin reuptake inhibitors **(SSRIs).** These drugs allow serotonin to stay in the synapse longer and prevent depression. Examples of SSRIs include Prozac, Zoloft, Paxil, and Viibyrd. Another category is the selective serotonin norepinephrine reuptake inhibitors **(SSNRIs).** These drugs allow both serotonin and norepinephrine to stay in the synapse longer to prevent depression. Examples of SSNRIs include the number one and two most prescribed antidepressants, Cymbalta and Pristiq.

A person diagnosed with depression and who is prescribed an antidepressant should see some improvement within just a few weeks. The hopelessness and despair should be significantly lessened. This improvement should give the person a clearer perspective on life and life's events.

Not only are antidepressants popular in treating depression, but some such as Paxil are popular in treating generalized anxiety feelings, including fear, overworry, overconcern, and panic. And since antidepressants influence neurotransmitters, they are often prescribed for conditions other than depression. Many people are able to prevent migraine headaches with antidepressants, and many others with chronic pain feel antidepressants decrease the intensity of pain they regularly experience.

Long-term use of antidepressants appears to be safe. On occasion a news article has focused on a bad side effect with Prozac or Zoloft, but upon further evaluation, there has not been enough evidence to pull the drug off the market. This doesn't mean that it won't eventually happen; it just means the problem that was observed could not be related to the use of antidepressants, or the effect happens in such a small number of users that closer patient monitoring is needed rather than pulling the drug from the market.

MINOR TRANQUILIZERS

Minor tranquilizers have been referred to as "anti-anxiety drugs." **Benzodiazepines** are the most commonly prescribed minor tranquilizers and include such drugs as Valium, Xanax, and Tranxene. These drugs are designed for short-term medication

SSRI is a selective serotonin reuptake inhibitor, which is used to treat depression.

SSNRI is a selective serotonin and norepinephrine reuptake inhibitor also used to treat depression.

Benzodiazepines are minor tranquilizers and include drugs such as Xanax, Valium, and Tranxene.

of anxiety and insomnia. They should not be used long term. If long-term medication is needed for anxiety, most physicians will cycle the person through the SSRIs to determine which one works best.

Minor tranquilizers are generally taken in pill form. The effects last a short time, and tolerance to these drugs can build quickly. When taken in conjunction with alcohol, the effect can be toxic.

MAJOR TRANQUILIZERS

Major tranquilizers are termed *antipsychotic drugs* because they can be effective in medicating people with serious conditions such as schizophrenia. Drugs from a category of major tranquilizers called *phenothiazines*, such as Thorazine, have made a positive difference in the lives of millions. Before the introduction of phenothiazines, most people who suffered from schizophrenia had to be institutionalized.

Lithium is another major tranquilizer. It is used to treat serious bipolar disorder, which has also been called *manic depression*. The benefits of major tranquilizers far outweigh the side effects.

DATE RAPE DRUGS

The common scenario for a date rape begins with a man dropping a drug into a woman's drink. About 20 minutes after consuming the drugged beverage, the woman feels light-headed and wants to go home. The man who put the drug in her drink assists her, but his motive is to rape her. Shortly after the onset of symptoms, she lapses into unconsciousness or dissociates herself from the environment, meaning that she is awake but not processing environmental stimuli. In this state, he rapes her, and later when she is conscious, she has no memory because the drug has induced amnesia.

A drug commonly used in date rapes is Rohypnol, a minor tranquilizer from the benzodiazepine group. Rohypnol is similar to Valium but 10 times more powerful. Rohypnol is illegal in the United States but is available in many other countries, so there are multiple sources for the drug.

Another date rape drug is gamma-hydroxybutyrate, or GHB. GHB was originally developed as a dissociative anesthetic, and like PCP, it was found to have negative side effects and so was never marketed. The precursor to GHB contains chemicals commonly used by bodybuilders, so smart chemists can purchase these chemicals at health food stores and cook up GHB. The effects of GHB include significant muscle relaxation, nausea, vomiting, and amnesia. A high dose can cause hallucinations, respiratory distress, seizures, and possible coma. When combined with alcohol, the effects are enhanced and potentially life-threatening.

✓ NEED TO KNOW

It is easy for a drug such as Rohypnol or GHB to be put into a drink. Always make sure that there is no possibility for someone to add something to a drink. Trust your instincts—if you feel unusually or excessively drowsy or light-headed after a drink, then be sure to have friends take you home.

Designer drugs and club drugs are not categories of drugs like stimulants. **Designer drugs** are those made a certain way, and **club drugs** are those used in nightclubs or raves. Designer drugs are chemical analogues—that is, drugs that are very similar chemically to another drug but not exactly the same.

For example, fentanyl is a pain reliever more powerful than morphine. In many cities, the heroin that is marketed is actually a designer drug derived from fentanyl that is processed to look like heroin. Just about any drug distributed in the illegal market could be a designer drug.

A more common designer drug is the amphetamine analogue called Ecstasy. Its effect is similar to an amphetamine in that it increases heart rate and respiration. Some users experience mild distortions of perception, interpreted as a tranquil effect, which often progresses to a feeling of trust in their social interactions. This has led to Ecstasy being referred to as the *love drug*. A purer crystalline powder form of Ecstasy called Molly (slang for molecular) has more recently been distributed and used.

There have been two waves of Ecstasy popularity—one in the mid-1980s and one currently. After the wave of use in the mid-1980s, the drug was discovered to destroy serotonergic neurons, those neurons that produce serotonin, and brain damage can result. For this reason, Ecstasy is considered a dangerous drug.

In addition to its negative effect on neurons, Ecstasy can throw off the body's thermostat, resulting in dehydration and, potentially, cardiac arrest. People do die from Ecstasy use because of this. Ecstasy users trying to game the system have been known to "front load" their water, or drink gallons of water before or immediately after consuming Ecstasy, so that they will not become dehydrated. This behavior can also be life-threatening because it can produce a condition called *hyponatremia*, in which too much water causes tissues to swell. In extreme cases death can result.

Ecstasy is also considered a club drug. Other club drugs include LSD, shrooms, and marijuana. These are drugs that have long-lasting effects, are used in club or rave settings, and are used to maximize the club or rave experience.

✓ **NEED TO KNOW**

Ecstasy is an extremely powerful chemical. It destroys nerve cells and disrupts the body's thermostat, resulting in extreme dehydration. People under the influence of Ecstasy don't feel thirsty, yet they need fluids. This loss of fluids can result in a heart attack. Some users recognize this and drink excessive amounts of water before experiencing the effects of Ecstasy. This also has some dangers because consuming excessive amounts of water can cause body tissues to swell, and if swelling occurs in the brain, brain damage or death can result.

Designer drugs are chemical analogues of other drugs.

Club drugs are powerful drugs used in the nightclub scene or raves.

➤ Drug Testing and Drug Treatment

Drug testing is a common practice to determine if a person has used certain drugs. The most common drugs tested for are opiates, cocaine, amphetamines, marijuana, Ecstasy, and barbiturates. Traces of these substances remain in urine for varying times after use. The typical window of time for a person's urine sample to test positive after use of opiates, cocaine, amphetamines, Ecstasy, and barbiturates is 24–48 hours. Marijuana can be detected for one week up to two months, depending on frequency of use, because THC is stored in the fat and released slowly.

DRUG TESTING PROTOCOLS AND PROCEDURES

There are three major drug testing protocols: random, for cause, and condition of employment. Random drug tests can be carried out at any time without a particular reason or suspicion. Most random drug screens are done in professions with a strong public-good emphasis where the employees should be drug-free, such as medicine, law enforcement, airlines, and the military. For-cause drug tests are given to employees because a problem or incident at work provokes suspicion of substance abuse. Drug testing as a condition of employment is done to screen out drug-using candidates before they are hired.

A urine test is the most common procedure in testing for drugs. It is simple and inexpensive. The urine sample is divided into two separate samples. The first one is subjected to an **immunoassay** test, where antibodies react to the drug being tested for. If the person tests positive, the second sample is subjected to a confirmation test, such as gas chromatography or mass spectrometry. This confirmation test is expensive, but it is precise in terms of confirming the immunoassay. There is also a possibility of a false positive, so the confirmation test is very important.

Another drug test uses hair samples. Not currently as popular as urine, the hair-sample test adds another dimension to testing because a drug is contained in the hair for a long time after ingestion, whereas urine tests detect only what has been in the system for a short period.

FALSE POSITIVES AND FALSE NEGATIVES

Drug testing is usually very accurate. However, some substances can interfere with the tests and make the results inaccurate. When a person tests positive to a drug but has not used it, this is called a *false positive*. Benadryl, a common antihistamine, can cause a false positive for amphetamines. Ibuprofen, an over-the-counter analgesic, can cause a false positive for marijuana. Poppy seeds can cause a false positive for opiates. This is why the confirmation test is so important. A gas chromatography or mass spectrometry will be able to determine if the person used Benadryl or amphetamines.

When a person has used a drug and tests negative, this is called a *false negative*. Generally a false negative results when the urine has been adulterated with a chemical that can deceive the immunoassay. Many products are sold in counterculture magazines and on the Internet that claim a false negative will result if the product

Immunoassay is the most basic drug test used as a part of the urine screen.

is ingested before a drug test. The most common way for a false negative to occur is if the urine is diluted to a point where the immunoassay cannot react to the drug.

STANDARD DRUG TREATMENT MODEL

The standard treatment model for substance dependence is detoxification, counseling, and support groups. This model was discussed earlier in the chapter with respect to treatment for alcohol dependence. The components are similar no matter what drug dependence is being treated. What is important for treatment is a three-pronged approach: medical detoxification, psychological counseling, and support groups that give reinforcement for staying clean and sober. If all three elements are not in place, then a person will be at high risk for relapse.

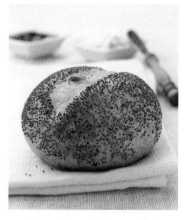

Certain foods, such as the poppy seeds on a roll or over-the-counter drugs such as Benadryl, can cause false-positive results in certain drug tests.

© Jupiterimages/Getty Images

Unfortunately, too few drug treatment programs are available in the United States. Many more resources are allocated to law enforcement than to treatment. Beyond the physical and mental difficulties of breaking from addictive behaviors, the cost of treatment is also a major hurdle. People who want to become clean and sober but who don't have good health insurance can find treatment and recovery a difficult road to navigate.

✓ NEED TO KNOW

Drugs can circulate through the body for long periods of time. Most drugs have about a 24- to 48-hour window of being detectable in the system. Marijuana (THC) is different—it is stored in the fat and slowly released into the blood. So THC can be detected for much longer periods of time—weeks or months depending on the extent of use. Drug testing will be a part of everyone's future—whether it be a condition of employment or health insurance.

connect Resources

ARTICLES

4.1 "The Academic Opportunity Costs of Substance Use During College." A Brief Report from the Center on Young Adult Health and Development. This concise report summarizes academic problems often faced by substance use during the college years. **www.cls.umd.edu/docs/AcadOppCosts.pdf**

4.2 "A Host of Trouble." *U.S. News & World Report.* When party hosts allow or excuse excessive drinking, they might be legally responsible for any problems that occur.

4.3 "Screening and Brief Intervention for Underage Drinkers." *Mayo Clinic Proceedings.* This piece gives contemporary information on alcohol-related screening, intervention, and referral for treatment for underage drinkers.

4.4 "Science Seeks to Unlock Marijuana's Secrets." *National Geographic.* This article highlights key issues surrounding the mainstreaming of marijuana focusing on what we actually do know about the drug.

SELF-ASSESSMENTS

4.1 Is Alcohol a Problem in Your Life?

4.2 How Much Do You Know about Marijuana?

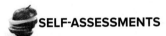

Website Resources

CASA—National Center on Addiction and Substance Abuse at Centers for Disease Control and Prevention **www.cdc.gov**

Columbia University **www.casacolumbia.org**

DanceSafe—Promoting Health and Safety Within the Rave and Nightclub Community **www.dancesafe.org**

Drug Enforcement Administration **www.usdoj.gov/dea/index.htm**

Drug Policy Alliance **www.drugpolicy.org**

National Institute on Drug Abuse **www.nida.nih.gov**

National Organization for the Legalization of Marijuana **www.norml.org**

Office of National Drug Control Policy: Media Campaign **www.whitehouse.gov/ondcp/anti-drug-media-campaign**

Substance Abuse and Mental Health Administration **www.samhsa.gov**

Knowing the Language

immunoassay, 144
inhalation administration, 115
lethal dose, 117
oral administration, 114
Oxycontin, 129
parenteral administration, 114
physical dependence, 116
psychological dependence, 117
rectal administration, 115

sedative-hypnotic, 129
set, 116
setting, 116
SSNRI, 141
SSRI, 141
tolerance, 117
transdermal
    administration, 115
vaping administration, 115

Understanding the Content

1. Distinguish between the different methods of drug administration and absorption.
2. Define the following terms: *drug use, drug misuse, drug abuse, set, setting, physical dependence, psychological dependence*, and *tolerance.*
3. Describe the effects of alcohol on the cerebrum, cerebellum, and medulla.
4. What are the differences between the different forms of marijuana?
5. What are the major dangers in designer and club drugs?
6. Describe the components of the standard drug treatment model.

Exploring Ideas

1. Use of alcohol, including underage drinking, is considered a rite of passage in college. At age 18, one can legally vote and serve in the military. Should the drinking age be lowered to 18? Why or why not?
2. How does someone know he or she may have a drug problem? What kinds of signs and symptoms should the person look for?
3. Are you concerned about recreational use of marijuana being legal in several states? If yes, why? If no, why not?
4. Some professionals feel that the more punitive the measures, the more compliant people will be with the law. With that in mind, should college students be randomly drug tested to determine the extent of drug use in this population?

Selected References

American Psychiatric Association. *Diagnostic and Statistical Manual of Mental Disorders* (4th ed.). Washington, DC: APA, 1994.

Arria AM, Caldeira KM, Bugbee BA, et al. The Academic Opportunity Costs of Substance Use During College. Center on Young Adult Health and Development, University of Maryland School of Public Health, May 2013.

Calabresi, M. The price of relief. *Time*, June 15, 2015, pp. 28–34.

Cerda M, Moffitt TE, Meier MH, et al. Persistent Cannabis Dependence and Alcohol Dependence Risks for Midlife Economic and Social Problems: A Longitudinal Cohort Study. *Clinical Psychological Science,* March 22, 2016, DOI:10.1177/2167702616630958

Drug Enforcement Administration. Drug Schedules. 2013. **www.usdoj.gov/dea/ pubs/scheduling.html**

Drug Enforcement Administration. Federal Trafficking Penalties. 2013. **www.dea.gov/druginfo/ftp3.shtml**

Firger, J. The Great Kentucky Hemp Experiment. *Newsweek,* October 11, 2015.

Firger, J. Marijuana use—and abuse—in the U.S. has doubled in the past decade. *Newsweek,* October 21, 2015.

Haroz R, Greenberg MI. New drugs of abuse in North America. *Journal of Laboratory and Clinical Medicine* 26: 147–164, 2006.

Johnston LD, O'Malley PM, Bachman JG, et al. *Monitoring the Future: National Survey Results on Drug Use, 1975–2013.* Volume I: *Secondary School Students* (NIH Publication No. 10–7584). Bethesda, MD: National Institute on Drug Abuse, 2014, 734 pp.

Kinney J, Leaton G. *Loosening the Grip: A Handbook of Alcohol Information* (7th ed.). New York: McGraw-Hill, 2003.

Maxwell, JC. *Patterns of Club Drug Use in the U.S., 2004.* Austin, TX: Center for Excellence in Drug Epidemiology, 2004.

National Center on Addiction and Substance Abuse at Columbia University. *Wasting the Best and Brightest.* New York: Columbia, March 15, 2007.

National Institute on Alcohol Abuse and Alcoholism. *College Drinking.* Bethesda, MD: National Institute on Alcohol Abuse and Alcoholism, December 2015.

National Institute on Drug Abuse. *Community Drug Alert Bulletin (Club Drugs).* Bethesda, MD: National Institute on Drug Abuse, May 2004.

National Institute on Drug Abuse. *Methamphetamine Abuse and Addiction.* Research Report Series. Bethesda, MD: National Institute on Drug Abuse, September 2006.

Office of Applied Studies, Substance Abuse and Mental Health Services Administration. *Prevalence of Substance Use Among Racial and Ethnic Subgroups in the U.S., 2005.*

Office of National Drug Control Policy. *Consequences of Illicit Drug Use in America.* Washington, DC: Office of National Drug Control Policy, April 2014.

Patrick ME, Schulenberg JE. Prevalence and predictors of adolescent alcohol use and binge drinking in the United States. *Alcohol Research: Current Reviews* 35 (2). Bethesda, MD: National Institute on Alcohol Abuse and Alcoholism, 2013.

Ruhm CJ. Alcohol policies and highway vehicle fatalities. *Journal of Health Economics* 15 (4): 435–454, 1996.

SIUC/Core Institute. Core Alcohol and Drug Survey, Long Form, Executive Summary. August 25, 2014.

Snyder LB, Milici FF, Slater M, et al. Effects of alcohol advertising exposure on drinking among youth. *Archives of Pediatrics and Adolescent Medicine* 160: 18–24, 2006.

Substance Abuse and Mental Health Services Administration. *Results from the 2001 National Household Survey on Drug Abuse.* Rockville, MD: SAMHSA, September 2002.

U.S. Department of Health and Human Services. *Alcohol Alert, Economic Perspectives in Alcoholism Research.* Rockville, MD: U.S. DHHS, 2001.

White A, Hingson R. The burden of alcohol use: Excessive alcohol consumption and related consequences among college students. *Alcohol Research: Current Reviews* 35 (2). Bethesda, MD: National Institute on Alcohol Abuse and Alcoholism, 2013.

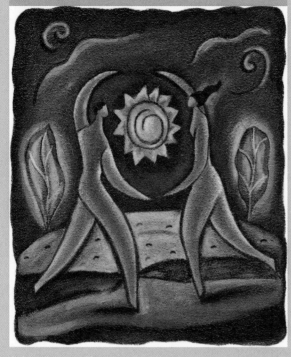

Familiarity breeds contempt—and children.

—Mark Twain

Chapter 5

RESPECT SEXUALITY

In Chapter 5, we cover a wide variety of topics related to both the physical and psychosocial aspects of human sexuality. Probably no other topic is as misunderstood as sexuality, from the details of reproductive anatomy to the range of behaviors. Most misunderstandings result from questionable sources of sexuality information. Friends, family, and media often communicate incomplete or incorrect information, and ignorance about the facts can lead to high-risk decisions. This chapter reviews the basics of sexual anatomy, reproduction, and contraception. It also discusses selected aspects of sexual dysfunction, sexual identity, sexual behavior, and relationships.

world. Having some control over births is central to control of property, wealth, and
lineage—in other words, power—for both individuals and societies. Before contraception existed, the only way to control births was to discourage certain segments
of the population, such as the very young and the unmarried, from having sex.
Abstinence was the only reliable birth control. Relatedly, the main activity of women
was childrearing, and families tended to be large.

The rules by which society operated changed with the development of reliable
contraception methods in the 20th century. Especially after the birth control pill
became widely available in the 1970s, consequences for various behaviors became
different. In turn, so did the behaviors of many Americans. People could engage
in sexual activity without a baby being a near-automatic part of the relationship.
Women could delay reproduction, have fewer children, or avoid motherhood altogether. This created opportunities for women to enter educational, professional,
and social circles that had once been exclusive to men. This so-called sexual
revolution in the late 20th century sometimes encouraged good outcomes, such as
more equality among men and women, but it also contributed to new challenges,
such as the rise of AIDS and other sexually transmitted infections (STIs).

Today sexuality is defined as much more than just fertility. It is something that
begins before birth and continues throughout life, influencing and shaping relationships at every age. In addition to anatomy, physiology, sexual development, and
reproduction, sexuality includes sexual orientation, gender identity, and people's
values and beliefs regarding these issues. To make good decisions regarding health
and relationships, adults must be educated in the full range of these issues.

➤ Female and Male: Genetics and Hormones

Healthy people are born with 46 chromosomes arranged in 23 pairs. It is the 23rd
pair of chromosomes that determines sex—females have an XX pair, and males have
an XY pair. Sexual development is genetically programmed to occur when children
reach the age of 12 or 13, and signs of maturation begin well before that. During
puberty, the reproductive system matures, secondary sex characteristics appear, and
masculine and feminine body features become refined.

Chemical messengers called **hormones** bring about puberty and rule sexuality.
The most important sexual hormones are estrogen, progesterone, and testosterone.
Estrogen controls female secondary sex characteristics such as breast development
and also plays a part in menstruation and ovulation. **Progesterone** is responsible for
building up the endometrial tissue lining a woman's uterus, a key step of the female
fertility cycle. In males, **testosterone** is responsible for both primary and secondary
sex characteristics, such as a deepening voice and sperm production. We tend to

Hormones are chemical messengers.

Estrogen is a female hormone responsible for female secondary sex characteristics.

Progesterone is a female hormone responsible for the development of
endometrial tissue.

Testosterone is a male hormone responsible for male secondary sex characteristics.

FIGURE 5.1 FEMALE REPRODUCTIVE SYSTEM

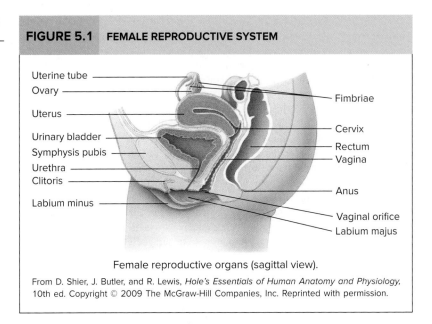

Uterine tube
Ovary
Uterus
Urinary bladder
Symphysis pubis
Urethra
Clitoris
Labium minus

Fimbriae
Cervix
Rectum
Vagina
Anus
Vaginal orifice
Labium majus

Female reproductive organs (sagittal view).

From D. Shier, J. Butler, and R. Lewis, *Hole's Essentials of Human Anatomy and Physiology*, 10th ed. Copyright © 2009 The McGraw-Hill Companies, Inc. Reprinted with permission.

classify estrogen as female and testosterone as male, but women actually have small amounts of testosterone in their bodies, and men have small amounts of estrogen. In addition to being important for secondary sex characteristics, estrogen and testosterone are necessary for brain functions, including the sex drive.

THE FEMALE REPRODUCTIVE SYSTEM

The female reproductive system includes both internal and external organs (Figure 5.1). The internal organs are the ovaries, fallopian or uterine tubes, uterus, cervix, and vagina. The **ovaries** are the female reproductive glands that produce ova (eggs), the female sex cells. They also produce estrogen and progesterone. When an ovary releases an egg, it is swept into the nearby **fallopian tube,** where fertilization can take place if the egg meets up with a sperm cell.

Whether fertilized or not, an egg travels down the fallopian tube and ends up in the **uterus,** an elastic, muscular organ designed to stretch to accommodate a growing baby. At the bottom of the uterus is a round, thick muscle called the **cervix.** The cervix connects the uterus to the **vagina,** where sperm are deposited during intercourse. The vagina

Ovaries are glands that produce ova and the hormones estrogen and progesterone.

Fallopian tubes are the structures into which a ripe ovum is released and where it is fertilized by a sperm.

The **uterus** is the organ in which a fertilized ovum implants and develops into a baby.

The **cervix** is the neck of the uterus, opening into the vagina.

The **vagina** is the passage between the cervix and the external sex organs and the female structure for sexual intercourse; it is also referred to as the *birth canal.*

FIGURE 5.2   MENSTRUATION HORMONES

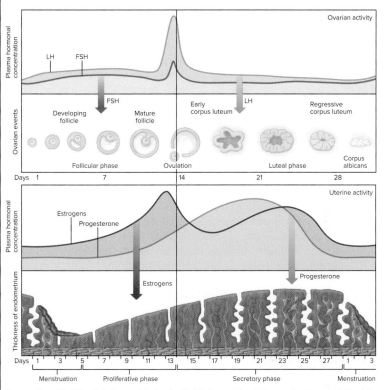

Source: From D. Shier, J. Butler, and R. Lewis, *Hole's Essentials of Human Anatomy and Physiology,* 10th ed. Copyright © 2009 The McGraw-Hill Companies, Inc. Reprinted with permission.

is also the route through which a woman's endometrial tissue sloughs off during menstruation, and it is the canal through which a baby enters the world during birth.

The external female genitalia, collectively referred to as the *vulva,* include the clitoris, labia majora, labia minora, and Bartholin's glands. The **clitoris** contains a dense nerve network that when stimulated results in an orgasm, the heightened pleasurable sensation that is the climax, or culmination, of sexual stimulation. The labia majora and labia minora are folds of tissues that cover the opening to the vagina. The Bartholin's glands, located inside the labia minora, secrete a lubricating substance during sexual arousal that results in less skin friction during intercourse.

The menstrual cycle (or fertility cycle) is typically about 28 days long (Figure 5.2). The first day of the menstrual cycle, or "period," is usually counted as day 1, with the menstrual period lasting about 5 days. After menstruation ends, the pituitary gland secretes follicle-stimulating hormone (FSH), which causes an ovum to ripen in an

The **clitoris** is composed of a dense nerve network and is important in female arousal and orgasm.

ovary. FSH also signals the ovary to secrete more progesterone, so the endometrial tissue in the uterus builds up in preparation for a potential pregnancy. The ovum reaches maturity around halfway through the cycle (approximately day 14), and at that point the pituitary gland secretes luteinizing hormone (LH), signaling the ovary to release the ripe egg into the fallopian tube. This is called **ovulation.**

An egg in a fallopian tube can survive 48–72 hours. If the ovum is not fertilized by a sperm during that time, it will break down and be reabsorbed into the body. At around day 28 of the cycle, a new period begins.

Some women experience physical and emotional discomfort before menses, referred to as premenstrual syndrome (PMS). Common PMS symptoms include acne, breast swelling and tenderness, bloating, headache, backache, tension, irritability, and anxiety or depression. If a woman is bothered by these symptoms, her physician may prescribe synthetic estrogen or progesterone to provide relief.

If fertilization occurs, cell division begins immediately. The fertilized egg leaves the fallopian tube and implants in the endometrial tissue in the uterus (Figure 5.3).

Females usually become fertile around age 13, when they get their first period. Women usually lose the ability to get pregnant in their late 40s or 50s. **Menopause** is the term for the process by which ovaries stop releasing eggs and monthly periods end. Menopause is a gradual process, but as the ovaries produce less and less progesterone and estrogen, many physical and emotional symptoms can occur as the body adjusts to the changes. Common symptoms include hot flashes, irritability, loss of libido, depression, muscle aches, and sleep problems.

THE MALE REPRODUCTIVE SYSTEM

Like the female system, the male reproductive system includes both internal and external organs (Figure 5.4). The internal organs are the testes, vas deferens, bulbourethral glands, prostate gland, urethra, and the glans penis. The external organs are the penis and the scrotum.

Testes are glands that produce sperm, the male sex cells, and the hormone testosterone. The epididymis is attached to the testes and is the place where sperm mature and are stored. Surrounding the testes is a sac of skin called the **scrotum.** The scrotum not only protects the testes but also maintains a lower-than-core-body temperature in the organs inside it, which is important for healthy sperm production.

After sperm are produced in the testes, they move to the **vas deferens,** where sperm are stored and provided with a route to the urethra, where during orgasm they will be ejaculated. As sperm travel down the vas deferens, they collect fluids from three major glands: the **seminal vesicles,** the **bulbourethral glands,** and

---

Ovulation is the release of a mature or ripe ovum.

Menopause is the cessation of the menstrual cycle.

Testes are glands that produce sperm and the hormone testosterone.

The **scrotum** is the sac of skin that protects the testes.

Vas deferens are structures that receive sperm from the testes and provide a route for the movement of sperm.

Seminal vesicles secrete a nutritive substance so that sperm can survive.

The **bulbourethral glands** secrete a lubricating substance to help sperm pass through the urethra.

FIGURE 5.3 FERTILIZATION

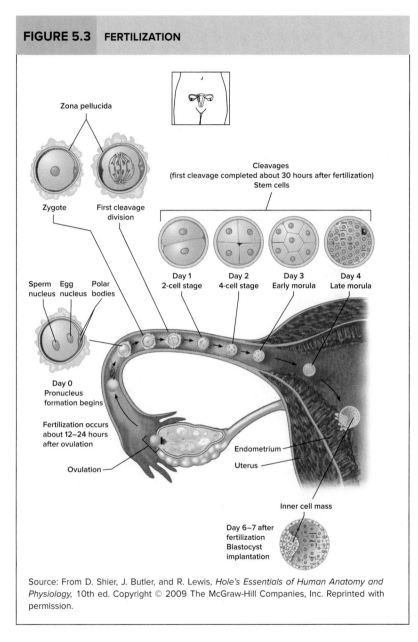

Source: From D. Shier, J. Butler, and R. Lewis, *Hole's Essentials of Human Anatomy and Physiology,* 10th ed. Copyright © 2009 The McGraw-Hill Companies, Inc. Reprinted with permission.

the **prostate gland.** The seminal vesicles secrete a nutritive substance so that sperm can thrive. The bulbourethral glands (also called *Cowper's glands*) secrete a lubricating substance that is believed to lubricate the urethra to facilitate the

The **prostate gland** secretes an alkaline substance that neutralizes the acid medium normally present in the vagina.

FIGURE 5.4 **MALE REPRODUCTIVE SYSTEM**

Urinary bladder
Pubic bone
Vas deferens
Urethra
Corpus cavernosum
Corpus spongiosum
Penis
Glans penis
Prepuce

Large intestine
Ureter
Seminal vesicle
Ejaculatory duct
Prostate gland
Bulbourethral gland
Anus
Epididymis
Testis
Scrotum

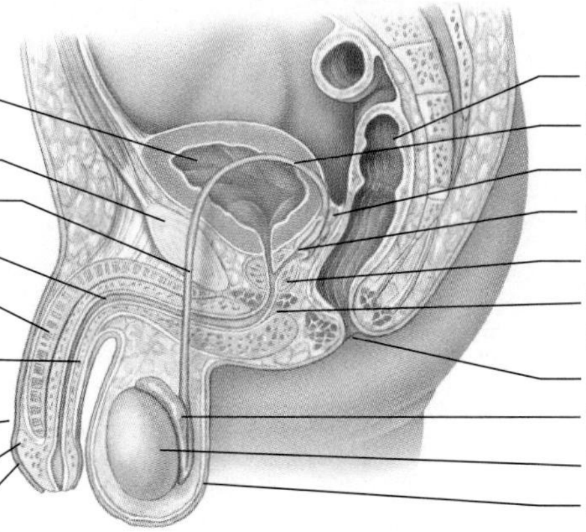

Source: From D. Shier, J. Butler, and R. Lewis, *Hole's Essentials of Human Anatomy and Physiology*, 10th ed. Copyright © 2009 The McGraw-Hill Companies, Inc. Reprinted with permission.

passage of sperm. The prostate gland secretes an alkaline substance that neutralizes the acidic environment in the vagina. Collectively, secretions from all these glands and the sperm are referred to as *semen*.

The urethra in males is located in the penis and transports both urine and semen, though not at the same time. (In females, the urethra is not part of the reproductive system; its sole purpose is to carry urine from the bladder.) The penis is the male external reproductive organ that contains the majority of the urethra. The head of the penis (or **glans penis**) has a dense nerve network that when stimulated can result in orgasm, inducing the involuntary ejaculation of semen.

During sexual activity, sperm move from the testes to the vas deferens and then pass through the seminal vesicles, bulbourethral glands, and prostate gland. The semen travels down the urethra, and if orgasm occurs, it is ejaculated. If ejaculation occurs during vaginal intercourse, sperm in the semen will attempt to move up through the cervix, uterus, and fallopian tubes. If the sperm comes into contact with a mature ovum in the fallopian tubes, then fertilization can occur.

DISORDERS

A variety of common disorders can affect both the female and the male reproductive systems. Effects of these disorders can range from mild discomfort to infertility.

The **glans penis** is the head of the penis and is a dense nerve network and the focal point for orgasm.

Female Disorders

Several fairly common irregularities can affect female fertility. **Menorrhagia** is heavy menstrual bleeding, or an excess flow of endometrial tissue. It is often caused by hormonal imbalances and can be treated with synthetic estrogen and/or proges-terone (in the form of birth control pills). Less often it is caused by uterine fibroids, which are benign tumors of the uterus.

Amenorrhea is the absence of menstruation. If the woman is not pregnant or breastfeeding, amenorrhea is usually caused by stress, being extremely underweight, or having an extremely low percentage of body fat. Excessive exercise and partici-pation in rigorous sports can lead to amenorrhea, as can eating disorders such as anorexia nervosa.

Dysmenorrhea is painful menstruation, characterized by severe cramping. It can be caused by high levels of body chemicals called *prostaglandins;* when this is the case, symptoms can often be relieved simply with ibuprofen. It can also have other causes, including *endometriosis,* a condition where endometrial tissue becomes implanted in the abdominal cavity outside the uterus; *ectopic pregnancy,* when a fertilized egg implants in the wrong location in the uterus or in the fallopian tube or ovary; and *pelvic inflammatory disease (PID),* a widespread infection of tissue in the pelvic area.

Menstrual problems require a physician's evaluation, and once the cause is iden-tified, there are usually interventions available to treat the condition. Medical inter-ventions can range from occasional use of pain relievers or taking birth control pills (which tend to make women's periods lighter) to, in severe cases, a surgery called *dilation and curettage (D&C),* which removes the endometrial tissue from the uterus.

Male Disorders

Several disorders for males are also relatively common. A hernia is a protrusion of an organ through a structure that contains it. Hernias can result from too much pressure or straining when lifting heavy objects. An inguinal hernia occurs when a loop of intestine has broken through the abdominal wall located above the scrotum (called the *inguinal wall;* Figure 5.5).

Hernias can be serious because the intestinal loop can push its way into the scrotum, causing a bowel constriction or even sterility. Physicians conducting phys-ical exams on male patients typically will place the index finger up under the pubic bone in the top part of the scrotum and ask the patient to cough. The coughing usually can exert enough pressure for the physician to feel if a hernia exists. Some-times surgery is needed to pull the loop of intestine back to where it belongs and suture the damaged inguinal wall.

Prostate problems are most common in older males, but infections such as STIs can cause prostate problems in younger men. If the prostate becomes infected, a man may have difficulty urinating or have a continual urge to urinate. The prostate is checked through a digital rectal exam whereby the physician inserts a finger into the rectum and feels the prostate for enlargement and for growths.

Menorrhagia is excessive menstruation.

Amenorrhea is the absence of menstruation.

Dysmenorrhea is painful menstruation.

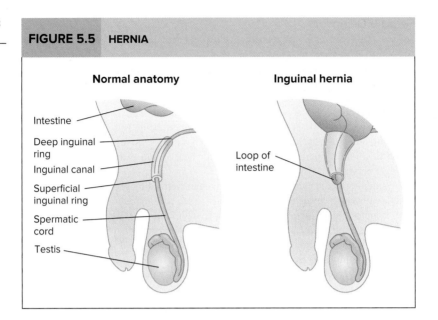

FIGURE 5.5   HERNIA

Normal anatomy

Intestine

Deep inguinal ring

Inguinal canal

Superficial inguinal ring

Spermatic cord

Testis

Inguinal hernia

Loop of intestine

In addition to some prostate problems, STIs can also cause pelvic inflammatory disease (PID) or infertility. Many of these problems are discussed in Chapter 11.

✓ NEED TO KNOW

Hormones are chemical messengers that represent the most basic language of sexuality. The female hormones include estrogen and progesterone. Estrogen and progesterone are the major hormones produced by the ovaries and are responsible for secondary sex characteristics in females. Testosterone is the major hormone produced by the testes and is responsible for secondary sex characteristics in males. Secondary sex characteristics begin to develop during puberty. The female and male reproductive systems are different in structure but similar in function: production of hormones and of female ova or male sperm. Some common problems in the reproductive systems are menstrual problems such as dysmenorrhea, menorrhagia, and amenorrhea in females and hernia and prostate problems in males. Medical interventions are available to treat these problems.

➤ Conception, Pregnancy, and Childbirth

Pregnancies typically last about 40 weeks and are divided into three phases of about three months (13 weeks) each, referred to as **trimesters.**

Trimesters are the three phases of pregnancy, each about three months long.

The first trimester lasts 12–13 weeks. During most of the first trimester, the ball of rapidly dividing cells is referred to as an **embryo.** From the 10th week onward, the unborn baby is called a **fetus.** Formation of all the vital organs, including the brain and spinal cord, occurs in the first trimester. The heart begins to beat, arms and legs grow, and the face and gender of the baby become distinguishable. In addition to the anatomical development, an organ called the *placenta* grows. Placentas allow unborn babies to obtain oxygen and nutrients and exchange waste products with their mother. At the end of the first trimester the baby is about 2–4 in. long and weighs 1–2 oz.

SECOND TRIMESTER

Weeks 14–26 are the second trimester of pregnancy. The organs that formed in the first trimester become more specialized and functional. The baby can swallow and digest, has waking and sleeping periods, and moves. Hair grows. At the end of the second trimester the baby is about 15 in. long and weighs 2–2½ lb.

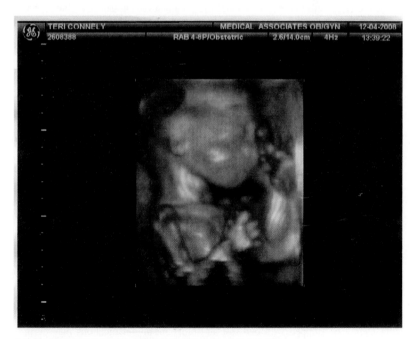

A 3-D ultrasound image of a male fetus aged 5 months.
© Jim Connely

An **embryo** is an unborn baby from conception through the eighth or ninth week of pregnancy.

A **fetus** is an unborn baby from about the 10th week of pregnancy to birth.

Weeks 27–40 are the final phase of pregnancy. During this period the fetus grows rapidly. Toward the end of the trimester the baby begins to change position in preparation for birth. Fetal lungs mature to the point that they will be ready to breathe air after birth, when the placenta stops providing oxygen. At birth an average baby weighs about 7–8 lb. and measures over 14 in. long. The third trimester culminates in labor and childbirth.

COMPLICATIONS OF PREGNANCY AND CHILDBIRTH

Although most pregnancies culminate in the birth of a healthy baby, complications can sometimes occur. For instance, gestational diabetes is a form of diabetes that occurs only during pregnancy. The pregnancy affects the woman's pancreas, which produces insulin, so that levels of blood sugar become uncontrolled. (For more information on diabetes, see Chapter 10.) Urinary tract infections are also common during pregnancy, and if undiagnosed and untreated, they can cause premature labor.

When a fertilized egg implants in a location other than the uterus, such as in the fallopian tube or on the ovary itself, the result is an **ectopic pregnancy.** In some cases, the body rejects the embryo and the pregnancy ends naturally, but in other cases the embryo may rupture the fallopian tube, causing life-threatening problems, including massive hemorrhaging. The embryo and sometimes the fallopian tube need to be removed surgically to save the mother's life.

Normally placentas develop above the cervix inside the uterus, but occasionally a placenta will cover the cervix as it grows. This condition is called *placenta previa,* and it can cause severe bleeding beginning at the end of the second trimester. Treatment for placenta previa can range from bed rest during pregnancy to blood transfusions. Vaginal delivery is considered too dangerous due to risk of hemorrhaging. So, if the mother has placenta previa at the end of pregnancy, the baby will be delivered via caesarian section (C section).

Placental abruption occurs when the placenta separates from the uterine wall before delivery, potentially depriving the baby of oxygen. Once the condition is diagnosed, depending on its severity, the treatment can include bed rest, hospitalization, or a caesarian section.

Preeclampsia is a condition characterized by high blood pressure, edema (the swelling of tissue from excess fluid), headaches, dizziness, vision problems, and stomach pain in the pregnant woman. It can also cause fetal distress and even fetal death. If not treated, preeclampsia can progress to *eclampsia,* which is characterized by seizures, coma, and sometimes death. If preeclampsia is severe enough, labor may be induced or an emergency C section may be performed to protect both mother and baby.

Premature labor is labor that occurs before 37 weeks of gestation. If premature labor cannot be stopped with bed rest and other means, medications may be prescribed to stop the contractions.

Postpartum depression is normally a mild depression that occurs three days to two weeks after delivery. Most times the depression ends naturally; however, there are some extreme cases where the depression requires counseling and medication.

Ectopic pregnancy occurs when a fertilized egg implants somewhere other than the uterus, usually in a fallopian tube.

Miscarriage is the expulsion of the embryo or fetus from the uterus before the middle of the second trimester. In most cases, a miscarriage is due to a problem with a lack of progesterone being produced during the first and second trimesters. During the first and second trimesters of pregnancy, significant amounts of progesterone are produced until the placenta matures. However, if the production of progesterone decreases before the placenta is mature, then a miscarriage can result.

✓ NEED TO KNOW

The female and male reproductive systems are very complex with the main functions being the production of hormones for secondary sex characteristics and production of female ovum or male sperm. When an ovum and sperm unite in the fallopian tube, conception or pregnancy is the result and the united ovum and sperm implants in the uterus. After healthy implantation and embryonic and fetal development over approximately a nine-month period, a baby is ready to be born. If conception doesn't occur, the endometrial tissue or lining of the uterus is sloughed off in what is termed menses or "period." Because the female and male reproductive systems are so complex, many problems can occur ranging from menstrual disorders to prostate problems. Between lifestyle changes and/or medical intervention, the problems can be effectively prevented or treated.

➤ Contraception

Unless you are actively trying to have a baby or would not object to an unexpected pregnancy, it is very important to use contraception whenever you engage in sexual activity. Table 5.1 details each of the contraceptive methods by type, failure rates, risk, availability, and convenience.

HORMONAL METHODS

Hormonal contraceptives such as injections, implants, birth control pills, and the contraceptive patch or ring are made from estrogen and/or progesterone (sometimes called by its synthetic form, progestin). These contraceptives biologically simulate pregnancy in the woman's body, thus suppressing ovulation. In addition, some of the hormonal methods thicken cervical mucus, which impedes the movement of sperm. Hormonal methods of contraception are very effective, with a failure rate of only 1–5 percent depending on the type of hormonal method used. In the United States they are available only by prescription. Usually a physician conducts a comprehensive physical evaluation to ensure that the woman does not have risk factors that would rule out their use.

Birth control pills come in a variety of dosages and strengths and are taken either daily or for three weeks each month, depending on the type of pill. Side

Hormonal contraceptives introduce progestin and/or estrogen into a woman's body in order to suppress ovulation.

The **birth control pill,** commonly known as "the pill," is a hormonal method of contraception in pill form.

TABLE 5.1 CONTRACEPTIVE DEVICES AND APPROACHES BY TYPE, FAILURE RATE, RISKS, AND AVAILABILITY

TYPE OF CONTRACEPTIVE	DESCRIPTION	FAILURE RATE (number of pregnancies expected per 100 women per year)	SOME RISKS	PROTECTION FROM SEXUALLY TRANSMITTED INFECTIONS (STIs)	AVAILABILITY
Male Condom Latex/ Polyurethane	A sheath placed over the erect penis blocking the passage of sperm.	18	Irritation and allergic reactions (less likely with polyurethane)	Except for abstinence, latex condoms are the best protection against STIs, including gonorrhea and AIDS.	Nonprescription
Female Condom	A lubricated polyurethane sheath shaped similarly to the male condom. The closed end has a flexible ring that is inserted in the vagina.	21	Irritation and allergic reactions	May give some STI protection; not as effective as latex condom.	Nonprescription
Diaphragm with Spermicide	A dome-shaped rubber disk with a flexible rim that covers the cervix so that sperm cannot reach the uterus. A spermicide is applied to the diaphragm before insertion.	12	Irritation and allergic reactions, urinary tract infection. Risk of toxic shock syndrome, a rare but serious infection, when kept in place longer than recommended.	None	Prescription
Spermicide Alone	A foam, cream, jelly, film, suppository, or tablet that contains nonoxynol-9, a sperm-killing chemical.	20–50 (studies have shown varying effectiveness rates)	Irritation and allergic reactions, urinary tract infections	None	Nonprescription

Method	Description		Risks/Side Effects	STD Protection	Availability
Oral Contraceptives— –Combined pill –Progestin-only minipill –91-day regimen (Seasonale)	A pill that suppresses ovulation by the combined actions of the hormones estrogen and progestin.	5	Dizziness; nausea; changes in menstruation, mood, and weight; rarely cardiovascular disease, including high blood pressure, blood clots, heart attack, and strokes	None	Prescription
Patch (Ortho Evra)	Skin patch worn on the lower abdomen, buttocks, or upper body that releases the hormones progestin and estrogen into the bloodstream.	5 Appears to be less effective in women weighing more than 198 pounds	Similar to oral contraceptives—combined pill	None	Prescription
Vaginal Contraceptive Ring (NuvaRing)	A flexible ring about 2 inches in diameter that is inserted into the vagina and releases the hormones progestin and estrogen.	5	Vaginal discharge, vaginitis, irritation. Similar to oral contraceptives—combined pill	None	Prescription
Postcoital Contraceptives (Preven and Plan B)	Pills containing either progestin alone or progestin plus estrogen	Almost 80 percent reduction in risk of pregnancy for a single act of unprotected sex	Nausea, vomiting, abdominal pain, fatigue, headache	None	Prescription
Injection –Depo-Provera	An injectable progestin that inhibits ovulation, prevents sperm from reaching the egg, and prevents the fertilized egg from implanting in the uterus.	Less than 1	Irregular bleeding, weight gain, breast tenderness, headaches	None	Prescription
IUD (Intrauterine Device)	A T-shaped device inserted into the uterus by a health professional.	Less than 1	Cramps, bleeding, pelvic inflammatory disease, infertility, perforation of uterus	None	Prescription

(Continued)

TABLE 5.1 CONTRACEPTIVE DEVICES AND APPROACHES BY TYPE, FAILURE RATE, RISKS, AND AVAILABILITY *(concluded)*

TYPE OF CONTRACEPTIVE	DESCRIPTION	FAILURE RATE (number of pregnancies expected per 100 women per year)	SOME RISKS	PROTECTION FROM SEXUALLY TRANSMITTED INFECTIONS (STIs)	AVAILABILITY
Periodic Abstinence	To deliberately refrain from having sexual intercourse during times when pregnancy is more likely.	20	None	None	Instructions from health care provider
Transabdominal Surgical Sterilization— Female −Falope Ring −Hulka Clip −Filshie Clip or −Essure System	The woman's fallopian tubes are blocked so the egg and sperm can't meet in the fallopian tube, preventing conception.	Less than 1	Pain, bleeding, infection, other postsurgical complications, ectopic (tubal) pregnancy	None	Surgery
Surgical Sterilization— Male	Sealing, tying, or cutting a man's vas deferens so that the sperm can't travel from the testicles to the penis.	Less than 1	Pain, bleeding, infection, other postsurgical complications	None	Surgery

Note: Failure rates are based on information from clinical trials submitted to the U.S. Food and Drug Administration (FDA) during product reviews. This number represents the percentage of women who become pregnant during the first year using a birth control method. For methods that the FDA does not review, such as periodic abstinence, numbers are estimated from published literature. For comparison, about 85 out of 100 sexually active women who wish to have a child and do not use contraception become pregnant within one year of first trying to conceive.

Source: Food and Drug Administration, April 2015.

effects include high blood pressure, headaches, diabetes, elevated cholesterol levels, and blood clots.

Contraceptive implants are surgically placed under the skin of the upper arm. The implants contain progestin and can suppress ovulation for up to five years. Implanon, consisting of a single capsule and providing protection for three years, was approved by the FDA in 2006 and is now available.

Injectable contraceptives are administered via a shot in the arm or buttocks and provide protection for approximately 14 weeks. The best-known injectable is **Depo-Provera,** but others are under development. Each injection is generally effective for three months.

The vaginal ring is a flexible plastic ring that contains low levels of hormones. It is inserted into the vagina and left in place around the cervix for approximately three weeks and then removed for one week for menstruation. A new ring is inserted every month.

The contraceptive patch contains hormones that slowly absorb into the body through the skin. The patch can be placed on the buttocks, upper arm, or upper torso and is changed once a week for three weeks and then not worn one week during menstruation.

Hormonal methods of contraception have the advantage of providing long-term, highly effective protection against pregnancy with little effort on the part of the woman. However, hormonal methods are not for all women because some of the side effects mentioned earlier can be significant and result in medical emergencies.

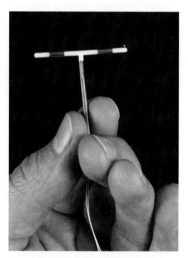

Intrauterine devices (IUDs) must be placed in a woman's uterus by a trained medical professional. They can remain in place and provide highly reliable contraception for 1 to 10 years.

© McGraw-Hill Education/Jill Braaten, photographer

BARRIER METHODS

Barrier methods of contraception include the intrauterine device (IUD), condom, sponge, diaphragm, and cervical cap. These methods work by blocking sperm from traveling through the cervix and into the uterus and fallopian tubes. Some of the barrier methods—such as the sponge, diaphragm, and cervical cap—also use a chemical that kills sperm (spermicide), making them even more effective.

An **IUD** is a small, T-shaped, plastic or copper device that is inserted into the uterus

Contraceptive implants, such as Implanon, are surgically inserted under the skin and can provide hormonal contraception for up to five years.

Depo-Provera is a hormonal method of contraception delivered in an injection.

An **IUD** (intrauterine device) is a barrier method of contraception in which a small plastic or copper unit is placed in the uterus. It is thought to function by affecting the movement of sperm and/or egg or preventing fertilization.

by a physician. Depending on the type, the IUD can be left in place for 1 to 10 years. There are two types of IUDs: copper (brand name ParaGard) and hormonal (brand name Mirena). In addition to being "T" shaped, they both release either a metal or a hormone, and the resulting action is a bit different. The copper released by ParaGard prevents sperm from reaching and fertilizing an egg. The progestin released from Mirena prevents the ovary from releasing an egg. ParaGard can stay in the uterus 5 to 10 years, and Mirena can stay in the uterus for up to 5 years. The effectiveness of the IUD as a contraceptive method is high, with a failure rate of only 1–2 percent. Some relatively rare side effects of IUDs include uterine perforations, cramping, and heavy bleeding.

A **diaphragm** is a thick, flexible concave rubber structure with a hard but flexible outer ring. It is inserted into the vagina and placed over the cervix, forming a barrier to sperm. A small amount of spermicide is placed in the diaphragm and around the rim to kill any sperm that penetrate the physical barrier. For maximum effectiveness, the diaphragm must be inserted before intercourse and be left in place for six hours afterward. The failure rate for the diaphragm can be as high as 15 percent. If the diaphragm is left in place for an extended period of time, there is a small risk of toxic shock syndrome, a dangerous bacterial infection.

The **cervical cap** is a small, flexible cap that is inserted into the vagina and placed over the cervix to form a barrier to sperm. Like the diaphragm, it is used with spermicide. It can be left in place for longer—up to 48 hours. The failure rate can be as high as 17–24 percent. As with the diaphragm, there is a slight risk of toxic shock syndrome if the cervical cap is left in place too long.

Sponges are round, soft foam devices that contain a spermicide. It is inserted into the vagina and covers the cervix. It can be worn up to 30 hours and can be inserted 24 hours before sex. Failure rates are between 12 and 24 percent.

Condoms are the most common and popular type of barrier contraception because they do not require a prescription, are available in many stores, and are fairly inexpensive and simple to use. Condoms are made and marketed for both males and females, but the more popular ones are male condoms.

The male condom is a tightly rolled latex sheath that is worn by unrolling it down over an erect penis. During intercourse, semen is ejaculated into the condom, thus preventing sperm from entering the vagina. The failure rate is approximately 18 percent. Male condoms not only help prevent pregnancy, but they also provide protection against sexually transmitted infections (STIs). They are available in a wide variety of brands, colors, and styles, with and without lubricants and spermicides. Condoms that contain the spermicide nonoxynol-9 (N-9) in some cases have been found to increase tissue irritation, which can increase the likelihood of STI transmission. (See this chapter's "Breaking It Down.")

The female condom is a polyurethane sheath with a flexible ring on each end. The ring on the closed end is inserted into the back of the vagina and the other ring

A **diaphragm** is a concave latex "cup" that is inserted into the vagina and serves as a barrier method of contraception.

Cervical cap is similar to the diaphragm, but smaller.

Sponges are a soft, foamlike barrier method of contraception.

Condoms are latex devices that either cover the penis (male condom) or line the vagina (female condom) and serve as a barrier to sperm.

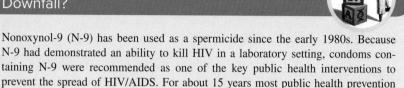
Nonoxynol-9 (N-9) has been used as a spermicide since the early 1980s. Because N-9 had demonstrated an ability to kill HIV in a laboratory setting, condoms containing N-9 were recommended as one of the key public health interventions to prevent the spread of HIV/AIDS. For about 15 years most public health prevention messages emphasized use of condoms containing N-9. However, now studies have found that N-9 is not only ineffective at stopping the spread of HIV, but it has actually increased risk of disease transmission. How could this have occurred?

The problem originated because officials and product manufacturers made a critical error: They assumed that if N-9 killed HIV in the laboratory, it automatically must be effective in real-world situations involving sex. Unfortunately, this proved untrue. The evidence against the effectiveness of N-9 was highlighted in a 2000 study of N-9 use among sex workers in South Africa and Thailand. A chief finding of this study was that the incidence of HIV was higher among women using N-9 than among those using a similar product without N-9. Even worse, some people who used N-9 frequently had problems with tissue damage. This led the Centers for Disease Control and Prevention and the World Health Organization to the following conclusions:

- N-9 is ineffective at killing the HIV virus and other STIs.
- When used vaginally multiple times a day, N-9 can cause genital lesions that may increase a woman's risk of acquiring HIV.
- Condoms lubricated with a small amount of N-9 are no more effective in preventing pregnancy than are lubricated condoms without N-9.

The case against N-9 was so strong that major condom manufacturers like Johnson & Johnson discontinued production of condoms containing N-9. The Planned Parenthood Federation of America also recommended that production of condoms containing N-9 be stopped.

N-9's plunge in popularity reflects an important principle in science and health. When new information from scientific studies discredits a "sound" prevention approach, then industry and society respond, and in this case they responded appropriately. It also shows how important it is for us to keep our health knowledge current. "Best practices" in all areas of health continue to evolve. What may have been the gold standard in treatment last decade could turn out to be less than optimal as scientific evidence builds.

---

remains outside the vagina. During intercourse, the sheath creates a barrier to sperm. The failure rate for female condoms is 20 percent, more than that for male condoms.

Spermicides are chemicals marketed in many forms: gels, foams, suppositories, and jellies. These chemicals are inserted into the vagina before intercourse. In theory, when sperm are ejaculated into the vagina, the spermicide kills them. To be effective, the spermicide should be placed in the vagina one hour before intercourse,

Spermicides are chemicals that kill sperm.

and if intercourse is repeated, more spermicide should be used. The failure rate is 20–30 percent.

Combining barrier methods can significantly decrease failure rate. For example, use of both spermicides and condoms can be 95 percent effective in preventing pregnancies.

SURGICAL METHODS

Vasectomy for men and tubal ligation for women are the two most common surgical methods of contraception. Neither procedure should have an effect on sex drive.

The **vasectomy** is a simple surgical procedure in which the vas deferens in each testis is cut, and the exposed ends are sealed by cauterization (burning with special instruments). After cauterization the exposed end is folded back and tied. Sperm are still produced and released but are not able to progress past the cauterized, tied end of the vas deferens. The vasectomy takes about 20–30 minutes and can be done in a physician's office under local anesthesia.

Tubal ligation is usually done in a surgical facility under general anesthesia, but the principle is similar. An incision is made in the lower abdomen, and the fallopian tubes are cut, cauterized, and tied back. Mature ova are still produced, and menstruation still occurs, but the egg that is released into the fallopian tube will travel only as far as the cauterized, tied end of the fallopian tube. Sterilization implants (brand name Essure) and the procedure are relatively new and involve placing a thin tube into each fallopian tube. After about three months scar tissue forms in the fallopian tube, which prevents movement of both the egg and sperm, resulting in sterilization.

Self
Assessment
5.1

Vasectomy, tubal ligation, and sterilization implants should be considered permanent. Although the procedures can be reversed in some cases, there is no guarantee that reversal will be successful.

NATURAL METHODS

Of course, the most natural method of birth control—complete abstinence from sexual intercourse—is also the most effective. But another **natural method** of birth control that is used by some sexually active women is referred to as *fertility awareness* or *periodic abstinence*. This method requires a woman to accurately predict when she is ovulating on the basis of body temperature and other signs and determine "safe" versus "unsafe" days for intercourse. Accurately monitoring body temperature is key—body temperature drops slightly just before ovulation and rises

Vasectomy is a surgical method of contraception for men, where the vas deferens are cut, cauterized, and tied to block movement of sperm.

Tubal ligation is a surgical method of contraception for women, where the fallopian tubes are cut, cauterized, and tied to block movement of both sperm and ova.

Natural methods of birth control are methods that are designed to reinforce abstaining from sexual intercourse. They include fertility awareness, or determining the days a women is most fertile (i.e., releasing an egg), and, if pregnancy is not desired, abstaining from intercourse on these days. Another method is withdrawal, or removing the penis from the vagina just before orgasm.

slightly afterward. A woman using the fertility awareness method takes her temperature with a special thermometer (called a *basal body temperature thermometer*) every morning before she gets out of bed. When her temperature drops and then rises, she can assume that ovulation is taking place. She abstains from intercourse on the 10–12 days per month she is fertile (from about 7 days prior to ovulation to about 3 days after). Since so much effort is required and the margin for error is great, periodic abstinence has a failure rate of 14–47 percent.

Withdrawal is also considered a method of natural birth control. With this method, at the point of orgasm the penis is removed from the vagina so that ejaculation occurs outside the vagina. But withdrawal is very ineffective for two reasons: first, some sperm are in the pre-ejaculate fluid and, second, withdrawal requires a significant amount of self-discipline.

EMERGENCY CONTRACEPTION

Emergency contraception can be used after unprotected sex or when contraception fails (such as a condom breaking). Emergency contraception usually consists of a "morning after" pill that contains enough hormones to cause a woman's period to come early. This "restarts" a woman's monthly fertility cycle, so that pregnancy does not occur.

Plan B One-Step is a widely available emergency contraception. The pill is taken no more than 72 hours after unprotected intercourse. It is available over the counter to women 18 years of age and older. Women under 18 need a prescription.

Ulipristal is another emergency contraceptive drug. It can be taken up to 5 days after sexual intercourse.

TERMINATION OF PREGNANCY

In everyday language the term **abortion** usually refers to ending a pregnancy by choice. But medically speaking, the word *abortion* is more generic, describing both "natural" losses, when the body rejects a developing embryo or fetus, as well as surgical or medical procedures that interrupt pregnancy. *Miscarriage* is the common term for a **spontaneous abortion** that occurs in the first half of a pregnancy. Death of a fetus after week 20 in a pregnancy is often referred to as *stillbirth*. And medically speaking, ending a pregnancy by choice is usually referred to as **artificial abortion.**

Pregnancies end via spontaneous abortion about 20 percent of the time, usually within the first 90 days of pregnancy. Many of these pregnancy losses are due to genetic problems in the developing fetus or from problems in the uterine environment. Often, levels of progesterone, which must be high the first 90 days of pregnancy until a placenta develops fully, decline suddenly and significantly. When levels get too low, the pituitary gland secretes a chemical called oxytocin, which causes the uterus to contract and expel the embryo or fetus.

Abortion is the expulsion of an embryo or fetus from the uterus before it has fully developed.

Spontaneous abortion, often called miscarriage, is the body's rejection of the embryo or fetus.

Artificial abortion is a medical procedure that is used when a woman chooses to terminate her pregnancy.

Methods for terminating a pregnancy by choice differ based largely on the stage of pregnancy during which they are performed. During the first trimester, a surgical procedure called dilation and curettage (D&C) may be used to remove the embryo from the uterus. The cervix is dilated, and a suction curette, a hollow tube, is inserted into the uterus; the contents of the uterus are then suctioned out. Another surgical procedure used during the first trimester is *manual vacuum aspiration*. This method is similar to suction curettage but can be performed earlier in pregnancy. Both procedures are performed under local anesthetic at a clinic or medical facility.

Drugs called *abortifacients* may also be used during the first trimester. They cause a change in the balance of hormones in the body and lead to uterine bleeding and expulsion of the embryo. RU-486, consisting of the two drugs mifepristone and misoprostol, is an example of an abortifacient.

The most common second trimester abortion method is *dilation and evacuation (D&E)*, a procedure somewhat similar to a D&C. Other options include labor and hysterotomy. In labor induction abortions, which are performed rarely, saline solution and prostaglandins are injected into the uterus, killing the fetus and inducing labor. The fetus is delivered 2 to 4 days after the procedure. Hysterotomy is a surgical procedure in which incisions are made in the lower abdomen and uterus and the fetus is surgically removed.

According to the Guttmacher Institute (2014), a prominent nonprofit organization that focuses on sexual health and public education, more than 1 million artificial abortions are performed in the United States each year. This is down 13 percent from 2008. Women in their 20s account for more than 50 percent of all abortions, with those 20–24 accounting for 33 percent of artificial abortions. Further, 88 percent of abortions are done during the first trimester, and fewer than 1 percent are performed after the 20th week of pregnancy.

Although there can be physical complications with abortions, the risk is minimal, especially if done early in the pregnancy. Psychological and emotional consequences are difficult to measure because it is such a deeply personal issue and very much grounded in morality and religious beliefs. Long-term, scientifically sound studies, while difficult, should be conducted to determine psychological and emotional consequences of abortion.

THE ABORTION CONTROVERSY

Abortion has become one of the most highly charged issues of modern times in American politics and society. Opponents of abortion, the so-called pro-life camp, base their opposition on the belief that human life begins at the moment of conception. According to this view, ending that life at any time, for any reason, is morally wrong and ought to be illegal. On the other side, the so-called pro-choice camp believes that women should have the right to choose the circumstances under which they have children. According to this view, the decision regarding whether to continue a pregnancy or end it is a personal one that (within certain limits) should stay a private matter that is not interfered with by the government.

Fetal viability, or the age at which a fetus can survive outside the uterus, has become a key issue in the abortion debate. By 24 weeks gestation, there is a 40 percent chance for survival outside the uterus, whereas by week 28 in a pregnancy (near the beginning of the third trimester), the chance of survival is 90 percent.

Health & the Media Pregnancy Prevention

Since 2000, the National Campaign to Prevent Teen Pregnancy has sponsored an annual contest with cash prizes for 13- to 21-year-olds to design a public service announcement (PSA). The assignment is to create a compelling magazine ad with a catchy slogan and image to spread the message of teen-pregnancy prevention. The top PSAs appear in magazines nationwide. This winning PSA reflects a realistic view of a teenager speaking to other teenagers. It suggests abstinence but also emphasizes contraception for those who have sex. The message clearly communicates responsibility without being preachy. The National Campaign is working to build a more coordinated and effective grassroots movement and to influence cultural values by teaming with the entertainment media and other influential sectors in society.

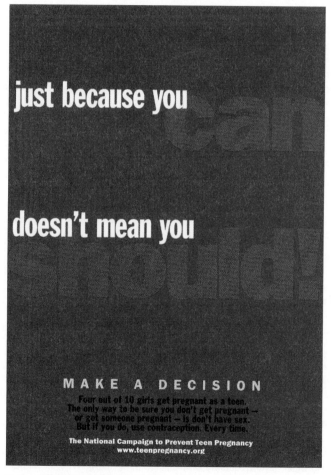

just because you can doesn't mean you should!

MAKE A DECISION

Four out of 10 girls get pregnant as a teen.
The only way to be sure you don't get pregnant —
or get someone pregnant — is don't have sex.
But if you do, use contraception. Every time.

The National Campaign to Prevent Teen Pregnancy
www.teenpregnancy.org

Source: The National Campaign to Prevent Teen and Unplanned Pregnancy.

Pregnancy can be prevented. Knowing the options regarding contraceptive methods and how those methods work is important in making the best individual choice. Abstinence is the only method of contraception that is 100 percent effective. Hormonal methods biologically simulate pregnancy through use of synthetic hormones, but they can have side effects. Barrier methods block movement of the sperm and prevent them from reaching the ovum. Surgical methods—vasectomy and tubal ligation— are invasive and should be considered permanent. The fertility awareness method requires careful body monitoring to determine the unsafe days for intercourse. When contraception fails, it is mostly due to human error. Choosing to terminate a pregnancy through abortion is a deeply personal and difficult decision. The invasiveness of the procedure depends on when in the pregnancy it is performed.

➤ Sexual Behavior

Article
5.1

Hormones influence not only reproductive processes but also how people experience and express their sexuality. Humans have a biological urge for sexual activity known as the *sex drive* (or libido), driven primarily by testosterone. The sex drive also has cognitive and emotional components. For example, a person can become sexually aroused just by thinking or fantasizing about sex and sexual images.

The sex drive usually becomes intense in both boys and girls at puberty. The libido is highest for men in their late teens and early 20s and for women in their mid-20s into their 30s.

The Centers for Disease Control and Prevention (CDC) have surveyed sexual behavior among Americans and have reported the following findings for adults aged 25–44 (Chandra et al., 2011):

- 97 percent of men and 98 percent of women have had vaginal intercourse.
- 90 percent of men and 89 percent of women have had oral sex with an opposite-sex partner.
- 44 percent of men and 36 percent of women have had anal sex with an opposite-sex partner.
- 12 percent of women and 5.8 percent of men aged 25–44 reported any same-sex contact in their lifetime.

The survey also showed there is a high percentage of sexual activity in younger age groups. Roughly 40 percent of adolescents report having sex for the first time between ages 15 and 17. Seventy percent of 18- and 19-year-olds reported having sex with the opposite sex.

Article
5.2

Sexual behaviors are influenced by a variety of factors, including individual biology and personality, personal values and beliefs, family and cultural influences, and the media. People often wonder if they are normal in terms of what is sexually arousing to them, how frequently they engage in sexual activity, how they express themselves sexually (e.g., through masturbation, intercourse, etc.), and so on. For better or worse, there is no real answer to the question, What is normal sexual

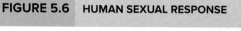

FIGURE 5.6 HUMAN SEXUAL RESPONSE

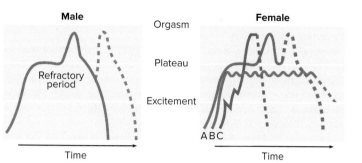

Note: A, B, and C represent three different female sexual responses.

Source: From William H. Masters and Virginia E. Johnson, *Human Sexual Response,*
Figures 1-1 & 1-2, p. 5. Copyright © 1966 by William H. Masters and Virginia E. Johnson.
Boston: Little, Brown and Company.

behavior? Sex drive and sexual behavior are deeply personal matters, and although
there are some universals, there is also tremendous variation. Further, sex drive
varies significantly over the course of the lifespan. To try to establish norms and
benchmarks is misleading and ultimately meaningless.

THE HUMAN SEXUAL RESPONSE MODEL

Although scientists have long understood human reproduction, the physiology of the
human sexual response was not well understood until the 1970s, when William
Masters and Virginia Johnson conducted their groundbreaking clinical research on
sexuality. Masters and Johnson studied the physiological changes that occur during
sexual activity and identified four major stages in human sexual response: excitement, plateau, orgasm, and resolution. They also identified differences between the
sexual response of men and women, adding to the body of knowledge about men's
and women's sexual health.

According to the **human sexual response model** (Figure 5.6), the first phase is
excitement, when both males and females become sexually aroused. Signs of arousal
include erection of the penis in men and vaginal lubrication and swelling of the
clitoris in women. Heart and breathing rates increase. As arousal intensifies, there
is a transition to the plateau stage, a leveling off of sensation just before orgasm.
Muscle tension increases, the penis increases in size, and the upper part of the
vagina expands. The third phase is orgasm, a reflex involving a massive discharge
of nerve impulses, causing muscle contractions in the genital area, sensations of

The **human sexual response model** is a four-stage model of the physiology
of sexual response; the four stages are excitement, plateau, orgasm, and
resolution.

intense pleasure, and, in men, the ejaculation of semen. The last phase is resolution, a return to a relaxed, pre-arousal state.

During the resolution phase, men experience a refractory period, during which blood vessels are constricted and the penis is flaccid so they are not able to experience another orgasm. The refractory period can last from minutes to hours. Women do not experience a refractory period.

As mentioned previously, women and men experience the sexual response differently. For example, the excitement and plateau phases tend to be longer for women than men—it generally takes women longer than men to become aroused. Another difference is that men experience one orgasm, and women can experience multiple orgasms. These are normal differences between the sexes that may or may not make any difference in a relationship.

When a sexual problem does occur in a relationship, it may take the form of a man experiencing excitement, plateau, and orgasm while the woman is still experiencing excitement. As a result he is sexually satisfied while she is still only aroused. The solution generally recommended is that there be more foreplay to increase the woman's arousal level. It is more natural physiologically for men to extend the excitement and plateau phases than for women to try to shorten these phases. Issues involving the human sexual response are often issues affecting couples, and couples need to work together to deal with them. Good communication skills are essential to satisfying sexual relationships.

SEXUAL DYSFUNCTION

At some point in their lives, most people experience sexual problems or dysfunctions. **Sexual dysfunctions** are usually categorized as disorders of desire or arousal, orgasm disorders, and pain disorders.

Sexual desire disorders, or lack of interest in sex, can affect both men and women, as can sexual arousal disorders. Both disorders can be related to hormone levels, the ability to relax, and, to a certain extent, wellness—that is, how well a person is functioning physically, mentally, and socially. Low levels of testosterone in men and estrogen in women can reduce desire and arousal, as can high levels of stress, emotional problems, worries and anxiety, and problems in the relationship. Certain medical conditions can also affect arousal, such as back pain, heart problems, endocrine disorders, or an enlarged prostate. Interventions for sexual desire and sexual arousal disorders include medications, relaxation techniques, and, if appropriate, counseling and education.

Sexual arousal disorder in men can result in erectile dysfunction (ED), also known as *impotence*. ED is the inability to achieve and/or maintain an erection long enough to have intercourse. ED is both a symptom of a condition and a condition itself. The causes of ED can range from low testosterone levels to depression and anxiety or vascular disease, including coronary artery disease. Sometimes medications that are used to treat a variety of conditions—including high blood pressure, diabetes, and depression and anxiety—can also cause ED as a side effect. The anxiety associated with ED can be emotionally damaging and can exacerbate the condition.

Sexual dysfunctions are common sexual disorders including sexual desire disorders, sexual arousal disorders, orgasm disorders, and sexual pain disorders.

There are interventions that treat the symptom of erectile dysfunction and allow a man to achieve and maintain an erection long enough for intercourse without treating the underlying problem. Medications like Viagra act directly on the blood vessels that carry blood to the penis. When these blood vessels relax and dilate, they allow the erectile tissue in the penis to become engorged, producing an erection. Viagra allows a man to have an erection even in the midst of anxiety.

In women, sexual arousal disorders can result in the inability to relax vaginal muscles long enough to allow intercourse, to produce enough vaginal lubrication, or to attain orgasm. Intercourse can then be painful or undesirable. Unlike ED, sexual arousal disorders in women are not easy to treat with a drug. However, the symptoms can be treated with a lubricant to make vaginal penetration by a penis less painful and with muscle relaxants or minor tranquilizers to induce relaxation of vaginal muscles and allow orgasm to occur.

Both women and men can experience orgasm disorders, although such problems are more common in women. The chief symptom is delayed or absent orgasm. In many cases, lack of orgasm is due to timing differences between men and women, as described earlier, and the issue is more likely one of couple communication. Other causes of orgasm disorder include psychological or emotional problems, lack of knowledge, problems in the relationship, and the use of drugs or medications.

Sexual pain, or pain during or after intercourse, known as *dyspareunia,* is an unusual disorder that can affect both men and women. In women, dyspareunia may be caused by vaginismus, involuntary contractions of the vagina that make penetration painful, or by lack of vaginal lubrication. Vaginismus can have physical causes (e.g., pelvic inflammatory disease), which should be treated by a physician, or psychological causes, which may call for relaxation techniques or counseling. Lack of vaginal lubrication can be addressed with longer foreplay or with commercial lubrication products. In men, dyspareunia is generally related to infections of the urethra or inflammation of the urethra or foreskin, in some cases caused by a sexually transmitted infection. Men experiencing pain during or after intercourse should see their physician.

✓ NEED TO KNOW

Human sexual response consists of excitement, plateau, orgasm, and resolution. This response is different for males and females. Males have shorter excitement and plateau phases, one orgasm, and resolution. Women experience longer excitement and plateau phases, can have multiple orgasms, and have a slower resolution. These natural biological differences can become problematic in a relationship, particularly for a woman, so good communication is needed to ensure mutual sexual satisfaction. Sexual dysfunctions can have physiological or psychological origins, and most are a combination of both. Sexual arousal disorders, erectile dysfunction, orgasm disorders, and sexual pain are examples of sexual dysfunctions that most often require medical intervention, which can range from medication to counseling or be a combination of the two. The dysfunctions are common and treatable.

Gender Identity and Sexual Orientation

Up to this point this chapter has focused on the anatomy and physiology of human sexuality. The second half of the equation is how people express their sexuality. As noted at the beginning of the chapter, biological sex is determined at the chromosomal level and physically manifested in the appearance of the external genitals. Gender, on the other hand, is a concept defined more by a particular culture. Gender consists of the traits that a culture ascribes to males and females, contributing to what are considered "masculine" and "feminine" attributes and behaviors. **Gender identity** is the sense a person has that he or she is male or female.

By 18–30 months of age, children have a clear sense of whether they are boys or girls. Between the ages of 5 and 7, children solidify their sense of gender identity and strive to be consistent with their identity by employing stereotypes as rules. Between the ages of 7 and 12, children achieve gender stability, which is the cognitive understanding that gender is permanent. Both gender identity and stability are normally well formed prior to puberty.

Self Assessment 5.2

In rare instances and for mostly unknown reasons, some individuals experience a conflict between their biological sex and their gender identity. Boys or girls may feel they are "really" the opposite sex, rather than the gender that their body has. Individuals who experience this sense of gender dysphoria may be considered to have gender identity disorder and may be referred to as *cross-gender identified* or *transgendered*. Gender identity is not the same as sexual orientation. In other words, a transgendered person may either be homosexual or heterosexual.

Sexual orientation is commonly defined as an enduring emotional, romantic, and sexual attraction to members of one's own sex or of the opposite sex. It is generally recognized that sexual orientation exists along a continuum, with interest in romantic relationships exclusively with members of the same sex at one end of the continuum (homosexuality) and interest in romantic relationships exclusively with members of the opposite sex on the other end of the continuum (heterosexuality). Being attracted to and interested in members of both sexes falls in the middle of the continuum (bisexuality).

People can fall anywhere along this continuum, although social pressures encourage most people to identify themselves as heterosexual. Chandra et al. and the National Center for Health Statistics (2011) reported that among men aged 18–44, about 90 percent think of themselves as heterosexual, 2.3 percent say they are homosexual (gay), 1.8 percent report being bisexual, 3.9 percent say "something else," and 1.8 percent did not answer the question. Among women in the same age group, about 90 percent say they are heterosexual, 1.3 percent identify as homosexual (lesbian), and 2.8 percent say they are bisexual.

It is not clear what causes a person's sexual orientation, but it is most likely an interaction of environment and individual biology, including genetics and hormonal factors. People do not choose their sexual orientation, although they can choose to express it or conceal it. Gay men and lesbians are often the targets of homophobia (fear of homosexuality) and may experience prejudice, discrimination, and even

Gender identity is a person's sense of being male or female.

Sexual orientation is emotional, romantic, and sexual attraction to people of the same or the opposite sex.

violence. Sometimes people experience so much conflict about their sexual orientation that they conceal it from themselves, which can lead to depression and other psychological problems.

Homosexuality is not a mental illness. Rather, it is a normal variation in one aspect of human experience. Abundant research indicates that gay men and lesbians are as mentally healthy as their heterosexual counterparts and equally competent at citizenship, parenting, and relationships.

✓ NEED TO KNOW

Gender identity and sexual orientation are different. Gender identity is one's sense of being male or female. A person who experiences a conflict between his or her biological sex and gender identity may be said to have gender identity disorder. Sexual orientation is enduring emotional, romantic, and sexual attraction to members of one's own or the opposite sex. Sexual orientation exists along a continuum from exclusive heterosexuality through bisexuality to exclusive homosexuality. Sexual orientation is influenced by both biological (genetic, hormonal) factors and environmental (family, societal, cultural) factors. People do not choose their sexual orientation.

➤ Healthy Relationships

Sexuality is an integral part of adult intimate relationships, but it is just one facet of relationships. Healthy relationships meet many more human needs than the sexual one. In his hierarchy-of-needs model, Abraham Maslow identified love and belonging as basic human needs; these needs can be met only in relationships. Besides love and belonging, intimate relationships offer such comforts as emotional intimacy, affirmation and acceptance, companionship, connection to others, and security for the future. Healthy relationships are central to wellness.

Article
5.3

COMMITTED RELATIONSHIPS AND MARRIAGE

Most Americans meet their emotional needs in committed partnerships, whether marriage or cohabiting relationship. As a highly sanctioned social institution, marriage offers a great number of benefits, including economic benefits. Approximately 74 percent of Americans marry at least once in their life, reflecting the importance placed on marriage by the majority of the population. Research studies indicate that marriage is also good for your health—married people live longer than unmarried people, score higher on assessments of mental health, have lower rates of certain illnesses, and report being happier. Strong and supportive relationships of all kinds can offer some of the same benefits.

It has been reported that about half of all couples marrying today in the United States will eventually divorce. This statistic can be misleading, however; a more realistic percentage may be 40 percent. According to a U.S. Census Bureau report, marriages "are most susceptible to divorce in the early years of marriage. After 5 years approximately ten percent of marriages are expected to end in divorce, and another ten percent divorce by the tenth anniversary" (Kreider & Fields, 2002). The remaining 20 percent of all divorces happen between the 11- and 50-year mark. This shows that after a couple's 10th anniversary, the likelihood of divorce greatly decreases.

HEALTHY AND UNHEALTHY RELATIONSHIPS

The most important elements of a healthy relationship are respect, trust, support, honesty, accountability, and shared responsibility. Respect is expressed by not constantly negatively criticizing or judging your partner's beliefs and actions and by performing helping behaviors that make his or her life easier. Trust, honesty, and support involve sharing open communication, willingness to admit mistakes, and the ability to take responsibility for your behavior. Shared responsibility means that work in the relationship, both emotional work and physical work, is shared equally.

In an unhealthy relationship, on the other hand, power is often unequal, and one partner tries to dominate or control the other. The Iowa Coalition Against Violence developed criteria to assess relationships. The following seven points summarize these criteria. In a healthy relationship, most answers will be yes.

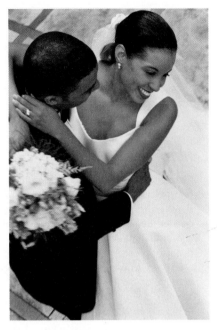

About **74** percent of Americans marry at least once in their lifetime, and research indicates people in committed relationships enjoy improved overall health compared to those who are not in committed relationships.

© Francisco Cruz/Purestock/Superstock

1. I can explain what I like and admire about my partner.
2. My partner is glad I have other friends, and has other friends himself/herself.
3. My partner is happy about my interests, accomplishments, and ambitions.
4. My partner has interests, accomplishments, and ambitions outside of me.
5. My partner has a good relationship with his/her family.
6. My partner takes responsibility for his/her actions and doesn't blame others for failures.
7. My partner talks about feelings, listens to me, and respects my opinions.

Article 5.4

COMMUNICATION AND CONFLICT RESOLUTION SKILLS

One way to improve relationships is by developing better communication and conflict resolution skills. Communication is key in both avoiding and resolving conflict. Conflict is simply disagreement between two people. Clear, open, and honest communication between people can cut down on conflict in relationships. Although some conflict is inevitable because people think and feel differently about things, it is very important not to allow conflict to become a contest where one must win at all costs. Differences in opinions are not contests. There is not a winner and a loser.

All the approaches to resolving conflict are intended to have a win–win outcome. In resolving conflict, it is important to (1) make sure communication is not hostile; (2) try to keep your emotions in check so that they don't get in the way of hearing what the other person is saying; (3) accept differences in opinions and feelings; (4) learn that it is OK to disagree; (5) listen to what is being said—don't be too quick to defend yourself; and (6) communicate in such a way that both of you feel that you have resolved the disagreement—even if you are not necessarily in agreement.

NEED TO KNOW

Healthy relationships are necessary to meet our basic needs of love and belonging. Committed partnerships are the most common way adults meet their emotional needs. All of us have flaws; we bring those flaws into relationships and it can cause many problems and result in some level of dysfunction. So it is very important that for a relationship to be healthy it must be grounded in respect, honestly, accountability, and shared responsibility along with good communication and conflict resolution skills.

connect Resources

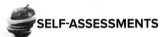 **ARTICLES**

5.1 "Hooking Up and Hanging Out: Casual Sexual Behavior Among Adolescents," University of Florida, IFAS Extension. This article examines current trends in adolescent and young adult sexual behavior.

5.2 "I Got Your Back: Friends' Understandings Regarding College Student Spring Break Behavior." *Journal of Youth Adolescence.* This piece examines the understanding of peers regarding high-risk sexual behaviors during spring break.

5.3 "Speed Dating." *Current Directions in Psychological Science.* Speed dating as a type of romantic attraction is trendy and might just lead to meaningful relationships.

5.4 "A Longitudinal Perspective on Dating Violence Among Adolescent and College Age Women." *American Journal of Public Health.* An analysis of physical assault in dating relationships and its co-occurrence with sexual assault from high school through college.

SELF-ASSESSMENTS

5.1 Sexual Health Assessment
5.2 Sexually Transmitted Infections Assessment

Website Resources

Alan Guttmacher Institute **www.guttmacher.org**
American Society for Reproductive Medicine **www.asrm.org**
Centers for Disease Control and Prevention (CDC) **www.cdc.gov**
CrisisPregnancy.com **www.crisispregnancy.com**
MSN Health Center **health.msn.com**
National Men's Health Network **www.menshealthnetwork.org**
National Women's Health Network **www.womenshealthnetwork.org**
Planned Parenthood **www.plannedparenthood.org**
Sexuality Information and Education Council of the United States **www.siecus.org**
WebMD (Pregnancy) **www.webmd.com/baby/**

Knowing the Language

Understanding the Content

1. Identify and briefly describe the structures in the male and female reproductive systems that have similar functions.
2. Discuss how each of the following methods of contraception work: hormonal, barrier, vasectomy and tubal ligation, and fertility awareness/periodic abstinence.
3. What is the difference between spontaneous abortion and artificial abortion? What are the major issues inherent in artificial abortion?
4. What are the implications of the phases of human sexual response for men and women?
5. Identify and briefly describe the major types of sexual dysfunction in both men and women.

Exploring Ideas

1. What is the relationship between physiology and sexuality? How can acknowledgment of this relationship help in making low-risk choices with respect to sexual issues?
2. What major issues should be considered in contraception?
3. Is it better to treat the symptoms of sexual dysfunction or to try to treat the causes of sexual dysfunction?

Selected References

Basson R. Are our definitions of women's desire, arousal and sexual pain disorders too broad and our definition of orgasmic disorder too narrow? *Journal of Sex and Marital Therapy* 28 (4): 289–300, 2002.

Blum D. *Sex on the Brain: The Biological Differences Between Men and Women.* New York: Viking Press, 1998.

Chandra A, Mosher WD, Copen C, et al. *Sexual Behavior, Sexual Attraction, and Sexual Identity in the United States: Data from the 2006–2008 National Survey of Family Growth.* Bethesda, MD: National Center for Health Statistics, 2011.

Guttmacher Institute. Facts on Induced Abortions in the United States. 2014. **www.guttmacher.org/sections/abortion.php**

Kinsey A, Pomeroy W, Martin C. *Sexual Behavior in the Human Female.* Bloomington: Indiana University Press, 1948.

Kinsey A, Pomeroy W, Martin C. *Sexual Behavior in the Human Male.* Bloomington: Indiana University Press, 1948.

Kreider RM, Fields JM. Number, timing, and duration of marriages and divorces: 1996. *U.S. Census Bureau Current Population Reports,* February 2002.

Masters W, Johnson V. *Human Sexual Response.* Boston: Little, Brown, 1966.

Masters W, Johnson V. *On Sex and Human Loving,* Vol. 1. Boston: Little, Brown, 1988.

Nelson A, Hatcher R, Zieman M, et al. *A Pocket Guide to Managing Contraception.* Dawsonville, GA: Bridging the Gap Foundation, 2005.

Oriel J. Sexual pleasure as a human right: Harmful or helpful to women in the context of HIV/AIDS? *Women's Studies International Forum* 5 (28): 392–404, 2005.

Potts A, Gaven N, Grace V, et al. The downside of Viagra: Women's experiences and perspectives. *Sociology of Health and Illness* 25 (7): 697–719, 2003.

Savin-Williams RC. Who's gay? Does it matter? *Current Directions in Psychological Science* (15): 1, 40–44, 2006.

Wincze J, Carey M. *Sexual Dysfunction* (2nd ed.). New York: Guilford, 2001.

Wolf N. *Promiscuities: A Secret History of Female Desire.* London: Chatto and Windus, 1997.

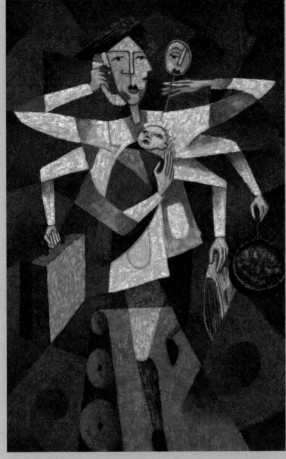

In the middle of difficulty lies opportunity.

—Albert Einstein

Chapter 6

MANAGE STRESS

Stress is part of life. Too much can be harmful, yet too little stress is unhealthy. In this chapter, we focus on understanding the concept of stress and how to recognize and deal with excessive stress. We describe a variety of proven stress management techniques and suggest new ways to think about stress.

Forbes, the flamboyant business-magazine publisher. This quotation captures the modern view of stress. It reflects the "life is hectic" sentiment, where people continually rush about trying to do everything. It is also a joking reference to life behind bars, which in reality would be dire. Forbes's tongue-in-cheek comment shows how easily stress can be found in all aspects of life. Common situations like waiting in line or being stuck in traffic can be stressful. Yet, in the larger picture, these are merely minor inconveniences that pale in comparison with truly grave situations involving mental anguish, unrelenting pain, or debilitating illness.

Stress is routinely mentioned in everyday conversations. Many Americans are still dealing with the effects of the Great Recession and continue to face bleak economic times and uncertainty about the future. Hardly a day goes by when we don't hear someone say, "I'm under a lot of stress" or "I'm really stressed out." As college students, you can easily list your top stresses. They arise from the challenge of balancing coursework and financial pressures with social life and family relationships. Many students have jobs too, which adds another significant factor to the equation.

Successfully coordinating all these activities along with resolving personal difficulties requires self-management skills. As we found with eating and exercise, a proven approach for improving a lifestyle behavior is to learn the basic concepts, chart a plan, and then develop the necessary skills and take action. In this case, the aim is to improve your ability to manage stress in a positive way.

Plainly, stress is part of living but highly variable. Much of the time we can control and manage the many demands and pressures in our lives. But it can be difficult. College students rank "dealing with stress" as a top concern. In this chapter, we examine the concept of stress through a broad, objective lens. You will find that stress can be a positive influence in your life, a force to be understood and reframed to your benefit, not simply something to be dreaded or avoided. We also review how to recognize excessive stress, and we present effective coping strategies.

➤ The Nature of Stress

The origin of the word *stress* can be traced to its use in physics, where it refers to the amount of force, pressure, or strain (load) put on an object to bend or break it. For example, when building a bridge or an airplane, engineers need to know the level of stress that component materials (woods, metals, plastics) can withstand before they break or fail. Decades ago, researchers in biology and medicine borrowed the term and applied it to the tensions and pressures that living organisms experience.

DEFINING AND DESCRIBING STRESS

At the onset, let's define a few basic terms, because *stress* and related words have multiple meanings even across the biological and social sciences. **Stress** refers to

Stress refers to a person's collective psychobiological responses to challenging situations, such as those which are tiring, threatening, exciting, or new. The situation, event, or factors that cause the stress response are known as stressors.

the collective psychobiological responses that occur when a person's natural balance is disrupted. Throughout the animal kingdom, organisms inherently strive to maintain physiological balance, or homeostasis. Any factor or force that disrupts homeostasis is technically known as a stressor.

A **stressor** can be physical or psychological, and both types are wide-ranging. Consider this scenario: You decide to go for a run—it's a cold morning and you misjudge a step, trip over a curb, and land full force on your knee. It's easy to imagine the pain and picture the bloody gash. In this hypothetical situation, several physical stressors can be identified: the exertion of the exercise, exposure to a low temperature, and the pain and tissue damage. There is also the momentary psychological stressor of the fall itself when you know you can't catch yourself and you're going down.

Let's extend the story. Later that day you complete a difficult math project (hallelujah!), participate in a student meeting that turns argumentative, and finally return to your dorm room ready for a quiet break after a trying day—only to discover your roommate has invited friends over. The psychological stressors include the mental challenge of the math assignment, followed by the relief of finishing it, and then frustrations with fellow students and the unwanted surprise of a packed dorm room. As in these examples, stressors are often multiple and overlapping, not just occasional, isolated events.

Stressors that deplete energy and cause a decline in performance or function lead to **distress,** or a negative stress condition. The word *stress* is typically used in this negative context, but technically, the correct term is *distress.* Conversely, stressors can also be positive. Stressors that motivate and result in improved performance or function lead to **eustress,** or a positive stress condition. Examples of eustress are a nice bonus for a job well done or the possibility of a new relationship with a person you find attractive. Stressors are not limited to threatening or unpleasant situations (distress) but also include those that are exciting or simply new (eustress).

Stress also can be categorized by its duration—as acute, episodic, or chronic. Acute stress is brief but intense. Examples include being called on unexpectedly in class or losing control of your car and narrowly avoiding an accident. Episodic stress is regular or predictable but intermittent. What are common examples of this type of stress? Patterns that meet the criteria are final exams and class projects at the end of every semester or a strained family situation that must be faced during visits home.

In contrast to acute or episodic stress, chronic stress is prolonged and continual. Military recruits experience this during boot camp. They are challenged physically and mentally with no letup throughout basic training. More common examples include unpleasant or unfulfilling jobs, or a high-stress job where one has large responsibility but little control. Arguably the most difficult type of chronic stress involves dealing with constant pain due to a health condition. The degree of distress is magnified if no viable options for relief are available.

Stressors disrupt a person's natural state of balance (homeostasis) and can be positive as well as negative.

Distress, or negative stress, is created by stressors that deplete energy and result in impaired performance.

Eustress, or positive stress, is created by stressors that motivate and result in improved performance.

FIGURE 6.1   GENERAL ADAPTATION SYNDROME

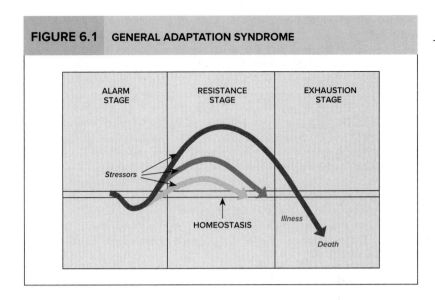

Before we review techniques for balancing and managing the stressors in our lives, let's briefly consider the concept of stress from two viewpoints—one biological, the other psychological. This background material will allow us to better understand the basis and rationale for different stress management techniques.

THE BIOLOGY OF STRESS: PHYSIOLOGICAL RESPONSES

The biological perspective is based on the principle that our responses to stress are regulated by the brain, which controls all body functions. The urge to act when threatened is rooted in our nervous and endocrine systems, whose coordinated stress responses provide the extra strength and energy needed to cope. These collective physiological responses—including an increase in heart rate and breathing, a tensing of muscles, and a focusing of attention—are known as the *fight-or-flight response.* The fight-or-flight response evolved as a survival mechanism in the early development of our species. Let's take a closer look.

Hans Selye, M.D. (1907–1982), known as the father of stress research, developed a model called the **general adaptation syndrome** to describe how animals, including humans, respond to stress. He defined a stressor as anything that disrupts homeostasis (physiological balance). In turn, he described the stress response as the body's adaptations designed to reestablish homeostasis.

In Figure 6.1, the general adaptation syndrome is shown as the time course of the body's resistance to a stressor (adaptive capacity). The baseline is the person's stable level of physiological balance (homeostasis). The three predictable stages are *alarm* (resistance is briefly lowered), *resistance* (the body mobilizes resources to

The **general adaptation syndrome** is a model that describes the body's physiological responses to stressors in three stages: alarm, resistance, and exhaustion.

increase resistance), and *exhaustion* (extreme or prolonged stress overrides the body's ability to adapt, leading to illness and sometimes death). This classic three-phase response to overwhelming stressors is represented by the red line. In general, though, our bodies readily adapt to stressors and return to homeostasis during the resistance stage (illustrated with dark orange and light orange lines). The specific time course of the stress response depends on the magnitude of the stressor and the individual's ability to adapt.

In the alarm stage, the brain's initial response to a stressor is to signal the **fight-or-flight response** throughout the systems of the body. This is achieved via the autonomic (involuntary) nervous system, the neuroendocrine system, and the voluntary nervous system. These complex systems can be thought of as a communication network that coordinates multiple physiological processes, some of which are activated while others are inhibited. For example, nutrients are released from energy stores to provide fuel for action, while blood vessels to the skin and digestive tract constrict to allow more blood to go to the muscles.

Many of these changes are mediated through the release of chemical messengers (neurotransmitters) such as epinephrine (adrenaline) and cortisol. These chemical messengers are commonly referred to as *stress hormones*. All physiological changes heighten awareness and ready the body for action—fight or flight. Routine sensations and feelings such as hunger, comfort, joy, and sorrow are simply overridden. The effect is rapid and intense.

If the stressor continues, the body enters the resistance stage and continues to mobilize energy and release stress hormones. In this stage, the body's physiological processes are aimed at both adapting to the stressor and regaining homeostasis. If additional stressors occur during this phase, the body will likely not be able to meet the challenge as all resources are already being tapped. In this sense, the body is particularly vulnerable during the resistance stage. If the body can adapt, homeostasis is regained. If, however, cumulative stress is too great or persists too long, the body moves into the exhaustion stage. In this stage, the stressor or stressors overcome the body's adaptive capacity, with subsequent exhaustion, illness, and death.

Visualize a lion stalking a gazelle and consider the biological alarm and cascade of effects that occur within the gazelle as it senses the presence of the lion (alarm stage). Due to a quick response and great speed, the gazelle may simply outrun the lion—the big cat is an intense but momentary stressor (short resistance stage). Alternatively, a brief encounter occurs, but the gazelle escapes with wounds that will heal (long resistance stage). Or perhaps the wounds do not heal and the gazelle struggles for days or weeks before dying (long exhaustion stage). The last option is that during the chase, the gazelle becomes exhausted and falls prey to the lion. In this case, the big cat is the final, lethal stressor and the gazelle succumbs quickly (brief exhaustion stage).

The fight-or-flight response is logical and purposeful as a means for dealing with short-term physical stress. Our ancestors regularly confronted wild animals. Just as with the gazelle, their ability to activate an innate emergency system was a key survival mechanism. Although this system has equipped humans for dealing with

The **fight-or-flight response** is the acute stress response in which the autonomic nervous system triggers a set of physiological changes that ready the body for action. The fight-or-flight response corresponds to the alarm stage of the general adaptation syndrome.

short-term physical stress, how well does it equip us for the unique mental and emotional stresses of modern life? As you can imagine, 21st-century stressors present a different set of challenges and require additional skills.

THE PSYCHOLOGY OF STRESS: MENTAL AND EMOTIONAL RESPONSES

Psychologists point out that although a biological perspective of stress is critical to our understanding, it alone does not present a complete picture. A limitation of the biological model is it does not explain the individual variability that we see in responses to stress. Research has shown that individuals do in fact respond differently to the same stressor because of differences in how they *perceive* and *interpret* the stressor.

Richard Lazarus, Ph.D. (1922–2002), a leading researcher on cognition and emotion, was among the first to propose that the interpretation of stressful events is more important than the events themselves. The ability of people to think about and assess future events—both the potential harms and challenges—makes them vulnerable in ways that other animals are not. Dr. Lazarus's research was primarily with humans, whereas the biological studies described in the previous section focused on laboratory animals. Research has confirmed that humans, due to their higher-level cognitive abilities, experience a wider range of mental and psychosocial stresses than do other animals.

Dr. Lazarus and his colleague Susan Folkman, Ph.D., defined stress as a particular relationship between the person and the environment. In their model, the individual appraises the environment as taxing or exceeding his or her resources and endangering his or her well-being. This definition is the basis of their **transactional model of stress and coping,** where stressful experiences are seen as person–environment interactions, or, using their term, transactions.

Two fundamental transactions are (1) a person's judgment about the significance of the stressor, and (2) the person's self-appraisal of his or her ability to successfully cope with the stressor. This psychological perspective on stress allows opportunities for management at several points: during the initial appraisal of the stressor, during self-assessment of one's ability to control or cope, and during implementation of coping behaviors. We will discuss specific stress management approaches in the last section of this chapter.

These psychological concepts of stress were dramatically brought to life during the classic Stanford Prison Study, conducted by researcher and social psychologist Philip Zimbardo and his colleagues in 1971. The intent of the experiment was to study the psychology of imprisonment by randomly assigning college men to roles as either prisoners or guards and then observing their interactions and behaviors for two weeks in a simulated prison environment. The unexpected occurred, conditions got out of control, and the study was shut down after six days **(www.prisonexp.org).**

The **transactional model of stress and coping** views stress as a transactional (person–environment) phenomenon dependent on the meaning of the stressor to the perceiver. The impact of the external stressor is first mediated by the person's appraisal of the stressor and then by the social and cultural resources at his or her disposal.

Even though the college students knew they were subjects in a study, the "prisoners" soon lost the ability to cope, with some showing signs of depression and extreme stress. Some "guards" became ruthless in their positions of authority. These surprising and controversial findings highlighted the importance of perception, control, and coping. The study demonstrated that the interactions between the person and the environment are malleable and dynamic—far more so than previously thought.

NEED TO KNOW

The nature of stress is highly variable. Stressors can be physical or psychological, and they can occur acutely, episodically, or chronically. Dr. Hans Selye, a pioneer in stress research, used animal studies to develop the general adaptation syndrome, a model depicting the biological effects of stress. His basic concepts are still used today to understand the broad array of stress-related disorders. Dr. Richard Lazarus, a leading psychologist of the 20th century, conducted complementary research with humans, examining the role of cognition and emotion on the experience of stress. He and other psychologists have shown that individual responses to stressful events not only are highly variable but also depend on one's perceptions both of the stressors and of one's ability to cope. Integrating biological and psychological perspectives provides a holistic view of the complex relationships among stress, behavior, and health.

➤ Stress and Illness

The role of stress, particularly chronic stress, in causing or contributing to illness and disease is one of the most studied topics in medicine. Although parts of the puzzle remain unsolved, fundamental knowledge about the sources of stress and resulting signs and symptoms of excessive stress are well established. An update on type A behavior as a risk factor for heart disease, the link of stress to obesity, and recent insights on the connection between social standing and well-being are highlighted to show the varied pathways in which stress may influence our health.

SOURCES OF STRESS

The main sources of stress in America today are associated with changes in personal relationships and occupation. (Of course, as a student your "job" is to make progress in school and eventually earn your degree.) Certain changes can be traumatic; examples include enduring the breakup of a close personal relationship, experiencing a major injury or illness, losing a job, or experiencing the death of a family member. As we now know, positive changes can also be stress-filled, such as graduating, getting married, having a child, or getting a job promotion.

Self
Assessment
6.1

In an effort to quantify the amount of stress a person is experiencing and the corresponding increased risk for stress-related illness, psychologists Thomas Holmes and R. H. Rahe developed their now-well-known Social Readjustment Rating Scale. Using a statistical analysis of responses from a large, diverse group of adults, they were able to assign values to a variety of events based on their perceived stressfulness. The resulting values indicate the relative impact of stressful events on health and

TABLE 6.1 EXAMPLES OF STRESSFUL EVENTS

LIFE EVENT	POINT VALUE
Death of a spouse	119
Divorce	96
Fired from work	79
Major injury or illness	74
Pregnancy	67
Birth of a child	66
Parents' divorce	59
Marriage	50
Change of residence to different city or state	47
Breakup of close personal relationship	47
Beginning or ending college	38
Making a major purchase	37
General work troubles	28
Change in personal habits	26
Vacation	24

Source: Based on Mark A. Miller & Richard H. Rahe, "Life changes scaling for the 1990s," *Journal of Psychosomatic Research* 43: 279–292, 1997. Used with permission of Richard H. Rahe, MD.

give a sense of the wide range of stressors in our lives. In Table 6.1, a few different events are listed to illustrate their findings. The events listed are representative. You could add items, many of them likely to carry high values.

Our environment also encompasses multiple sources of stress, many of which are seemingly omnipresent. Most Americans are city dwellers and encounter crowding, pollution, and noise in their daily lives. Separately, and even more so in combination, these stressors can harm health, particularly mental health. Collectively referred to as *urban press,* such negative environmental stressors are often beyond personal control. Conversely, positive environmental stressors can be found in the community via the arts, sports, museums, and parks. These can be sought out for excitement and enjoyment by individuals and groups.

SIGNS AND SYMPTOMS OF EXCESSIVE STRESS

Recognizing major life-changing events, such as those at the top of the stress scales, is not a problem. However, recognizing our *responses* to these events is not always so straightforward. Identifying the subtler combination or accumulation of less dramatic daily or episodic stressors and our responses to them requires a higher level of awareness and analysis. We should be alert to clues. The following 10 questions capture common signs and symptoms of excessive stress:

- Have you become anxious and easily depressed?
- Have you become indecisive and generally apathetic?
- Have you become irritable and easily angered?
- Have your memory and concentration deteriorated?

- Have you experienced an increase in headaches or digestive problems?
- Has your blood pressure become elevated?
- Has your sleep pattern changed (insomnia/excessive sleep)?
- Have your eating habits changed (appetite loss/binge eating)?
- Have you increased your use of alcohol or drugs?
- Have you developed any nervous habits or phobias?

If you answered yes to one or more of these questions, reassess the stressors in your life. First, can you identify them? Is it likely that they are causing the signs and symptoms? And if so, are you taking the time to address both the stressors and your responses to them? (See "Breaking It Down" on the topic of sleep.) A discussion of stress management, including practical strategies and techniques, is provided later in this chapter.

If you currently face demanding or distressing situations that tax your ability to make it through the day, or if you show signs of stress that are not subsiding, see a counselor or health care specialist at your counseling center or student health center. These professionals are there to assist you, so don't hesitate to make an appointment and meet with them.

CHRONIC STRESS AND HEALTH

The body's response to stress can be lifesaving in a crisis, but paradoxically may be harmful in the long run. From an evolutionary perspective, our stress response equips us to face emergencies with speed and strength. But times have changed. In the 21st century our stressors are more psychosocial than physical, and more chronic than acute. Continual and long-term activation of the stress response can have detrimental effects on the body's major systems. When anxiety and worry about work and relationships don't let up, stress hormones continue to circulate throughout the body in high levels, never leaving the blood and tissues.

Simply put, persistent stress can damage the same physiological systems activated or affected by the stress response in the first place. At the head of the list are the nervous, endocrine, cardiorespiratory, metabolic, immune, and gastrointestinal systems. Over time, unrelenting stress and the accompanying biochemical responses translate into an increased risk for a vast array of disorders and diseases. Stress can both cause diseases and worsen existing ones. Heart disease, obesity, and depression are three of the most common stress-related conditions.

Stress can accelerate the aging process, too. Think of recent presidents George W. Bush and Barack Obama and how they aged during their terms. Aging expert Michael Roizen of the Cleveland Clinic believes the nonstop and high-pressure demands of being president of the United States or a top CEO ages a person at about twice the normal rate. In Figure 6.2, the toll of the presidency is captured in the face of Barack Obama.

Stressful Behavior: Type A Behavior and Hostility

In the 1960s, two cardiologists, Meyer Friedman and R. H. Rosenman, developed the concept of **type A behavior** and identified it as a psychological risk factor for heart disease. They found individuals with classic type A personality continually put themselves in stressful situations, which over time resulted in far more heart attacks than happened to those who were not type A.

Today we are familiar with type A behavior and easily recognize it in others. Such individuals are competitive, aggressive, and time-driven; they never seem to

FIGURE 6.2 — THE PRESIDENCY AND PREMATURE AGING: BARACK OBAMA IN 2007 AND 2011

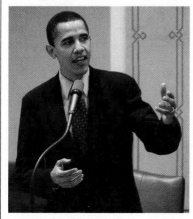

© Seth Perlman/AP Images

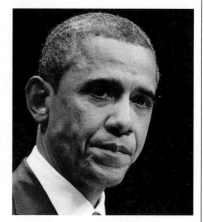

© Kevork Djansezian/Getty Images

miss a step. In contrast, type B individuals are methodical, move at a slower pace, and are generally easygoing. In reality, most of us fall somewhere in between the classic type A (driving, impatient) and type B (unhurried, calm) dispositions.

Further research on type A behavior and heart disease yielded additional important findings. Type A traits can be broken down into three components—excessive competitiveness, time-urgency, and **hostility**—and the hostility component is the primary culprit behind the continual activation of the stress pathways that lead to disease. Hostility—a combination of anger, aggression, and cynicism—may be a better predictor of heart disease than traditional risk factors like cigarette smoking, hypertension, and high cholesterol. Take the 10-question questionnaire and see how you score.

Self Assessment 6.2

Stress and Obesity

Connections between chronic stress and seemingly unrelated conditions continue to be uncovered. The role of chronic stress in the current obesity epidemic is one example. As researchers unravel how the body's stress response system is regulated, the details of the actions and interplay between the brain and multiple chemical messengers are becoming clearer. It is now known that caloric input, energy stores, and body weight are intertwined with the chronic stress response network.

Type A behavior is characterized by excessive competitiveness, time-urgency, and hostility. People with this profile tend to engage their stress response systems on a chronic basis.

Hostility is a combination of anger, aggression, and cynicism. It appears to be the main trait that puts people at risk for the development of heart disease and other stress-related medical conditions.

Breaking It Down   Update on Sleep

The need for sleep is as fundamental to life as the need for food and water. We literally cannot live without sleep. In fact, forced sleep deprivation is used as a means to break down prisoners during interrogation. Despite extensive research, scientists have yet to understand why sleep is so vital—this essential question remains a mystery. However, they do know a great deal about the characteristics of sleep—for example, the types of sleep (shallow vs. deep) and its structure (sequence, organization) and how these aspects change from infancy to old age.

Of particular interest is how normal sleep patterns are affected by sleep disturbances such as insomnia, sleep apnea (breathing interruptions during sleep), and narcolepsy (daytime "sleep attacks"). Sleep-related problems affect about one out of three Americans of all ages, races, and socioeconomic classes. More and more physicians are being trained in sleep medicine, a specialization offered through the American Boards of Internal Medicine, Pediatrics, Otolaryngology (ear, nose, throat), and Psychiatry and Neurology. Patients with sleep problems can see a specialist at one of more than 2,000 accredited sleep centers in the United States.

The relationship between sleep and stress is reciprocal. Stressors can definitely disrupt sleep—we've all had nights when emotional turmoil or a major deadline has kept us up. And, conversely, not getting enough sleep is also a stressor, so the potential for a vicious cycle exists. For college students, the effects of inadequate sleep on learning are especially relevant. Sleep loss results in impaired cognition—that is, poorer attention, memory, and problem solving. Studies in which sleep was actively restricted or optimized showed a corresponding worsening or improvement in learning and academic performance.

Establishing a healthy sleep routine depends on recognizing and then eliminating or minimizing sleep disrupters:

Caffeine consumption—avoid coffee, sodas, pills, and, yes, chocolate too within a few hours of bedtime.

Exercise—by all means engage in regular exercise, but complete your workout a few hours before bedtime.

Indigestion—avoid problem foods and have antacids on hand just in case.

Reaction to medicines—be aware of active ingredients that may interfere with sleep, and find substitutes.

Avoidance of naps, especially in the afternoon—if you can't fall asleep at bedtime, eliminate even short catnaps.

Other sleep disrupters—such as pain, emotional upset, or illness—can be more difficult to deal with but are still generally manageable. Thankfully, in most cases, these are short-lived. If you have recurring or chronic sleep problems, see a health care professional at the student health or counseling center. Depending on your situation, you may be referred to a sleep medicine specialist for a complete sleep-disorder evaluation.

Even though today's high-tech world seemingly runs 24/7, humans are still subject to the biological control of circadian (daily) rhythms that dictate our need for regular restful sleep. Sleep deprivation interferes with our ability to learn and function, and thus hinders our ability to cope. The opposite is true as well:

maintaining healthy sleep habits goes a long way in helping us deal with stressors that are beyond our control.

For more information on the science and medicine of sleep and tips for getting restful sleep, go to:

National Sleep Foundation
https://sleepfoundation.org

American Academy of Sleep Medicine
www.sleepeducation.com

The details of these interactions are exceedingly complex and require specialized study to fully understand. The essence is that problematic eating behaviors, including overconsumption of so-called comfort foods (pleasing foods typically high in carbohydrates and fat), may be stimulated by elevated levels of stress hormones. These surplus calories tend to be stored in the belly and over time result in abdominal obesity. This type of obesity is strongly related to type 2 diabetes, heart disease, and stroke.

Emotional eating—consuming high-calorie foods when under stress, even when not hungry—is a behavior we've experienced firsthand at one time or another. To prevent weight gain during stress, get a handle on your stress by using effective strategies. When you feel less stressed and more in control, you will find it easier to stick to healthy eating and exercise routines. This chronic stress–obesity connection is another example of the dynamic interactions among physiological systems, emotions, and coping methods.

Social Standing and Health Status

It should come as no surprise that the most disadvantaged among us face more stress-related illness. A daily struggle for life's necessities (food, clothing, housing), discrimination, and limited access to health care highlight their plight. These difficult living conditions exist even though government and private-sector agencies work diligently to reduce inequities.

Recent research in public health has produced a finding with wide-reaching implications. Based on longitudinal analysis of demographic, psychological, and health variables in large population studies, a British research team led by Michael Marmot, M.D., at University College, London, found it's not socioeconomic level per se that determines health (quality of life, longevity) but the underlying and related factors of individual autonomy and social participation. These psychosocial factors are at work not just among the poor but across the entire socioeconomic spectrum.

Article
6.1

Dr. Marmot labels this the **status syndrome.** Higher status usually affords more opportunities for individual control and meaningful relationships. Lower status

Emotional eating refers to consuming large quantities of foods—usually "comfort" or junk foods—in response to negative feelings (for example, when stressed, angry, or sad) instead of hunger.

The **status syndrome,** a recent concept in public health, refers to the effect of social position on a person's quality of life and longevity beyond that accounted for by education and income; it appears that risks for stress-related health problems are mediated through the opportunity for, or lack of, individual autonomy and social participation.

means that external forces are more likely to determine one's fate. In other words, a person's health appears to be tied more to his or her place in the social gradient—beyond those defined by income, level of education, health behaviors, and genetic predisposition. The take-home message is that individual control and opportunities for social engagement are critical for lessening the risk of stress-related disorders and maximizing well-being and longevity.

STRESS—THE "BIG PICTURE"

This is an opportune time to step back and reconsider the "big picture" about stress, health, and disease. As described earlier, there are two complementary views. The first is the mainstream medical view where connections between stress and health are explained as physiological processes. The second is anchored in a mind–body view where psychosocial factors are of paramount importance. The reality is that each view is incomplete without the other. We've shown that elements of both views underpin the phenomena of type A behavior, emotional eating, and status syndrome. Another more recent finding provides an even better example of the convergence of the biological and psychological perspectives.

In 2000, researchers reported that women appear to display an alternative stress response that they dubbed the **tend-and-befriend response.** It turns out that the classic fight-or-flight stress response was based largely on studies of male laboratory animals. When similar studies were conducted with female animals, their stress responses—which are in part mediated by sex-specific hormones—were, not surprisingly, somewhat different from the stress responses of males.

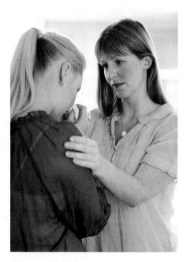

Females demonstrated an added dimension of protecting offspring and seeking the companionship of others. When stressed, females—both lab animals and humans— exhibit nurturing-of-children behavior and seek social support, especially from other females. Indeed, clinical and social psychologists know that women are more likely than men to seek out and provide social support when facing difficult situations.

Researchers are careful to note that the tend-and-befriend response is not a universal female phenomenon but rather is a general gender-related behavioral tendency. The tend-and-befriend finding is another step forward in understanding variability in how

When stressed, women often display "tend-and-befriend" behavior as a way of coping.

© Juli Balla/Getty Images

The **tend-and-befriend response** is a behavior pattern of protecting and caring for offspring and seeking social support exhibited by humans (and some other animals) when under threat. This type of stress response appears to have both biological and psychological underpinnings.

we respond to stressors. Moreover, it illustrates the power of understanding stress from a holistic perspective that unifies biological and psychosocial knowledge.

Finally, let's not forget the essential role of stress in living a full life. Because uncontrolled chronic stress is clearly linked to a variety of health problems, it's easy to forget that stress is primarily a positive force in our lives. Think of stress in the context of excitement, challenges, and new experiences. Stress is not just good or bad but an undulating blend of positive and negative stressors. This motley assortment of forces and events that we dub stress is not optional. Rather it's an unavoidable part of living and personal growth.

In times of high stress, we often say we long for a stress-free life, when in fact we actually mean a life with a manageable level of stress. Certainly, after a prolonged period of hard work or difficulty, a few days of carefree living are welcomed and can be restful and restorative—but then it's back to a routine with roles, responsibilities, and expectations. In a matter of days or weeks, a truly stress-free life would become boring, as many discover when they retire. As long as we focus on goals and challenges, a healthy level of stress will be part of the equation. The key is to recognize stress and manage it to our benefit when we can. In many situations, we can use stress to reach our goals, whether at school or work or with family and friends.

✓ NEED TO KNOW

Excessive stress can cause or worsen a wide range of illnesses. The primary sources of stress include significant changes in personal relationships, responsibilities, or daily routine. Excessive stress often produces signs and symptoms that should alert you to assess your situation and take action. Recent research findings about type A behavior and hostility, stress and obesity, and social standing and health status illustrate the diverse ways in which stress can impact our health. Yet, not all stress is negative. Stress is a varied blend of positive and negative stressors that enriches life and helps define who we are.

➤ Managing Stress

Many adults are quick to tell college students to enjoy themselves. They often add that their college years were the best times of their lives. Whether this is selective memory or wistful longing for a time with fewer responsibilities is open to speculation. What we do know is that for increasing numbers of students today, the college years are not carefree, joyful times but rather full of anxiety and stress.

Mass media brings news of corruption, violence, wars, and natural disasters to us—every day, all day. While cell phones allow us to stay in touch with family, the constant flow of depressing news may be difficult to process for those living far from home. Moreover, for some students, family support systems are in transition—as more parents struggle with their own economic and personal crises.

As college costs and student loans continue to rise, financial worries among students are common. More students are working part time to help pay for school. And then there are looming questions about life after graduation. For many majors, employment prospects are bleak. Add these concerns to the traditional sources of student distress—homesickness, difficulty making friends, poor grades, broken romances, easy access to drugs and alcohol, and sleep deprivation—and you have a situation that can be challenging to even the most resilient students.

Despite these challenges or perhaps because of them, the college experience is a time of growth filled with opportunities. These years provide a special juncture for personal development and transition to independent living. With planning, exploration, and follow-through, you can find your place, succeed in college, and, yes, have fun along the way.

With background on its biology and psychology, and knowledge of its signs and symptoms, let's consider how to successfully control stress. There are three key aspects to successful stress management. The first relates to the importance of using time management to reach your goals and avoid unnecessary stress. The second focuses on understanding your own personality and temperament and how you perceive and respond to stress. And the third deals with identifying healthy coping strategies—including specific stress management techniques.

TIME MANAGEMENT

The transition from high school to college presents various challenges. For many students, the greatest challenge is learning to manage their time effectively. Going to college means greater personal independence and less parental oversight of day-to-day activities. With increased freedom comes more responsibility for routine tasks previously handled by parents, such as those associated with meals, laundry, paying bills, and scheduling appointments. When these new duties are suddenly added to a student's normal college activities—attending classes and labs, completing assignments, studying for tests, making new friends, and participating in extracurricular activities—it's easy to become overwhelmed. Commuting and part-time jobs are often part of the mix as well. Even for the best prepared, the transition to college life requires adjustment and flexibility. Given these factors, it should come as no surprise that poor time management is a root cause of many stressors college students face.

Article
6.2

Time management simply means the planned efficient use of one's time. It is the prioritization, scheduling, and execution of responsibilities to one's personal satisfaction. Everyone has the same amount of time in a day, so it's up to each of us to make the best use of it. We certainly don't want to squander time, the very currency of life. The good news is that time management does not have to be complicated. It can be boiled down to three steps: perform a time audit, prioritize activities, and develop an action plan.

Perform a Time Audit

Analyze how you use your time. Write down all your activities on several representative days and make a chart showing the time allocation over the 24-hour periods. Next, categorize your activities into committed time (e.g., classes, work, family), maintenance time (e.g., personal hygiene, eating, exercising, necessary chores, sleeping), and discretionary time, which is free time to use as you wish. Identify blocks of time that could be better used. For example, are small blocks of time being lost that could be rearranged to be used more efficiently?

> **Time management** is the prioritization, scheduling, and execution of responsibilities to one's personal satisfaction.

Prioritize Your Activities

First things first. Organize your activities by importance and urgency into four categories: (1) urgent and important, (2) not urgent but important, (3) urgent but not important, and (4) not urgent or important. For example, studying for an exam may be both urgent and important, whereas spending time with family and friends is not urgent but important. Attending a sale may be urgent but not important, while watching a TV sitcom is neither urgent nor important. The aim is not to forgo all activities that fall into category four; fun and recreation have their place too! Rather, the lesson is that prioritizing is time well spent. Not prioritizing leads to stressful situations because the most important activities are not given the special consideration they deserve.

Develop an Action Plan

Create a plan and execute. Based on your time audit and prioritization of activities, develop a schedule and to-do list. Many students use print versions of daily planners or similar features on smart phones. Both are fine because they allow you to translate the first two steps into action by having a planned schedule and a timeline for tasks and projects. Execution is the final phase—the act of carrying out or completing the tasks you set out to accomplish. All the analysis and planning is for nil if you don't roll up your sleeves and actually do the work. A large part of time management is the drive to get tasks done and do them well. When you reach this point, your system for time management is in place. With time and practice, the steps will eventually become second nature.

Few of us learn time management as part of our formal education, yet it is fundamental to being productive and preventing negative stressors. Indeed, poor time management is recognized as the primary factor contributing to low graduation rates (only 5 in 10 college students graduate within six years). Colleges now recognize the importance of time management to student success and routinely cover this topic in first-year student seminars. Other noncredit, short courses are often offered periodically through student services. If you feel your time management skills need sharpening, investigate what's offered on campus and get a refresher course.

KNOW THYSELF

How we view our level of personal control in the world can have a major bearing on our response to stress. To better understand this personal control–human behavior connection, clinical psychologist Julian Rotter, Ph.D., developed the concept of **locus of control** and devised a scale to measure it. Locus of control is simply a set of beliefs about the relationship between behavior and subsequent outcomes. These beliefs are described in one of two ways—an **internal control orientation** or an **external control orientation.** For most people, one orientation dominates their view and approach to living.

> **Locus of control** is a psychological concept referring to a person's beliefs about the underlying causes of events in his or her life.
>
> An **internal control orientation** is a view of the world in which an individual believes that outcomes are contingent on his or her actions.
>
> An **external control orientation** is an outlook of the world in which an individual believes that outcomes are determined by events or forces outside his or her personal control.

Those with an internal control orientation believe that outcomes of their actions depend on what they do. These "internalizers" presume that they chart their own course and control their destiny. They believe they are autonomous and, as masters of their fates, also bear responsibility for what happens to them. In contrast, those with an external control orientation believe outcomes are based on events outside their personal control and they have little influence. That is, outcomes are determined by powerful others, by luck or fate, or are simply unpredictable. These "externalizers" believe they are subject to external forces, and their actions often show that they feel little or no responsibility for what happens to them.

Self
Assessment
6.3

A major difference between these attribution styles is that people with an internal locus of personal control know how to act to get their desired outcomes, whereas people with an external locus of personal control seem not to have this knowledge. Externalizers tend to wait passively for whatever comes their way. Yet, we should be mindful that various factors can shape our sense of autonomy—it's not simply a matter of choice. For example, those who face discrimination—because of poverty, lack of education, race, religion, gender, age, or other factors—may have learned from experience that what they do doesn't have much effect.

Locus of personal control plays a major role in our motivation, expectations, self-esteem, and risk-taking behavior, and in so doing can influence our actions and their outcomes. How we view the world certainly relates to how we perceive and cope with stressors. Clearly, an internal locus of control is more conducive to behavior change including stress management.

Locus of control is unequivocally linked to the stress–health relationship. Knowledge about this dimension of our personality can be revealing and instructive. Our responses to stress and our coping methods are shaped by many factors, including personal experience, family background, social and societal influences, and the specific situational context. While not all factors are within an individual's control, one's approach to planning and self-determination can be changed.

As suggested earlier, if you are concerned about a self-assessment score, a troublesome trait, or if your level of stress is so high it's difficult getting through the day, make an appointment with a counselor at the campus counseling center or student health center. You will find professionals who understand and are ready to help you cope with your experiences. They will be glad to talk with you and provide guidance and resources.

STRESS MANAGEMENT TECHNIQUES

Stress management focuses on techniques to help us deal with challenges that are surmountable. These approaches are effective *within limits*. The distress faced by a refugee, a homeless person, a terminally ill person, or the victim of a violent crime is in a different realm from the routine stressors we face every day. Standard stress management techniques will not solve dire situations, nor were they developed with that in mind. Disastrous conditions and traumatic experiences require special expertise and resources.

As a side note, a sincere effort to consider our personal crises in light of those faced by people who lack the most fundamental needs can add perspective. A further step would be to assist those with greater needs. Whether it's volunteering at a homeless shelter or aiding an elderly neighbor with a project, a simple act of service and kindness to others can provide a restorative break from our own personal struggles.

Most of us can benefit from stress management. As referred to earlier when discussing Lazarus and Folkman's transactional model of stress and coping, accurate appraisal of the stressor followed by effective coping is central to successful stress control. First, a judgment is made about the stressfulness of an event. How stressful is it? Is it manageable, positive, or irrelevant? Next is an appraisal of our coping options and resources. What options are available to me? Can I apply reasonable steps to manage the stressor?

Clearly, coping with modern-day stressors is not automatic. Fight-or-flight is rarely the appropriate response. Indeed, coping is a process that's always changing. It's a learned pattern that requires effort. And remember that coping is an effort to *manage* the situation—complete control and mastery are not necessary (or possible) in most cases. Successful coping is dependent on your overall health and energy, a positive belief, problem-solving skills, and social support.

To reinforce and complement the stress management suggestions from psychologists Lazarus and Folkman, we provide the following strategies from neuroscientist Robert Sapolsky, Ph.D.:

- *Learn to accurately recognize signs of stress.* This is the important first step. We must learn to recognize the signs and to identify the circumstances most responsible for the stress response. As noted earlier, it's important to "know thyself."
- *Find an enjoyable outlet and practice it regularly.* Take part in an activity or hobby that helps you release frustrations, and set aside time to do it regularly. The type of activity is not critical as long as it's one you enjoy and is not stressful to others.
- *Seek control in the face of stress, but be realistic.* A can-do outlook is important. We generally have options to control stressors in a positive manner. Gather information, make a plan, and take action, but be realistic. We cannot control events that have already occurred, nor should we try to control future events that are uncontrollable.
- *Develop social support through strong relationships.* Nurture your social network. We are social creatures and long to be part of something larger than ourselves, whether it's a family unit or other kind of group. This is true even for the most independent and individualistic. Yet remember, strong relationships work both ways—they are reciprocal and dynamic. To have a good friend, you must be a good friend.

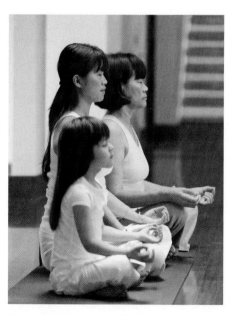

In addition to these general strategies, specific stress management techniques are available. A few of the best known are described briefly below. The first four—deep

Deep breathing or meditation can alleviate symptoms of stress.

© Ariel Skelley/Blend Images, LLC

Article
6.3

breathing, progressive muscle relaxation, visualization, and meditation—are based on inducing a relaxation response in which one consciously focuses on countering or reducing the natural physiological stress responses (e.g., increases in breathing rate and muscle tension). In contrast, physical activity dissipates stress by simulating the body's call to action inherent in the fight-or-flight response.

All stress management techniques have been shown to be effective for some people, but no single technique works well for everyone. Consider these like choices on a menu. Depending on your personal characteristics, preferences, and experiences, some will appeal to you more than others. The key is to find an approach that meets your needs and fits your lifestyle.

The only way to find out which technique works for you is through trial and error. Nearly all colleges provide a variety of courses and workshops on stress management techniques. Take a class. Experiment with different techniques. Reading about them is not enough. We learn by doing. Listen to your own reactions and trust your instincts. You will be able to tell which techniques really work for you.

Deep Breathing

Deep breathing is a simple technique that is easily mastered and requires only a few minutes. Sit or lie down in a comfortable position with a straight spine. Begin by breathing deeply, using the full capacity of the lungs. Expand the chest and abdomen with each deep inhalation and then empty the lungs with a complete exhalation. Don't strain; this should be done comfortably. Allow the chest to rise and fall with each breath. The breathing rate should be slower than normal. Attempt to balance the time of the inhalation (a few seconds) with that of the exhalation. Deep breathing is most effective if practiced daily for 5 to 10 minutes.

Progressive Muscle Relaxation

Progressive muscle relaxation is a technique in which one systematically contracts and relaxes different muscles in a sequential order coupled with deep breathing exercise. It can be performed in a seated or supine position. To try this technique, begin with the muscles of the right foot. Inhale deeply, contract the muscles, then exhale and release the contraction, relaxing your foot completely. Notice how relaxation in this part of your body feels and enjoy the sensations. Next, go to the calf of your right leg, and proceed similarly through the major muscle groups in the rest of your body. The process takes about 10 minutes and promotes relaxation by dissipating peripheral tension. Remain still and enjoy the effects afterward.

Visualization

Creative visualization, or the use of imagery, can be an effective stress reduction technique. It is generally done in conjunction with deep breathing or progressive muscle relaxation, but can be practiced by itself. Find a quiet place and make yourself comfortable—sit or lie down, with legs uncrossed and spine straight. Close your eyes and visualize a peaceful scene in nature—for example, a perfect, undisturbed place on a beach, an island, or a mountain or in a forest or a garden. It may be an actual place you recall or a place you are simply imagining. Immerse yourself in this beautiful, peaceful place by focusing on the details of the setting—see the colors and textures, hear the sounds, smell the fragrances, feel the breeze. With 5 to 10 minutes of visualization, you can create a mini-vacation and have a real break from the daily grind.

Health & the Media Humor as a Stress Buster

"A clown is like an aspirin, only he works twice as fast."

—Groucho Marx

When we think of stress, our images are nearly always negative, reflecting distress. Conflict, sickness, grief, frustration, or sadness are part of the angst of the human condition. Certainly, perspective is important in dealing with stress. Our doubts and worries can sometimes run wild. Chuckling at this cartoon should remind us that humor is a most useful stress buster. By poking fun at the absurdity or incongruity of life's situations—from small annoyances to dire situations—humor can facilitate coping and healing. As Bob Newhart once said, "Laughter gives us distance. It allows us to step back from an event, deal with it, and then move on." Many hospitals now use clowns as a regular part of their care systems. Look for mirth in those stressful situations, as your sense of humor is a valuable tool for maintaining positive mood and overall well-being.

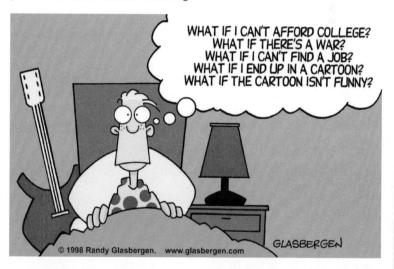

Meditation

Practiced in Asia for millennia, meditation has found a worldwide following over the past century. In the 1970s, Harvard cardiologist Herbert Benson studied people who practiced transcendental meditation and noted their remarkable ability to reduce blood pressure and heart rate. He became a leading proponent of mind–body medicine and made meditation accessible to Americans in his book, *The Relaxation Response*. He distilled meditation down to its essential elements, removing them from their Eastern religious context. Nearly all types of meditation involve adopting a passive attitude toward one's thoughts as they come and go. Find a quiet environment and sit comfortably with your eyes closed. Focus on your breathing, or silently repeat a word or phrase with each exhalation. As your mind wanders (and it will), simply notice it and bring your attention back to your breathing. Practice for 15 to 20 minutes daily, or at least three or four days a week. Like deep breathing, progressive muscle relaxation, and visualization, meditation induces the relaxation response.

Physical Activity

Physical activity is a natural way to reduce stress. During exercise, we process (metabolize) stress chemicals and lessen the damaging effects associated with their accumulation. As discussed in Chapter 3, regular physical activity imparts many health benefits, including an immediate reduction in tension and anxiety. Physical activity is convenient and readily available—when you are really stressed out, just put on your sneakers and go for a walk or a jog. You might be surprised by how effective 20 to 30 minutes of exercise can be in helping you deal with even the most difficult situations. The type of exercise is not critical. Nearly all types of physical activity reduce stress. The key is to find an activity that you enjoy, can maintain, and will engage in regularly.

In this section, we have provided both overall strategies and specific techniques to assist you in managing stress. A central theme woven throughout this chapter is the importance of balance. That is, to effectively deal with stress, we must strive to balance our lifestyle behaviors (nutrition, exercise, sleep) with work, family, and social responsibilities. Simply put, good lifestyle behaviors better equip us to face stressors of all kinds, from the unexpected or uncontrollable to the minor annoyances in everyday life. Moreover, self-knowledge, along with a healthy lifestyle, provides the basis for the ongoing development of self-management skills that enable us to set and reach goals and overcome obstacles.

Article
6.4

The college years are an opportune time to hone these life skills. Be proactive, seek answers, and use campus resources. Stress is part of life, and to a great degree

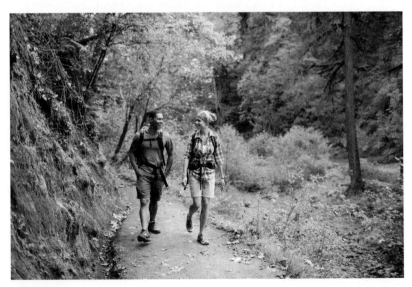

Regular exercise has many benefits—stress relief among them.
© Isaac Koval

we have the ability to control stressors and our responses to them. Stress need not be dreaded—rather, it should be welcomed. Separate the wheat from the chaff—the daily hassles from more significant events—and realize that in most cases, stress can be a positive force in your life.

✓ NEED TO KNOW

The college years present different challenges for different people. For many, the rough patches seem to dominate. To prevent unnecessary stress, use time management to reach goals. To manage excessive stress, understand how you perceive and respond to stress (locus of control). Based on self-knowledge and time-tested recommendations, develop a set of coping strategies. Find a stress management technique that works for you and practice it on a regular basis. Tailor a constructive approach to stress management. And be aware that colleges provide resources, from specific courses to professional counseling, to assist students in dealing with excessive stress.

connect Resources

 ARTICLES

6.1 "Strong Medicine Speaks: Recollections from the Matriarch of a Once Hidden Tribe." Smithsonian.com. Stress is not just an individual phenomenon; it can affect groups too, often as a function of race, ethnicity, or culture. In this article the matriarch of a Native American tribe reflects on the struggles for survival and identity.

6.2 "Professors' Guide: Top Ten Secrets to College Success." *U.S. News & World Report.* Tips from professors to incoming students on how to flourish in college.

6.3 "Change in Lifestyle Is the Best Kind of Cure." *Milwaukee–Wisconsin Journal Sentinel.* When counseling and medication do not do enough to improve anxiety and depression, science turns back toward the basics—diet, exercise, nature, and spirituality—to further improve patients' lives.

6.4 "Unraveling Beliefs." *Edge.* Understanding how personal beliefs are set and become familiar and how established beliefs can be changed are big steps toward understanding behavior and human nature.

 SELF-ASSESSMENTS

6.1 Recent Life Changes Questionnaire
6.2 Hostility Questionnaire
6.3 Locus-of-Control Questionnaire

Website Resources

American Academy of Sleep Medicine **www.sleepeducation.com**
American Institute of Stress **www.stress.org**
American Psychological Association: Stress **www.apa.org/topics/stress**
Jed Foundation: Emotional Health **www.jedfoundation.org/students**
National Institute of Mental Health **www.nimh.nih.gov**
National Sleep Foundation **www.sleepfoundation.org**
University of Chicago: Stress Management **https://wellness.uchicago.edu/page/stress**
University of Georgia: Managing Stress **www.uhs.uga.edu/stress**
U.S. News: Education **www.usnews.com/education**

Knowing the Language

1. Define and provide examples of common physical and psychological stressors.
2. Discuss both the general adaptation syndrome model and the transactional model of stress and coping and then contrast them.
3. Describe the signs and symptoms of excessive stress. What steps should a person take if he or she is experiencing these signs or symptoms?
4. Describe several stress management techniques and how they relieve stress.

Exploring Ideas

1. How do modern-day stressors differ from those our ancestors faced several thousand years ago? Consider how our society is organized differently today and the impact of technology on our daily lives.
2. The stress–illness relationship is reciprocal. Excessive stress can lead to or worsen disease, and, conversely, dealing with an illness can compound a person's level of distress. Have you experienced this firsthand with family or friends? Describe circumstances that show how stress can be both a cause and a consequence of illness.
3. Explain the concept of locus of control. Using yourself or someone you know well, describe and discuss how a person's locus of control positively or negatively impacts his or her ability to assess and cope with stress. How can one move along the locus-of-control continuum from more external to more internal control?

Selected References

Benson H. *The Relaxation Response.* New York: Morrow, 1975.

Covey SR. *The 7 Habits of Highly Effective People.* New York: Simon & Schuster, 1989.

Curio G, Ferrara M, DeGennaro L. Sleep loss, learning capacity and academic performance. *Sleep Medicine Reviews* 10: 323–337, 2006.

Dallman MF, Pecoraro N, Akana SF, et al. Chronic stress and obesity: A new view of "comfort food." *Proceedings of the National Academy of Sciences* 100 (20): 11696–11701, 2003.

Diener E, Biswas-Diener R. *Happiness: Unlocking the Mysteries of Psychological Wealth.* Malden, MA: Blackwell, 2008.

Friedman M, Rosenman RH. *Type A Behavior and Your Heart.* New York: Knopf, 1974.

Holmes TH, Rahe RH. The social readjustment rating scale. *Journal of Psychosomatic Research* 11: 213–218, 1967.

Jacobs L, Hyman J. *The Secrets of College Success* (2nd ed.). San Francisco: Jossey-Bass, 2013.

Kabat-Zinn J. *Full Catastrophe Living.* New York: Bantam, 2013.

Lazarus RS, Folkman S. *Stress, Appraisal and Coping.* New York: Springer, 1984.

Lovallo WR. *Stress and Health: Biological and Psychological Interactions* (3rd ed.). Thousand Oaks, CA: Sage, 2015.

Marmot M. *The Status Syndrome: How Social Standing Affects Our Health and Longevity.* New York: Henry Holt, 2004.

McEwen BS, Lasley EN. *The End of Stress as We Know It.* New York: Dana Press, 2002.

Miller MA, Rahe RH. Life changes scaling for the 1990s. *Journal of Psychosomatic Research* 43(3): 279–292, 1997.

Rotter JB. Generalized expectancies for internal versus external control of reinforcement. *Psychological Monographs* 80 (whole no. 609), 1966.

Ruark J. Positive psychology: An intellectual movement for the masses. *Chronicle of Higher Education,* August 3, 2009.

Sapolsky RM. *Why Zebras Don't Get Ulcers* (3rd ed.). New York: Henry Holt, 2004.

Selye H. *Stress in Health and Disease.* Boston: Butterworth, 1976.

Selye H. *The Stress of Life.* New York: McGraw-Hill, 1956.

Society for Neuroscience. *Brain Facts.* www.brainfacts.org

Taylor SE. Tend and befriend: Biobehavioral bases of affiliation under stress. *Current Directions in Psychological Science* 15(6): 273–277, 2006.

Williams R, Williams V. *In Control: No More Snapping at Your Family, Sulking at Work, Steaming in the Grocery Line, Seething in Meetings, Stuffing Your Frustration.* New York: Rodale, 2006.

Zimbardo PG. Stanford Prison Study: A Simulation Study of the Psychology of Imprisonment Conducted at Stanford University. **www.prisonexp.org**

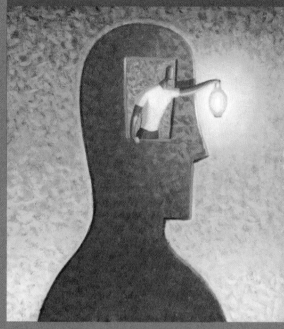

You can handle depression in much the same way you handle a tiger. . . . If depression is creeping up and must be faced, learn something about the nature of the beast. You may escape without a mauling.

—R. W. Shepherd

© Rob Colvin/Stock Illustration Source/Getty Images

Chapter 7

MENTAL HEALTH AND DISORDERS

Until recently, mental illness was often kept secret. But today more people seek treatment openly, as anyone watching television will note upon seeing the frequent ads for anti-anxiety and antidepression drugs such as Paxil, Zoloft, and Cymbalta. This openness is fortunate, given that mental illness is fairly common. Twenty percent of the U.S. population is affected by it, according to the Centers for Disease Control and Prevention. Depression is the most common mental illness, and it is also the leading cause of disability and suicide. In Chapter 7 we explore the concept and characteristics of mental health and common problems related to mental health; we then discuss mental illness and options for seeking help.

The Association for University and Counseling Center Directors (2013) reports that in a survey of college counseling center directors, 95 percent reported that the number of students with significant psychological problems is a growing concern. In addition 70 percent of directors felt that the number of students with severe psychological problems on their campus has also increased. Other reported findings include that among college students:

- 41.6 percent reported that anxiety is the top presenting concern.
- 36.4 percent reported depression.
- 35.8 percent reported relationship problems.
- 24.5 percent were taking psychotropic medications.
- 19 percent reported that availability of psychiatric services on their campus is inadequate.
- 21 percent of counseling center students present with severe mental health concerns and 40 percent with mild mental health concerns.

Further, the National Alliance on Mental Illness (2013) reports that:

- 1 in 3 students reported prolonged periods of depression.
- 1 in 4 students reported having suicidal thoughts or feelings.
- 30 percent of students reported problems with schoolwork due to a mental health issue.
- 50 percent of students rated their mental health below average or poor.
- 50 percent of students received no education on mental health issues prior to college.
- 1 in 7 students reported engaging in abnormally reckless behavior.

The behaviors associated with depression, suicide, and related alcohol abuse can greatly affect a student's academic and personal life.

Knowing the signs and symptoms of mental disorders, as well as the available treatments, is important for any student today. Most people will experience anxiety, depression, and difficulty adjusting to life's circumstances at some point. For some people these are short and self-correcting problems, but for others they can be long-term and significantly interfere with daily life.

Article 7.1

Not that long ago there was little understanding of the physiology related to mental disorders, and there were not many treatments. But as the role of brain chemicals called *neurotransmitters* was unraveled, new drugs were developed in addition to the many counseling approaches already available. Further, since the underlying physical causes of disorders such as anxiety and depression are now better understood, people tend to view these illnesses as the physical diseases they are. The stigma of admitting to suffering from depression or anxiety has diminished greatly. There has never been more effective help available to those suffering with mental illness or disorders than there is today. Truly, there is no good reason for anyone to suffer in silence anymore.

Article 7.2

➤ Mental Health

Maintaining good mental health is as important to good quality of life as is maintaining good physical health. We gauge **mental health** by assessing several factors, including how fulfilling people's relationships are, how well they adapt to or cope with adversity, the level of their communication skills, their resilience, and their self-esteem.

FIGURE 7.1   INTERACTION OF BODY, MIND, AND ENVIRONMENT

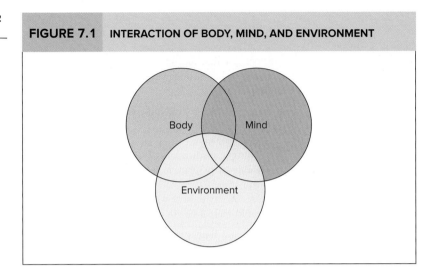

MIND, BODY, AND CULTURE

The interdependence of the physical, mental, social, and spiritual dimensions of health are emphasized throughout *iHealth*. This notion remains true in regard to mental health. The word **psychosomatic** refers to the mind's influence on the body. In Chapter 6 the body's physical reaction to stress was discussed. Biology and emotions also influence each other, as shown in Figure 7.1.

When we are angry, our body responds by secreting certain types of chemical messengers called *hormones* that, in turn, influence neurotransmitters in the brain that relate to mood. When our body produces too little of certain neurotransmitters, depression can result. Just as the body has a fight-or-flight response to danger or stress (see Chapter 6), it also may respond to thoughts and feelings with back or chest pain, changes in appetite, constipation, high blood pressure, insomnia, upset stomach, weight loss, or weight gain.

Culture can also influence our mental health. When society emphasizes the importance of something an individual member of that culture can't attain, it causes conflict and potentially negative mind–body outcomes. Conversely, some institutions and organizations (such as religious or support groups) can greatly improve mental health and one's sense of well-being. This influence of culture is hard to measure but is nonetheless an important factor that individuals must include in making decisions regarding mental health.

BASIC MENTAL HEALTH DEFINITIONS AND THEORIES

When discussing mental health, there are a few basic terms you should know. *Behavior* is how someone acts. **Motivation** is something that leads to a behavior.

Mental health is the successful performance of mental functions resulting in productive activities.

Psychosomatic refers to the influence of the mind (*psyche*) on the way the body (*soma*) functions.

Motivation is the state of being energized to perform a task.

Self-concept is a set of core beliefs and values that you feel describes yourself. **Self-esteem** is how you feel—either positively or negatively—about your core qualities and attributes. And finally, *assertiveness* is being very open and honest about declaring your rights, whereas *aggressiveness* is forceful behavior with the intent to dominate.

Maslow's Hierarchy of Needs

Abraham Maslow's (1970) hierarchy of needs is a model that describes the motivation for behavior. As shown in Figure 7.2, Maslow's contention is that people display behaviors in order to meet needs. Further, he describes five levels of needs. The first level represents the most basic physiological needs—for food, water, and shelter.

Once our physiological needs are satisfied, we need to meet the psychological needs of feeling safe and secure. If these two basic levels of needs are met, then people tend to be motivated by needs higher in Maslow's hierarchy, such as the desire for love and belonging or for self-esteem. Successful people who seem to be

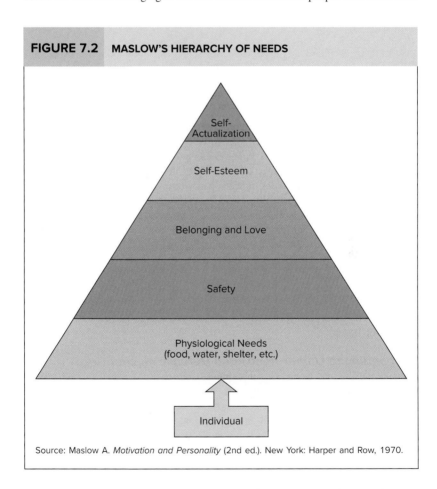

FIGURE 7.2   MASLOW'S HIERARCHY OF NEEDS

Self-Actualization

Self-Esteem

Belonging and Love

Safety

Physiological Needs
(food, water, shelter, etc.)

Individual

Source: Maslow A. *Motivation and Personality* (2nd ed.). New York: Harper and Row, 1970.

Self-concept is a stable set of beliefs about one's qualities and attributes.

Self-esteem is how one feels, good or bad, about one's qualities and attributes.

FIGURE 7.3   SIMPLE BEHAVIOR PARADIGM

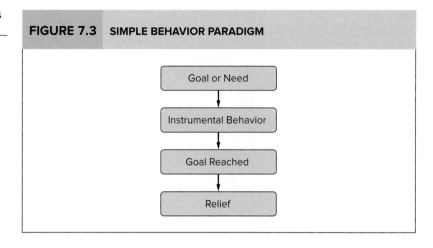

living life to its fullest might be seen as reaching the level of self-actualization, though some say this level is questionable, since we can never really know what our full potential is.

Simple Behavior Paradigm

Using Maslow's hierarchy of needs as a reference point, we can conclude that our behavior is either need-directed or goal-oriented. A simple paradigm to describe behavior is presented in Figure 7.3. The needs referred to in this figure can be the needs identified by Maslow (physiological needs, safety and security). Once the need is identified, people display an instrumental behavior to meet the need. If the behavior leads to achieving the goal, we get relief.

We discover early in life that the real world is rarely as simple as what Figure 7.3 describes. That is, our behaviors don't always result in a need being met. Often we display a behavior, and the need is not met; the goal is not reached. The result of a need not being met is displayed in Figure 7.4. Basically, we experience tension, frustration, and conflict, and then we respond. For example, we often interpret family expectations and personal expectations for success as needs or goals. When the expectations are not met or the goal is not reached, how we respond can result in relief or in no relief, in which case the tension, frustration, and conflict can either increase or lessen.

Responding to Unmet Needs and Defense Mechanisms

When a need is not being met, the simplest response is anger. Another way to respond is to be assertive and challenge something (or someone) to try to get the need met. If anger and assertiveness do not work, then people often become aggressive, which involves either verbal or physical domination. It is not a good approach for resolving conflict and often is counterproductive, especially if the aggressiveness is extreme or violent.

Another common way we respond to unmet needs is to protect or defend our ego, our conscious state of how we perceive ourself; hence, these responses are called *defense mechanisms*. One such mechanism is rationalization, or making excuses for our need not being met. Another defense mechanism is denial, or simply not acknowledging that there is any frustration or conflict. Displacement is

FIGURE 7.4   ALTERNATIVE BEHAVIOR PARADIGM

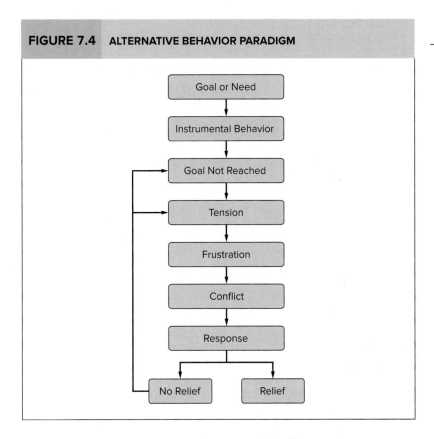

expressing our frustration by attacking another target—for example, a person has a bad experience with a coworker but takes out her frustration on her spouse. Repression, or selective forgetting, is another defense mechanism—we refuse to think about the event that led to the frustration. Reaction formation is displaying behaviors that are the opposite of the ones that we are actually feeling. Finally, projection formation is accusing another person of the same unacceptable behaviors that we have displayed.

Use of defense mechanisms is normal. However, they can be harmful if they are overused to the point where the individual never deals directly with the problem.

CHARACTERISTICS OF GOOD MENTAL HEALTH

The National Mental Health Association has identified 10 characteristics of people who are mentally healthy:

1. They feel good about themselves.
2. They do not become overwhelmed by emotions such as fear, anger, love, jealousy, guilt, or anxiety.
3. They have lasting and satisfying personal relationships.
4. They feel comfortable with other people.
5. They can laugh at themselves with others.
6. They have respect for themselves and for others even if there are differences.

Self
Assessment
7.1

7. They are able to accept life's disappointments.
8. They can meet life's demands and handle problems when they arise.
9. They make their own decisions.
10. They shape their environment whenever possible and adjust to it when necessary.

These characteristics have some common themes that are related to Maslow's hierarchy of needs, the behavior paradigm, and the use of defense mechanisms. These themes include a positive self-image, good communication skills, a sense of humor, a healthy response to unmet needs, and good problem-solving skills. It makes sense that people who display the characteristics of good mental health are well balanced, good problem solvers, and accept personal responsibility for their behavior.

NEED TO KNOW

Good mental health allows people to cope with the stresses and challenges of life. People's behaviors are motivated by their physical and emotional needs. According to Maslow's hierarchy, the most basic needs are the body's needs for food and shelter. Once those needs are met, people attempt to fill the most basic emotional needs, including a need for feeling safe and secure. When a need remains unmet, frustration results. Often people cope with unmet needs by using defense mechanisms such as denial, displacement, repression, reaction formation, and projection formation.

➤ Personal and Social Problems Related to Mental Health

Since mental health involves judgment, coping, communication, relationships, biology, and feelings, it is easy to see how most personal and societal problems are related to mental health. Some examples of social and personal problems related to mental health include suicide, drug abuse, violence, and eating disorders.

SUICIDE

Suicide is the tenth leading cause of death in the United States and the third leading cause of death among 15- to 24-year-olds. We know that depression is usually a precursor to suicide and that depression has a strong biological basis. So to say that suicide is "just" a mental health problem would be wrong.

Suicide can be examined in the context of the behavior paradigm discussed earlier. For example, when a need (food and shelter, safety and security, love and belonging, self-esteem) is not met, and tension, frustration, and conflict continue, then suicide can be the response. In the late 1800s sociologist Emile Durkheim identified three types of suicides. An egoistic suicide is ending one's life as a response to not being able to assimilate into a group or society—for example, a student taking his life after having severe difficulty fitting into the college environment. By contrast, an altruistic suicide is taking one's life to advance a cause or an ideal. Last, anomic suicides occur when the person or group that provided a sense

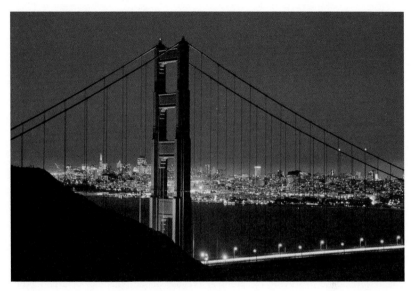

Some places, such as the Golden Gate Bridge in San Francisco, attract people contemplating suicide. Suicide hotline phones have been installed on bridge walkways to help prevent people from jumping.
© Larry Brownstein/Getty Images

of security no longer exists. The loss of a social network can cause such persistent frustration, conflict, and depression that a person may choose suicide. An example of an anomic suicide would be an elderly man who kills himself after his wife dies.

Notice in all of these descriptions that the person chooses suicide. Life becomes so difficult that the person perceives suicide as the only remedy. Suicide as a choice represents the ultimate personal defeat.

Unfortunately, most suicides are preceded by warning signs that may go unnoticed. Such warning signs include feelings of hopelessness, withdrawing from family and friends, sleeping too much or too little, feeling tired most of the time, acting compulsively, losing interest in most activities, giving away prized possessions, isolating oneself socially, feeling depressed, acting irrationally, being preoccupied with death, behaving recklessly, abusing alcohol or drugs, and being unable to concentrate. Many of the warning signs for suicide are also symptoms of depression, which is strongly related to suicide.

There are steps you can take to prevent suicide if you notice warning signs:

- Always take suicidal comments seriously.
- Try not to act shocked by what a suicidal person might say.
- Do not handle the situation by yourself—get assistance from a health professional.
- Listen attentively to everything that the person has to say.
- Comfort the person with words of encouragement.
- Let the person know that you are deeply concerned.
- If you perceive the person is at high risk of suicide, do not leave him or her alone.
- Talk openly about suicide.

- If the person talks about committing suicide with a firearm that he or she owns, call the police so that they may remove the firearm.
- Don't be judgmental.
- Be careful about statements you make.
- Listen; be gentle, kind, and understanding.
- Let the person express emotion in the way that he or she wants.

It takes time and patience, but you must understand that the suicidal person is in pain and sees few other options. With medical intervention, the crisis can end, and through therapy the person can recover.

DRUG ABUSE

Much information regarding drug abuse is discussed in Chapter 4. Here it is important to note that attempting to modify one's mood is a common response to tension, frustration, and conflict. The extent to which one binge drinks can be directly related to coping problems. Also, stimulants, depressants, and hallucinogens can serve as chemical Band-Aids that exert a psychoactive effect to lessen the intensity of the response to tension, frustration, and conflict. However, this is a quick fix, and it is counterproductive to solving the problem because of the potential for a new problem: drug dependence.

In some ways it is understandable that drug misuse and abuse is such a common problem related to mental health. The effects are immediate and can be powerful enough so that one's problems just don't seem as bad—that is, until the effects of the drug wear off. When that happens, the problems are still there, and some people respond immediately by modifying their mood to feel better once again. It's not long before using drugs as a coping mechanism creates compound problems—first, not only having to cope with the initial problem, but second, now having to deal with a drug problem.

VIOLENCE

According to a Centers for Disease Control and Prevention study, the cost in the United States of medical care, rehabilitation, and loss of productivity due to violence is estimated at more than $224 billion a year. In 2013 the CDC reported that homicide claimed the lives of over 16,121 Americans, whereas suicide was responsible for the deaths of over 33,000 Americans. Homicide is the second leading cause of death for people between 15 and 34, and it is the leading cause of death for African Americans in this age group. There were nearly 11,208 firearm-related deaths in 2013, and more than 2 million nonfatal violence-related injuries occurred in the United States.

Violence is a serious mental health issue and is largely preventable. Violent behaviors and mental illness are not necessarily related—that is, only a small percentage of those who are diagnosed as mentally ill are violent. The causes of violence are related to larger social problems such as stress, dangerous environments, unemployment, drugs, and poverty. Like many other topics we will cover in this chapter, violence represents a choice, and this choice can be the response to tension, frustration, and conflict described in the earlier paradigm.

Violence enacted by active shooters is a serious problem in the United States. *Active shooter* is a term used by law enforcement to describe a situation in which a shooting is in progress and an aspect of the crime may affect the protocols

Article
7.3

Breaking It Down   Predicting Violent Behavior

In April 2007, Seung-Hui Cho, a senior at Virginia Polytechnic Institute and State University, shot to death two students near their campus dormitory rooms. A short time later Cho chained the doors of a classroom building and systematically murdered 30 additional students and faculty before committing suicide as police approached him. The so-called Virginia Tech Massacre is the most deadly school shooting in U.S. history.

The biggest question is what motivated Cho to murder so many? A Governor's Task Force report could not find definitive explanations for Cho's actions. However, it uncovered many warning signs that indicated Cho might be a threat either to himself or to those around him.

Cho appears to have been a lonely young man with poor social skills. Students taunted and bullied him in high school, most likely because he was Korean and had poor English language skills. Not being able to express himself well, he internalized this rejection and became an introvert with an undisciplined fantasy life. He fantasized about committing violent acts. Cho sent a video manifesto to *NBC News* the morning of his attack at Virginia Tech. These actions reflected a stoic, determined, irrational man who wanted to make people pay the ultimate price for his problems. His victims were simply in the wrong place at the wrong time.

In the years leading up to the massacre, some people noticed that Cho needed help. He was referred and evaluated for psychological care, but sadly, he was never made to continue with therapy. Cho's violent fantasies and sense of alienation from people around him worsened. That, combined with the easy ability to buy weapons, resulted in the tragedy.

Several lessons can be learned from the Virginia Tech Massacre. A key point is that Cho fit the profile of a lonely, ostracized person who was capable of acting out violently. Unfortunately, the people around him were not networked in such a way that the full threat could become obvious before Cho acted out. When Cho was referred to counseling and didn't follow through, there was no mechanism to track what was happening with him. Strict privacy laws helped create a situation where Virginia Tech staff and faculty had no comprehensive record of the incidents that the faculty and staff at his high school had reported. If there had been such a record, perhaps when several female college students accused Cho of stalking them, charges might have been pressed, and Cho might have been forced to get help. Instead, Cho's brushes with mental health authorities and the criminal justice system remained slight, so he wasn't flagged in the gun dealers' database as a person who should not be allowed to purchase firearms. Without guns, the scope of whatever Cho chose to do would have been greatly diminished.

It should be noted that most people with Cho's apparent history of mental disorders and social problems do not resort to lashing out at others. If they act out, usually they turn their anger inward and take their own life. However, suicide has great cost not only to the person but also to the person's family and friends. Although stopping people from acting out violently on innocent bystanders is extremely important, preventing suicides is also an important goal, and it can be achieved with the same steps that can minimize the chance of another school massacre.

(*continued*)

The Virginia Tech Massacre shows that individuals, both teachers and students, often have good instincts about pinpointing people who could benefit from counseling, psychiatric medications, and, in some cases, hospitalization to prevent violent acts. The challenge is to track at-risk individuals so that they don't fall through the cracks like Cho did. With a good tracking system, easing of the privacy laws in situations like these, and the right people involved in discussions about the behaviors they are observing and the appropriate interventions, horrible incidents like this one can be prevented.

used in responding to and reacting at the scene of the incident (USDOJ, 2014). The United States Department of Justice (USDOJ) in its study of active shooter incidents in the United States between 2000 and 2013 found that there were 160 active shooter incidents resulting in 486 deaths and 557 wounded. Further, the USDOJ found that from 2000 to 2006 there was an average of 6.4 incidents each year and from 2006 to 2013 this increased to an average of 16.4 a year—a notable increase. Finally, 70 percent of active shooter incidents occurred in a commerce/business or educational environment and 60 percent of the incidents ended before police arrived.

EATING DISORDERS

As discussed in Chapter 2, the eating disorders anorexia nervosa and bulimia nervosa cause people to starve themselves or engage in binge-and-purge eating behavior. Eating disorders can be a response to unmet needs relating to self-esteem or perception of body image. According to the National Eating Disorders Association, the causes of eating disorders are psychological, interpersonal, and social. Psychological factors include low self-esteem, feelings of inadequacy or lack of control in life, and depression, anxiety, anger, or loneliness. Interpersonal factors include troubled family and personal relationships, difficulty in expressing emotions and feelings, history of being teased or ridiculed based on size or weight, and history of physical or sexual abuse. Social factors include cultural preferences that glorify thinness and place value on obtaining the "perfect body," narrow definitions of beauty that include only specific body weights and shapes for women and men, and cultural norms that value people on the basis of physical appearance and not inner qualities and strengths. These psychological, social, and cultural factors are all related to the Maslow model and the behavior paradigm described earlier.

Clinically, according to the American Psychiatric Association, **anorexia nervosa** has the following symptoms:

- Fear of being fat when at or below normal weight.
- Restricting eating so weight falls more than 15 percent below what is considered healthy.
- Distorted body image that creates a sense of obesity even when overly thin.
- In women, the absence of at least three consecutive menstrual cycles.

Anorexia nervosa is an eating disorder characterized by self-starvation, excessive thinness, and a distorted body image.

Bulimia nervosa, according to the American Psychiatric Association, is character-ized by binge eating and inappropriate compensatory methods to prevent weight gain, such as self-induced vomiting or misuse of laxatives and diuretics. Bulimia has the following symptoms:

- Recurrent episodes of binge eating (at least twice a week for three months).
- Complete loss of control during eating binges.
- Persistent overconcern with body shape and size.
- Regular self-induced vomiting or use of laxatives or diuretics to prevent weight gain.
- Strict dieting, fasting, or exercising to prevent weight gain.

Binge eating disorder is a relatively new classification of eating disorders. It is characterized by overeating as a response to frustration and conflict. Unlike bulimia, binge eating disorder does not involve purging after overeating.

Eating disorders have serious physical consequences. Anorexia nervosa can result in low blood pressure, reduction of bone density, muscle loss and weakness, and kidney failure. Bulimia nervosa can result in gastric rupture, inflammation of the esophagus, tooth decay, peptic ulcers, and pancreatitis. Eating disorders when extreme can result in death. No one knows how many deaths each year are related to eating disorders, primarily because official statistics of cause of death, such as kidney failure or suicide, do not show whether there is a link to an eating disorder. However, studies of anorexic patients have reported death rates from 4 to 25 percent.

NEED TO KNOW

Many personal and social problems are related to mental health, includ-ing violence against others, suicide, binge drinking, drug use, and eating disorders. While each of these problems may have a biological compo-nent as a cause, they all also relate to the psychological, social, and cultural factors described by both the Maslow hierarchy of needs and the behavior paradigm model.

➤ Mental and Personality Disorders

Mental disorders are perhaps the most misunderstood kind of illness. We often use terms like *schizophrenic, bipolar,* and *obsessive-compulsive* to describe people, but in reality these are clinical terms that are used to identify profound disorders. Med-ical and psychodynamic perspectives are used in discussing abnormal behavior. The medical perspective is grounded in the physiological reasons for a condition, and the psychodynamic perspective contends that these disorders are a result of psychologi-cal conflicts and represent a means of coping with these conflicts. There is ample

Bulimia nervosa is an eating disorder characterized by binge eating and compensatory methods to rid the body of food.

Binge eating disorder is characterized by excessive overeating.

evidence supporting each perspective as well as a combination of perspectives—that is, both medical and psychodynamic factors interact—and the consequence is a condition that can be diagnosed.

ANXIETY DISORDERS

Anxiety is excessive worry and concern that is extremely unpleasant and involves apprehension, fear, and panic. Symptoms of anxiety disorders include trembling, jumpiness, inability to relax, racing heart, irritability, hyperactivity, insomnia, and apprehension. There are several classifications of anxiety problems. **Generalized anxiety disorder (GAD)** is constant and uncontrollable worry and concern about everything. When anxiety comes on after a traumatic event—anything from a violent attack to an accident or the sudden death of a loved one—**posttraumatic stress disorder (PTSD),** where persistent frightening thoughts, feelings, and memories interfere with one's life, may result. **Panic disorders** are sudden, overwhelming attacks of fear. Usually the attacks are short but frequent. A person experiencing a panic attack has uncontrolled thoughts of impending doom for themselves or someone else, experiences intense anxiety symptoms, and may even pass out.

Phobias are fears of specific events, objects, or situations. There are many different kinds of phobias. Examples are autophobia (fear of being alone), pharmacophobia (fear of taking medicine), musophobia (fear of mice), microphobia (fear of microbes), hydrophobia (fear of water), acrophobia (fear of heights), and claustrophobia (fear of being in closed spaces). The number of potential phobias is infinite. The response to a phobia can be intense anxiety symptoms like those in panic attacks. People who have claustrophobia and find themselves in an enclosed area such as an elevator or closet may experience panic attack symptoms.

Finally, **obsessive-compulsive disorder (OCD)** is a condition characterized by repetition of the same act over and over again (compulsion) as a response to persistent unwanted thoughts or images (obsession). The behavior is acted out in a ritualistic manner. Examples of OCD symptoms include constantly checking a door to make sure it is locked or constantly washing one's hands.

Self
Assessment
7.2

MOOD DISORDERS: DEPRESSION AND MANIA

Mood disorders are serious and disabling instabilities in emotions. The extremes of mood disorders are depression and mania.

Anxiety is excessive worry and concern.

Generalized anxiety disorder (GAD) is constant and uncontrollable worry or concern about everything.

Posttraumatic stress disorder (PTSD) is an anxiety disorder that can occur after experiencing a frightening event in which physical harm may have occurred.

Panic disorders are sudden, overwhelming attacks of fear.

Phobias are fears of specific objects or events.

Obsessive-compulsive disorder (OCD) is repetition of an act over and over again as a response to unwanted thoughts.

Depression is feelings of worthlessness, indecisiveness, guilt, sadness, and apprehension. We wouldn't be human if we didn't experience depression at points in our lives because of deaths, disappointments, and conflicts. Usually, however, the intensity of these feelings wanes, and the depression naturally lifts. But sometimes depression is a long-lasting state rather than a passing mood. In this case, depression can cause many personal, professional, and relationship problems. **Mania** is characterized by an elevated mood in which the person appears extremely excitable and hyperactive, makes grandiose and incomprehensible statements, and has rambling thoughts.

There are three types of depressive illness: major depression, dysthymia, and bipolar illness. According to the National Institute of Mental Health, symptoms of major depression include:

- Sadness, irritability, excessive crying, anxiety, or hopeless feelings.
- Decreased energy and feelings of fatigue.
- Loss of interest or pleasure in usual activities.
- Appetite and weight changes.
- Sleep disturbances.
- Thoughts of death or suicide attempts.
- Difficulty concentrating, making decisions, remembering.
- Chronic aches and pains not explained by any other physical condition.

Dysthymia is a form of depression that is long-term and less severe than major depression, but it still impairs functioning to some degree. **Bipolar disorder,** which sometimes is referred to as *manic-depressive illness,* includes two states: extreme elation (mania) followed by the extreme low of depression. If the symptoms of depression are experienced only during a specific season, such as winter, when the days are short, the diagnosis may be **seasonal affective disorder (SAD).**

Article
7.4

Depression is a serious college health issue and certainly an impediment to academic success. It is important for anyone who experiences five or more of the symptoms of depression for two weeks or longer to seek some help from a health professional.

A person in a manic episode is hyperactive, believes he or she can do anything, and often talks in a rambling, incoherent manner. Although elation can be a symptom some people actually enjoy, a manic episode can make people delusional, and their actions can badly disrupt their life and relationships. Symptoms of mania include repeatedly starting new tasks, outbursts of inappropriate anger, grandiose sense of knowing more than others, extravagant spending, and energetic exercise. Hospitalization may be required to stabilize the person's mood in severe cases.

Depression is characterized by feelings of worthlessness, indecisiveness, guilt, sadness, and apprehension.

Mania is characterized by an extremely elevated mood and subsequent hyperactive behaviors.

Dysthymia is a form of depression that has long-term but less severe effects than major depression.

Bipolar disorder (sometimes referred to as *manic-depressive illness*) involves swings between mania (extreme elation) and depression.

Seasonal affective disorder (SAD) is when symptoms of depression are experienced during a specific season of the year.

Personality disorders are groups of persistent behaviors that impair social, academic, or professional functioning or cause personal distress. Common personality disorders include paranoid personality disorder, schizoid personality disorder, and schizotypal disorder.

A person suffering from **paranoid personality disorder** is excessively distrustful and suspicious of others, expects to be abused by others, doesn't confide in others, and may be extremely jealous. Schizoid personality disorder can result in extreme detachment from social situations and limited emotions in interpersonal relations. Finally, a person with a schizotypal disorder is usually socially isolated, exhibits bizarre behaviors and beliefs about the world, and is suspicious of others.

SCHIZOPHRENIA

Schizophrenia is a severe personality disorder that involves distorted thoughts and perceptions, atypical communication, inappropriate emotion, abnormal motor behavior, and social withdrawal. There are five types of schizophrenia.

Paranoid schizophrenics experience delusions and auditory hallucinations. They trust no one and are constantly on guard because they are convinced that others are plotting against them. Catatonic schizophrenia is characterized by excessive inactivity. The person can retain the same posture for long periods of time and may alternate between violent behavior and being immobile and totally unresponsive to the outside world. Disorganized schizophrenics experience extreme delusions, hallucinations, and have inappropriate patterns of speech, mood, and movements. Extreme laughing and crying at unsuitable times are hallmark signs of disorganized schizophrenics.

A schizophrenic who experiences delusions, hallucinations, and disorganized behavior but lacks other specific symptoms is classified as an undifferentiated schizophrenic. Finally, residual schizophrenia is a condition in which at least one episode of schizophrenia has occurred, but there are currently no prominent psychotic symptoms.

✓ NEED TO KNOW

Mental disorders are some of the most misunderstood illnesses. When people's behavior appears different, often it is incorrectly interpreted as a disorder. Mental disorders, like physical disorders, have common sets of symptoms that are characteristic of those having the disorder. The symptoms can range from mood disorders to severe disorders such as anxiety disorders, mania, and schizophrenia.

Paranoid personality disorder is characterized by excessive distrust and suspicion of others.

Schizophrenia is a severe mental disorder that involves distorted thoughts and perceptions, atypical communications, inappropriate emotion, and abnormal motor behavior. Forms of schizophrenia include paranoid, catatonic, disorganized, undifferentiated, and residual.

➤ Treatment

Psychotherapy and biomedical therapy are two approaches used to treat many of the disorders described in this chapter. In most instances a combination of both psychotherapy and biomedical therapy is used.

Psychotherapy is performed by a psychotherapist. A psychotherapist can be a psychologist, psychiatrist, a psychiatric nurse, or a counselor. In all instances there are licensure and certification requirements for people performing psychotherapy. (See Chapter 12 for a more detailed explanation of the educational backgrounds of various health professionals.)

The psychological techniques employed in psychotherapy include such approaches as psychodynamic, humanistic, person-centered, gestalt therapy, existential therapy, and behavior therapies, systematic desensitization, implosive therapy, flooding, biofeedback, aversive conditioning, token economy, cognitive therapy, rational-emotive therapy, feminist therapy, and group therapy. See Figure 7.5 for a summary of the different techniques.

The biomedical approach involves the use of drug therapies to treat the disorder. In general the drugs used in treating these disorders include anti-anxiety drugs, antipsychotic drugs, antidepressant drugs, lithium, and electroconvulsive therapy. (Some of these drugs were discussed in Chapter 4.) Anti-anxiety drugs are minor tranquilizers such as Valium and Xanax. These drugs are designed to be used short-term. Antipsychotic drugs are major tranquilizers that are used long term and are capable of acting on the psychotic process itself. Antidepressant drugs such as Prozac, Zoloft, Paxil, and Cymbalta act on the neurotransmitters norepinephrine and/or serotonin. These medications have been very successful in treating depression and have made a major difference in people's lives. Lithium is used to control the swings in bipolar mood disorders.

Electroconvulsive therapy (ECT) is a procedure in which electrodes administer shocks to the patient, who experiences a seizure and then lapses into unconsciousness. When conscious, the patient feels better because the ECT has affected nerve cells and the root physiological causes of depression. Exactly what happens neurologically after ECT is unclear, but it provides relief for some people. Because it has some serious risks, ECT is normally used only when all other treatments have failed. ECT can speed or slow the heartbeat and cause memory loss. When psychotherapy and biomedical therapy are not effective in keeping a person functional, institutionalization may be the only remaining option, especially for people who are dangerous to themselves or others.

✓ NEED TO KNOW

People who suffer from mental or emotional problems should be encouraged to know that interventions can help. After the condition is properly diagnosed, the appropriate treatment can be prescribed. Treatment can include counseling or medication or both. There have been tremendous advances in medications used to treat mental and emotional conditions. Medications such as anti-anxiety drugs and antidepressants have made a positive difference in many lives. Even people with profound mental problems might not need to be institutionalized as they were years ago. There are many options both in medications and counseling.

FIGURE 7.5 APPROACHES TO PSYCHOTHERAPY

Aversive conditioning: Client experiences unpleasant stimuli (shock, verbal insults) after behaving undesirably.

Behavior therapy: Principles of social learning are used to assist people in forming accurate perceptions of their feelings and themselves.

Biofeedback: Monitoring of body functioning provides feedback to the client.

Cognitive therapy: Client is taught to understand the irrationality of his or her thoughts or behaviors.

Encounter groups: Confrontational strategies are used to allow members to express true feelings.

Existential therapy: Emphasis is placed on free will and using the free will to develop insight and self-understanding.

Family therapy: This form of group therapy is directed at families.

Feminist therapy: Focuses on role of society and the role of discrimination in daily life.

Flooding therapy: Client is placed in a real situation that he or she fears, normally accompanied by the therapist.

Gestalt therapy: An approach that employs role-playing and confrontation.

Group therapy: Psychotherapeutic principles are applied to a group.

Humanistic therapies: The focus is on conscious thoughts and present times as opposed to psychodynamic (unconscious thoughts and past experiences).

Implosive therapy: Clients imagine and deal with their worst fears in a safe environment with a therapist.

Marital therapy: Husbands and wives receive therapy together to assist them in a more productive relationship.

Modeling: Client watches another person perform the feared behavior and with the help of the therapist copies that behavior.

Person-centered therapy: A warm, supportive environment is created where a person feels accepted and can reveal true feelings.

Psychodrama: Role-playing strategies are used including role reversal.

Psychodynamic therapies: Freudian insight therapies are used and involve free association and dream analysis; can be focused on the unconscious and past experiences.

Self-help groups: These support groups assist people in displaying behaviors to reduce risk of recidivism to a previous problem behavior (alcohol dependence).

Sensitivity groups: Strategies are used to promote self-awareness and trust of others.

Systematic desensitization: Principles of relaxation and visualization are used.

Token economy: Tokens are given as rewards for behavior in an effort to shape the behavior.

Health & the Media Advertising Antidepressants

Zoloft is a selective serotonin reuptake inhibitor (SSRI), one of the most widely prescribed antidepressants among that category of drugs. Drugs like Zoloft have made a positive difference in many people's lives. However, in 2004 Zoloft advertisements contained a cartoon character that asked, "Are you sad or anxious? Tired all of the time? Not sleeping well? Losing interest in things and people you love? Do these feelings stop you from enjoying life? These could be the signs of depression. When the cause is unknown, Zoloft can help." The ads were deemed misleading by the Food and Drug Administration (FDA) and pulled because the possible risks and side effects from taking Zoloft were not adequately described. The issue of whether drug companies should advertise to consumers directly—in effect, asking them to go to their doctor to get a specific drug, rather than going to the doctor with a problem and allowing the physician to evaluate prescription needs—remains controversial today.

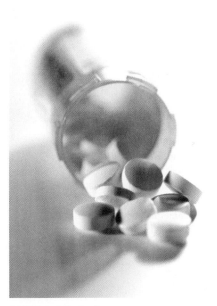

© Thinkstock/Jupiter Images

connect Resources

ARTICLES

7.1 "A Nation of Wimps." *Psychology Today.* Parents are making wimps of their children, resulting in mental health problems when the child reaches college.
7.2 "Mental Health Service Utilization Among College Students in the United States." *Journal of Nervous and Mental Disease.* A comprehensive examination of service utilization and help-seeking behavior for mental health problems among college students in the United States.
7.3 "Conceptualizing the Engaging Bystander Approach to Sexual Violence Prevention on College Campuses." *Journal of College Student Development.* The "engaging bystander" is an approach to prevent sexual violence including rape and can be a viable intervention to decrease sexual violence on college campuses.
7.4 "Sleep Debt and Depression in Female College Students." *Psychiatry Research.* The relationship between sleep habits and depressive symptoms among female college students is examined in this study.

 SELF-ASSESSMENTS

7.1 Are You on the Correct Path to a Healthy Self-Esteem?
7.2 Test Anxiety Questionnaire

Website Resources

Anxiety Disorders Association of America **www.adaa.org**
Centers for Disease Control and Prevention **www.cdc.gov**
Internet Mental Health **www.mentalhealth.com**
Jed Foundation **www.jedfoundation.org/students**
Mental Health America (formerly National Mental Health Association) **www.nmha.org**
National Eating Disorders Association **www.nationaleatingdisorders.org**
National Institute of Mental Health **www.nimh.nih.gov**
Obsessive-Compulsive Foundation **www.ocfoundation.org**
Substance Abuse and Mental Health Services Administration **www.samhsa.gov**
Suicide.org: Suicide Awareness, Prevention, and Support **www.suicide.org**

Knowing the Language

1. What is Maslow's hierarchy of needs and what does it have to do with mental health?
2. What can happen when needs are not met? What is the range of responses to tension, frustration, conflict?
3. What are the characteristics of good mental health?
4. What are the differences between mood disorders and personality disorders?
5. What are the common treatments used in treating mental disorders?

Exploring Ideas

1. How does one know the difference between someone who is different and someone who is mentally ill?
2. How can a clear understanding of mental health lessen the personal and social problems related to mental health?
3. Why is it so hard for people to admit they are having mental health problems? What can be done to help create a better environment for people to seek help?

Selected References

American College Health Association. *National College Health Assessment: Reference Group Summary.* Baltimore, MD: American College Health Association, 2010.

American Psychiatric Association. *Diagnostic and Statistical Manual of Mental Disorders* (4th ed.). Washington, DC: APA, 2000.

American Psychiatric Association. *Let's Talk Facts About Eating Disorders.* Washington, DC: APA, 2005.

Association for University and College Counseling Center Directors. *The Association for University and College Counseling Center Directors Annual Survey.* 2013. **files.cmcglobal.com/Monograph_2012_AUCCCD_Public.pdf**

Centers for Disease Control and Prevention. *Violence Prevention.* January 27, 2009. **www.cdc.gov/violenceprevention**

Durkheim E. *Suicide: A Study in Sociology* (trans. Simpson G, Spaulding JA). New York: Free Press, 2000.

Glanze W. *Mosby's Medical and Nursing Dictionary* (5th ed.). St. Louis, MO: Mosby, 2002.

Kadison R, diGeronimo T. *College of the Overwhelmed.* San Francisco: Jossey-Bass, 2005.

Kitzrow M. The mental health needs of today's college students: Challenges and recommendations. *NASPA Journal* 41(1): 165–183, 2003.

Marano H. A nation of wimps. *Psychology Today* 40: 25–32, 2004.

Maslow A. *Motivation and Personality* (2nd ed.). New York: Harper & Row, 1970.

Narrow WE, Rae DS, Robins LN, et al. Revised prevalence estimates of mental disorders in the United States. *Archives of General Psychiatry* 59(2): 131–145, 2002.

National Alliance on Mental Illness. *College Students Speak: A Survey Report on Mental Health.* 2013. **https://www.nami.org/About-NAMI/Publications-Reports/Survey-Reports/College-Students-Speak_A-Survey-Report-on-Mental-H.pdf**

National Institute of Mental Health. *Eating Disorders.* Bethesda, MD: National Institute of Mental Health, 2002.

National Institute of Mental Health. *Facts about Anxiety Disorders.* Bethesda, MD: National Institute of Mental Health, 2003.

Shortell S, Kaluzny A. *Health Care Management: Organizational Design and Behavior.* Albany, NY: Delmar, 2000.

Sontag D. Who was responsible for Elizabeth Shin? *New York Times*, April 28, 2002.

Steers RM, Porter LW. *Motivation and Work Behavior.* New York: McGraw-Hill, 1987.

Taylor S. *Health Psychology* (5th ed.). New York: McGraw-Hill, 2003.

United States Department of Justice. *A Study of Active Shooter Incidents in the United States Between 2000 and 2013.* Washington, DC: FBI, 2014.

U.S. Department of Health and Human Services. *Healthy People 2010.* Washington, DC: U.S. DHHS, 2000.

U.S. Public Health Service. *Mental Health: A Report of the Surgeon General.* Washington, DC: U.S. PHS, 2002.

Wrobel G. Accessing Medicaid Funding for School Based Mental Health Programs. Presented at the National Association of School Psychologists, Washington, DC, February 10–12, 2001.

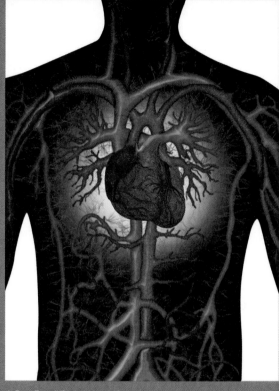

Eating a vegetarian diet, walking (exercising) everyday, and meditating is considered radical. Allowing someone to slice your chest open and graft your leg veins in your heart is considered normal and conservative.

—Dean Ornish, M.D.

© Don Farrall/Digital Vision/Getty Images

Chapter 8

HEART DISEASE AND STROKE

In this chapter, we focus on coronary heart disease (CHD) and stroke, the two most common types of cardiovascular disease. We discuss the underlying disease process of atherosclerosis and review the signs, risk factors, and treatments for CHD and stroke. Prevention measures are highlighted.

IN THE YEARS following World War II, America was buzzing. Families reunited, new families began, suburban communities around cities mushroomed, and the economy boomed. Life was upbeat. Americans were optimistic about their health, too. In contrast to the hard times of the Great Depression and World War II, people living in the postwar period benefited from major advances in health and medicine. Public health systems ensured cleaner water and sanitary-waste disposal, while the advent of antibiotics brought major killers like tuberculosis and pneumonia under control.

Yet, these good times were overshadowed by the rise in death and disability due to cardiovascular disease. The growth of desk jobs and the popularity of labor-saving devices such as the washing machine and the motorized lawn mower meant people were getting much less physical activity than their parents had. The typical American diet changed to one where whole milk, butter, and red meats were commonplace rather than special occasion foods. And in 1950 the world was unaware of the dangers of tobacco and about half of American adults smoked.

Although heart disease had been increasing since the late 1930s, doctors had little advice for their patients on the treatment or prevention of heart conditions. Doctors thought atherosclerosis was an inevitable part of the aging process and that blood pressure increased to enable the heart to pump blood through an older person's narrowed arteries. The standard treatment for those who survived a heart attack was four to six weeks of bed rest. Today, following a heart attack or heart surgery, patients are encouraged to get up and walk within hours.

In the 1950s, researchers began to investigate the potential roles of smoking, a high saturated fat diet, and physical inactivity on the increased rates of cardiovascular disease. By the 1970s, a growing body of scientific studies provided strong evidence that these lifestyle habits contributed to the rise in heart attacks and strokes. Today, complex surgeries and powerful drugs are available to treat the many forms of cardiovascular disease. But an advancement as important as medical treatments is our understanding that cardiovascular disease can be prevented. Exercising, not smoking, and smart eating greatly reduce our risk of what remains the number one cause of death in the United States.

Article 8.1

This chapter focuses on the two most common types of cardiovascular disease: coronary heart disease (CHD) and stroke. The underlying disease process of atherosclerosis is reviewed, followed by a synopsis of CHD and stroke, including their signs, risk factors, and treatments. The cardiovascular risk factors that are modifiable, along with preventive lifestyle behaviors, are emphasized throughout.

➤ Cardiovascular Disease

Cardiovascular disease is a general term that encompasses a broad array of diseases of the heart (*cardio-*) and blood vessels (*-vascular*). Cardiovascular disease has been the number one killer in the United States for decades. More than 600,000 Americans die from cardiovascular disease each year. That's about one in every four deaths from all causes. Coronary heart disease (CHD) and stroke are the two most common types, together accounting for about two-thirds of all cardiovascular deaths. Other cardiovascular deaths are attributable primarily to high blood pressure or hypertension (8 percent); heart failure, a decline in the heart's pumping capacity (7 percent); and peripheral arterial disease (3 percent). The remaining cardiovascular deaths are caused by a variety of less common heart and blood vessel disorders. Less than 1 percent of deaths are due to congenital cardiovascular defects.

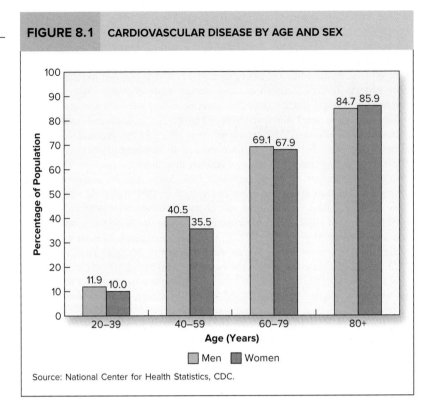

FIGURE 8.1   CARDIOVASCULAR DISEASE BY AGE AND SEX

Source: National Center for Health Statistics, CDC.

The prevalence of cardiovascular disease in adults by age and sex is shown in Figure 8.1. In this analysis, cardiovascular disease includes coronary heart disease, stroke, high blood pressure, and heart failure. Two points are important to highlight: (1) cardiovascular disease is not uncommon in young adults, and (2) its prevalence is similar for males and females across age.

A disease process called **atherosclerosis** causes both CHD and stroke. The term derives from the Greek words *athero-,* meaning "gruel" or "paste," and *-sclerosis,* meaning "hardness." Atherosclerosis is the buildup of patchy deposits—primarily fatty substances, cholesterol, cellular waste products, and calcium—inside the arteries. These deposits are collectively referred to as *plaque.* As the plaque accumulates, the arteries thicken and harden, becoming less elastic.

The process of plaque deposition is not uniform or equally distributed within an artery, but rather it is irregular and scattered. As plaque accumulates within an artery, blood flow is increasingly restricted as the inner diameter of the vessel becomes rougher and smaller. The combination of less elasticity of vessel walls and increased pressure within vessels weakens arteries and makes them vulnerable to rupture.

Atherosclerosis is the process in which the inner layers of arteries become irregular and thick due to accumulation of plaque (fatty deposits); over time, this process can lead to obstructive buildup within the arteries and weakening of the arterial walls.

As atherosclerosis develops, it becomes more likely a blood clot will form, blocking a narrowed artery. A clot can form within a narrowed artery (thrombus), or a clot can form in another part of the body and migrate to a narrowed artery (embolus). Complete obstruction of an artery or, less frequently, the bursting of an arterial wall can occur. If this occurs in the heart, we call it a *heart attack.* If it occurs in the brain, we call it a *stroke.*

Atherosclerosis may also occur in arteries far from the heart or brain—in the legs or pelvis, for example. This condition is known as *peripheral arterial disease.* It is much less common than heart attack or stroke as a cause of death, but it can be painful and limit one's activities. Cramping and fatigue in the legs while walking are early symptoms.

Atherosclerosis is a process that occurs throughout the body, although it may progress at different rates from one site to another. With that in mind, it's clear that a person at risk for any one of these three conditions—heart attack, stroke, or peripheral vascular disease—is also at risk for the other two. Moreover, atherosclerosis is often an underlying or contributing factor to hypertension and heart failure.

Until the 1990s, atherosclerosis was chiefly considered a disease of midlife and beyond. New research findings over a decade shifted this view. We now know atherosclerosis can progress more rapidly and earlier in life, even in people in their 20s. Furthermore, older people who have controlled their cardiovascular risk factors have relatively low rates of heart disease and stroke. Such evidence indicates age by itself is not as strong a determinant of atherosclerosis as was once believed. These findings provide a powerful incentive to reduce one's risk factors regardless of age.

Atherosclerosis is initiated by inflammation with subsequent scarring and calcification of the innermost layer of the artery (endothelium). Substantial evidence demonstrates that premature onset or accelerated atherosclerosis is caused by tobacco smoke, high blood pressure, high cholesterol, physical inactivity, obesity, and diabetes—all of which are largely modifiable. These and other risk factors are discussed later in the chapter. In the next sections, we present key terms and concepts about heart disease and stroke.

CORONARY HEART DISEASE

Do you wonder what it feels like to have a heart attack? In the opening paragraphs of her book *Heartsounds,* Martha Weinman Lear tells the true story of her physician husband having a heart attack:

> He awoke at 7 A.M. with pain in his chest. The sort of pain that might cause panic if one were not a doctor, as he was, and did not know, as he knew, that it was heartburn.
>
> He went into the kitchen to get some Coke, whose secret syrups often relieve heartburn. The refrigerator door seemed heavy, and he noted that he was having trouble unscrewing the bottle cap. Finally he wrenched it off, cursing the defective cap. He poured some liquid, took a sip. The pain did not go away. Another sip; still no relief.
>
> Now he grew more attentive. He stood motionless, observing symptoms. His breath was coming hard. He felt faint. He was sweating, though the August morning was still cool. He put fingers to his pulse. It was rapid and weak. A powerful burning sensation was beginning to spread through his chest, radiating upward into

his throat. Into his arm? No. But the pain was growing worse. Now it was crushing—"crushing," just as it is always described. And worse even than the pain was the sensation of losing all power, a terrifying seepage of strength.

On some level he stood aside and observed all this with a certain clinical detachment. Here, the preposterous spectacle of this naked man holding a tumbler of Coke and waiting to die in an orange Formica kitchen on a sunny summer morning in the 53rd year of his life.

I'll be damned, he thought. I can't believe it.

Coronary heart disease (CHD)—also referred to as *coronary artery disease*—is a condition in which the blood supply to the heart muscle (myocardium) is partially or completely blocked due to atherosclerotic narrowing of one or more coronary arteries. CHD causes about one out of every seven deaths in the United States. CHD was once thought to be a disease of men, and even today many people still believe this. But statistics show this is false. CHD is the single largest killer of American males *and* females, with the total number of deaths about evenly split between men and women.

On average, men develop CHD about 10 years earlier than women because, until menopause, women are somewhat protected from the disease by their higher levels of estrogen. For this reason, heart disease is often considered an "older woman's disease." It is the leading cause of death among women aged 65 years and older. However, heart disease is also the third leading cause of death among women aged 25–44 years and the second leading cause of death among women aged 45–64 years. With regard to race/ethnicity, the prevalence of heart disease for people aged 18 and older is similar for Whites (11 percent) and African Americans (10 percent) and lower for Hispanics (8 percent) and Asians (6 percent).

CHD is a chronic, progressive condition. As the plaque builds up in the coronary arteries, the blood flow channels become more restricted (Figure 8.2). If the artery becomes completely blocked, the likely outcome is chest pain or **heart attack.** The medical term for chest pain is *angina pectoris,* or more commonly just **angina.** Angina is uncomfortable pressure, squeezing, or pain in the chest, and it can vary widely in intensity.

Angina often occurs when the heart needs more blood to meet the demands of physical exertion such as when climbing a flight of stairs. It may also occur when experiencing strong emotions. Some people may have unstable angina in which chest pain occurs unexpectedly at rest. Nitroglycerin is the drug most often used to treat angina. This drug is a coronary vasodilator. It causes the blood vessels to relax and thus allows the channels inside the vessels to open up and improve blood flow.

A heart attack, or myocardial infarction, occurs when one or more of the coronary arteries are blocked. This can happen when plaque tears or ruptures, creating

Coronary heart disease (CHD) is a condition in which the coronary arteries are narrowed or blocked, usually because of atherosclerosis.

Heart attack is tissue death (infarction) to part of the heart muscle (myocardium) due to an insufficient blood supply when a coronary artery becomes blocked. The medical term for heart attack is *myocardial infarction.*

Angina, or *angina pectoris,* is the medical term for chest pain or discomfort caused by a restricted blood supply to the heart.

FIGURE 8.2 HEALTHY VERSUS DISEASED CORONARY ARTERY

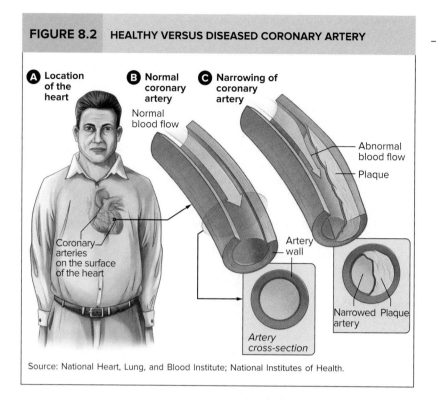

Source: National Heart, Lung, and Blood Institute; National Institutes of Health.

a snag where a blood clot forms and completely blocks the artery. If the blood supply is cut off for more than a few minutes, the cardiac muscle cells suffer permanent damage and die. Depending on the severity of heart damage, consequences can vary from a minor heart attack to sudden death. About half of all men and women who died suddenly had *no previous symptoms* of the disease. This is a sobering statistic. You may know of someone who died this way.

STROKE

Stroke is a disorder in which an artery to the brain becomes blocked or ruptures, resulting in death of brain tissue. When counted separately from other cardiovascular diseases, stroke ranks fourth among all causes of death, behind heart disease, cancer, and chronic lower respiratory disease. Stroke accounts for about 1 out of every 20 deaths in the United States. More women than men die from stroke. Stroke is also the second most common cause of disabling neurologic damage after Alzheimer's disease.

A **stroke** is brain-cell injury caused by a blockage or rupture of a blood vessel in the brain. Stroke is characterized by loss of muscle control, mental function, vision, sensation, and/or speech and other symptoms that vary with the extent and severity of brain damage. The medical term for stroke is *cerebrovascular accident.*

In adults over 60, the lifetime risk for stroke is about one in six. Women have a higher risk than men, perhaps due to their longer lifespan. With regard to race/ethnicity, African Americans are more likely than Whites, Asians, or Hispanics to have a stroke and die from it. Although stroke is much more common in older people than in younger adults, they do sometimes occur in younger individuals, especially if there is uncontrolled high blood pressure.

Most strokes are due to atherosclerosis, the same underlying disease process that leads to heart attacks. In a stroke, a carotid artery that supplies blood to the brain is affected (Figure 8.3). For this reason, strokes are sometimes referred to as *brain attacks.* The medical term for stroke is *cerebrovascular accident,* so called because the disorder affects the blood vessels (-*vascular*) to the brain (*cerebro-*).

There are two types of stroke: ischemic and hemorrhagic. The term *ischemic* refers to decreased blood flow due to constriction or obstruction of an artery. Most strokes (87 percent) are ischemic. In these cases, an artery has become blocked. Deprived of their blood supply and thus oxygen and nutrients, the affected brain cells can be permanently damaged.

A transient ischemic attack, sometimes called a *mini-stroke,* is a less serious variation of the ischemic stroke. In a transient ischemic attack, blood supply to part

FIGURE 8.3   HEALTHY VERSUS DISEASED CAROTID ARTERY

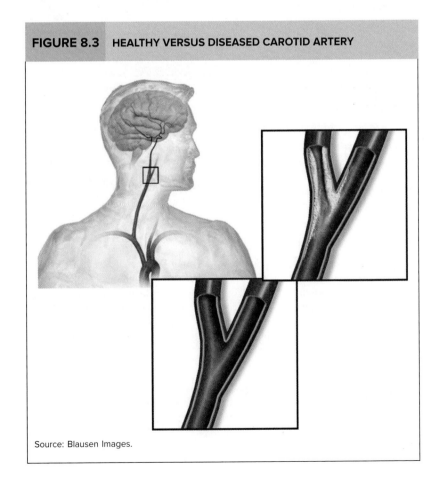

Source: Blausen Images.

of the brain is compromised but only for a brief time. In this case, normal blood flow reestablishes quickly, and brain tissue does not die. However, a transient ischemic attack may be a warning of an impending ischemic stroke. So, it's also an opportunity to take steps to prevent stroke.

Hemorrhagic strokes are less common (10 percent of all strokes) but are more dangerous than ischemic strokes. In this type of stroke, a blood vessel ruptures where the arterial wall has weakened. This not only prevents normal blood flow but also results in blood leaking into or around brain tissue, which in turn leads to life-threatening complications. Hemorrhagic strokes are more lethal than ischemic strokes.

When a stroke occurs, the resulting brain injury causes a loss of muscle control, mental function, vision, sensation, or speech, or a combination of these functions. Strokes usually damage only one side of the brain. Because nerves cross in the brain, symptoms appear on the side of the body opposite the injured side of the brain. Strokes affect people in different ways, depending on the type of stroke (ischemic vs. hemorrhagic), the specific area of the brain, and the extent of the brain injury.

✓ **NEED TO KNOW**

Cardiovascular disease includes all diseases of the heart and circulatory system. Coronary heart disease (CHD) and stroke are the two major types of cardiovascular disease and are the first and fourth leading causes of death in America, respectively. Atherosclerosis, a chronic progressive process of obstructive plaque buildup and weakening of the arterial walls, is the underlying cause of both CHD and stroke.

➤ Symptoms

Every adult in America should be able to recognize the symptoms of heart attacks and strokes and know the steps to take to activate the emergency medical system. *Onset of symptoms should trigger an immediate response.* You may be the only person available to provide assistance. Remember that emergency therapy for heart attack and stroke is critical for saving lives and reducing disabilities. The cardinal signs of a heart attack and of a stroke and the appropriate actions to take are presented in the next sections.

HEART ATTACK—KNOW THE SIGNS

In the opening to this chapter's section on heart disease, Dr. Lear struggles with disbelief and pain as he experiences a heart attack (described in the excerpt from *Heartsounds*). As a doctor, he knows the signs, yet he denies them. The thought that it must be something else—it *cannot* be a heart attack—is a typical initial response, even for knowledgeable adults. Many people experiencing a heart attack are not sure what's wrong and wait too long to get help. Know the signs—not only for your sake but for the sake of others who may be indecisive about getting emergency care.

What are the classical signs of a heart attack? Many think a heart attack is sudden and intense, like the Hollywood portrayal where the actor suddenly clutches his chest in anguish and falls over dead after an intense physical effort or emotional crisis. A heart attack can occur this way, but the truth is that two out of three people who have heart attacks experience warning symptoms a few days or weeks beforehand. A person may notice only mild pain or discomfort from time to time. Or chest discomfort (angina) may become more frequent and occur with less and less physical exertion. Even those who have had a heart attack may not recognize their symptoms, because the next heart attack can have entirely different ones.

The most recognizable symptom of a heart attack is chest pain that may spread to the back, neck, jaw, left arm, both arms, or abdomen. The pain can range from slight discomfort or pressure to an unbearable squeezing or crushing sensation. It may persist, or go away and return. Location of the pain can vary—it may occur in one or more of these sites and not in the chest at all. The chest pain of a heart attack is similar to the pain of angina but is generally more severe, lasts longer, and is not relieved by rest or nitroglycerin. Pain in the abdomen is sometimes mistaken for indigestion. Shortness of breath often accompanies chest discomfort. Other symptoms may include breaking out in a cold sweat, nausea, or light-headedness.

HEART ATTACK WARNING SIGNS

- Chest discomfort or pain.
- Upper body discomfort—one or both arms, back, neck, jaw, or stomach.
- Shortness of breath.
- Cold sweat, nausea, or light-headedness.

It's worth repeating that women are as vulnerable to a heart attack as men. Heart disease is the number one killer of both women and men, and women account for about half of all heart attack deaths. There is an average age difference, with women being about 10 years older than men when they have a heart attack.

As with men, women's most common symptom is chest pain or discomfort. But women are more likely than men to experience some of the other symptoms, particularly shortness of breath, nausea/vomiting, and back or jaw pain. Be forewarned: women are less likely than men to believe they're having a heart attack and more likely to delay seeking emergency treatment.

STROKE—KNOW THE SIGNS

Unlike those of a heart attack, the signs of stroke are not widely recognized. In a study by the Centers for Disease Control and Prevention, less than half of American adults knew the major symptoms. Strokes are most common in older people, but they are not rare among young adults. A stroke can occur in a young, fit person if risk factors are not controlled.

Symptoms vary widely depending on the exact location of the blockage or bleeding in the brain. Each area of the brain is supplied by specific arteries. For example, if an artery supplying the area controlling movement of the right arm is blocked, then the right arm becomes weak or paralyzed. Similarly, a loss of vision, speech, movement, or mental function can be the sign of a stroke, depending on the area of the brain affected.

The most common early symptoms of an ischemic stroke are sudden numbness, weakness, or paralysis of the face, arm, or leg on one side of the body; sudden confusion with difficulty speaking or understanding speech; sudden dimness or loss of vision, particularly in one eye; loss of balance or coordination, leading to falls; and sudden, severe headache. Symptoms of a transient ischemic stroke are the same but usually disappear within minutes.

Symptoms of a hemorrhagic stroke are largely the same as those of an ischemic stroke. However, sudden severe headache may be more common along with nausea and vomiting, temporary or persistent loss of consciousness, and very high blood pressure. Remember, a common characteristic of stroke whether ischemic or hemorrhagic is the sudden onset of symptoms.

STROKE WARNING SIGNS

- Paralysis or numbness of face, arm, or leg—especially on one side of the body.
- Trouble speaking or understanding.
- Trouble seeing in one or both eyes.
- Trouble walking, loss of coordination.
- Severe headache.

A final point: A person does not have to experience multiple symptoms to be having a stroke. Even if only one symptom is present, seek medical attention right away. It's tempting to ignore symptoms if they last only a few minutes. Yet, such a decision is a high-risk gamble—with much to lose. Transient ischemic attacks often signal that a major stroke is on the way. People who have a transient ischemic attack should see a doctor immediately.

ACT IN AN EMERGENCY

Starting medical treatment as soon as possible is critical when a person is experiencing a heart attack or stroke. The sooner emergency care is begun, the lower the risk of death or disability. There are clot-dissolving drugs and procedures that can open blocked arteries, but they must be delivered quickly—within the first one to three hours—to be effective.

It's critical to take action. Throughout the country, a call to 9-1-1 will activate emergency medical service and ensure quick arrival by paramedics. Be sure to note as much of the following information as you can for the paramedics and emergency room team:

- What are the symptoms?
- What time did the symptoms begin?
- Does the person have any medical conditions?
- What drugs, if any, does the person take?

The paramedics will be able to start medical treatment, monitor the patient on the way to the hospital, call ahead to prepare the emergency team, and provide the quickest possible transport.

In the unusual instance where 9-1-1 is not available, drive the person to the nearest hospital emergency room. Call ahead if possible and alert them that you are coming. People who may have had a heart attack or stroke should not attempt to drive themselves. An impaired driver is a hazard to everyone on the road.

You may face resistance to taking action—primarily from the person you are trying to assist! Many reasons can surface to delay calling 9-1-1. People can't believe a heart attack or stroke is happening to them. Symptoms are not what they expected. People wait to see if the symptoms will go away. They want to treat the symptoms themselves. They call a family member for advice. They call the doctor and wait for a return call. They try to make arrangements for children or other dependent family members before seeking emergency care. They fear large medical bills. Although these are rational reasons, none of them are good enough to postpone *emergency* treatment. A delay can result in death or lifelong disability.

If the symptoms turn out to be related to a less serious problem, consider that as good news. The paramedics and emergency room team will not fault you for your quick and decisive actions to known signs of a heart attack or stroke. Unfortunately, their dilemma is often just the opposite. They are sometimes unable to effectively treat people who waited too long before coming. In some cases, the time-sensitive window for using the most successful treatments may have closed.

Breaking It Down   Defibrillators—From the Emergency Room to the Shopping Mall

You've seen automated external defibrillators (AEDs) conspicuously mounted in all types of places, from shopping malls and airports to sports arenas and office towers. The aim is to have AEDs available in public and private settings where large numbers of people gather. AEDs save lives. But how did the defibrillator come from the emergency room to the shopping mall?

We've seen the scene depicted on TV many times. The patient suddenly loses consciousness and has no pulse. It's a case of cardiac arrest, and a "Code Blue" is called for immediate response by a trained team of nurses and doctors. The resuscitating team continues advanced cardiac life support until the patient recovers or dies. The good news—on TV and in real life—is that cardiac arrest is often reversed by the electric discharge of a defibrillator.

Nearly a quarter of all deaths in the United States are attributed to sudden cardiac arrest, which results from disturbances in the electrical activity of the heart—most commonly, ventricular fibrillation. During this abnormal heart rhythm, the ventricles begin to quiver—visualize a bowl of writhing worms—rather than contract in unison. This failure of the heart's ventricles to circulate blood and provide oxygen to the brain (cerebral hypoxia) causes victims to lose consciousness and stop breathing. If left untreated, cardiac arrest invariably leads to death within minutes.

Most of these deaths are due to underlying heart disease and associated with a heart attack. Sudden cardiac arrest occurs primarily in middle-aged and elderly people, though some victims are much younger. For many, there is no previous history of heart problems. Sudden cardiac arrest is often the first symptom and it can occur anytime, anywhere. By its very nature, sudden cardiac arrest is unpredictable.

The AED is a computerized medical device that can check a person's heart rhythm and advise the rescuer. If the heart can be shocked—called *defibrillation*—a normal heart rhythm may be restored. Learning to use an AED is surprisingly simple. Many report it's easier than learning CPR. AED courses last about three or four hours and include hands-on practice. Training is offered through several organizations, including the American Heart Association and the American Red Cross.

The key to successful treatment is to be quick. The shorter the time from collapse to defibrillation, the better the chances of survival. If defibrillation is delayed for more than 10 minutes, survival rates drop to less than 5 percent. The challenge is to respond within the first 5 to 7 minutes.

To summarize, *cardiac arrest* warning signs are sudden loss of responsiveness and no normal breathing. If the signs of cardiac arrest are present, tell someone to call 9-1-1 and get an AED, and begin CPR immediately. Use an AED as soon as it arrives. If you are alone, call 9-1-1 and get an AED if possible before you begin CPR.

CPR—STAY UP TO DATE

For 50 years, cardiopulmonary resuscitation (CPR) was taught to millions of people using the simple memory prompt of A-B-C for the steps of airway, breathing, and compressions. This changed in 2010 when the American Heart Association revised the guidelines and rearranged the three steps from A-B-C to C-A-B.

The revised approach begins with (chest) **C**ompressions, followed by (check) **A**irway, and then (rescue) **B**reathing. These guidelines apply to adults, children, and infants. The previous approach caused delays in chest compressions, which are crucial to keep blood circulating.

A simpler version of CPR known as Hands-Only CPR can be life-saving in many instances of cardiac arrest. Namely, it is recommended for use on teens or adults whom you see suddenly collapse. It consists of two easy steps: (1) call 9-1-1, and (2) push hard and fast in the center of the chest. Rate of compressions should be about 100 per minute. See the instructional video: **heart.org/handsonlycpr.**

Hands-Only CPR can double or even triple a victim's chance of survival. But also note that conventional CPR (with compressions *and* breaths) is recommended for infants and children and victims of drowning, drug overdose, or people who collapse due to breathing problems.

Take a course and learn (or renew) CPR and AED skills. If you needed help, you would hope that a bystander would know what to do. It may well be that you will be the bystander, not the victim, so be prepared.

NEED TO KNOW

Know the warning signs of a heart attack and those of a stroke and how to activate the emergency medical system in your area. The sooner emergency care is begun, the lower the risk of death or disability. Practice potentially life-saving skills by learning CPR (cardiopulmonary resuscitation) and how to use an AED (automated external defibrillator).

➤ Risk Factors

With the rapid rise in cardiovascular disease during the first half of the 20th century, the U.S. Public Health Service decided to undertake a large-scale study to investigate why. Researchers wanted to learn which biologic and environmental factors were responsible. They agreed on an epidemiological study, a new approach at the time, to learn how and why those who developed heart disease differed from those who remained disease-free.

In 1948, the town of Framingham, Massachusetts, was selected as the study site, and 5,209 healthy residents (30–60 years of age, men and women) were enrolled. Each underwent a detailed medical history, physical examination, and comprehensive laboratory tests. Every two years, participants returned for similar exams. In 1971, another group was recruited for the "offspring study": 5,124 children (and spouses) of the original group. Currently, the "third generation" (children of the offspring group) are being enrolled and will be studied for a better understanding of how genetic factors relate to cardiovascular disease.

It was the pioneering work of the Framingham Heart Study that led to the identification of the major risk factors. In fact, it was the first to coin the term *risk factor* in 1961. Findings from this longitudinal study laid the groundwork for today's emphasis on early detection and treatment of cardiovascular disease risk factors. In the years ahead, look for reports from the Framingham study as researchers continue to update our knowledge about the causes, prevention, and control of cardiovascular disease.

Since the 1970s, risk factors for heart disease and stroke have been described as one of two types: nonmodifiable or modifiable. Risk factors that *cannot* be modified or changed are age, gender, and heredity. Increasing age is a risk factor. Men are at greater risk than women. And a family history of early cardiovascular disease— particularly in parents, siblings, or grandparents—is a risk factor. Early or premature disease is usually defined as occurring before age 65.

Risk factors that *can* be modified, treated, or controlled include six major factors and other contributing factors. Many of you are aware of the three classic risk factors of smoking, high blood pressure, and elevated blood cholesterol. But you may not know that physical inactivity, obesity, and diabetes are also major risk factors. In the next few pages, we'll take a closer look at these six risk factors because they are the ones under our control.

CIGARETTE SMOKING

A smoker's risk is directly related to the number of cigarettes smoked daily. The nicotine and carbon monoxide in tobacco smoke reduce the amount of oxygen carried in the blood. These and other substances in tobacco smoke reduce HDL ("good") cholesterol, damage blood vessel walls causing plaque to build up, and may trigger the formation of blood clots. In addition to increasing one's chances of having a heart attack or stroke, smoking causes cancer and lung disease, is the strongest risk factor for peripheral arterial disease and sudden cardiac death, and harms the fetus during pregnancy. Moreover, constant exposure to the tobacco smoke of others (secondhand smoke) can be as harmful as smoking.

Cigarette smoking is the single most preventable cause of disease and death in the United States. Despite the multiple harmful effects of tobacco and large-scale efforts to curb its use, millions of Americans still smoke. The latest figures indicate nearly one in five Americans over the age of 18 smokes. Smokers have twice the risk of heart attack and stroke as nonsmokers. Yet, remarkably, a large portion of a smoker's risk disappears two years after stopping; by 10 years, a former smoker's risk is similar to a nonsmoker's. If you smoke, the single best step you can take to improve your health is to stop. Also, think of family and friends who smoke and what you can do to help them quit. See resources at: **www.smokefree.gov.**

High blood pressure, or **hypertension,** is a condition in which blood pressure is consistently elevated over repeated readings on different days. Blood pressure is the force with which the blood pushes against the walls of the arteries. If blood pressure is continuously high, the heart is working harder than it should, and over time this will damage both the heart and the blood vessels.

When blood pressure is measured, two values are recorded. The higher value, or systolic pressure, reflects the highest pressure in the arteries as the heart contracts. The lower value, or diastolic pressure, reflects the lowest pressure during the relaxation phase following a contraction. Blood pressure is written as systolic pressure/diastolic pressure; for example, 120/80 mm Hg (millimeters of mercury). This reading is referred to as "120 over 80." Although blood pressure today is often measured with automated monitors, it's useful to understand the standard method on which it's based.

Conventionally, blood pressure is measured with an inflatable cuff with a gauge (sphygmomanometer) to measure the pressure of blood flowing through the main artery in the arm. With a stethoscope placed over the artery below the cuff, a clinician inflates the cuff until it temporarily stops blood flow. Then the cuff is gradually deflated. When the pressure in the cuff equals the maximum pressure in the artery, the artery opens, and the sound of blood rushing through is amplified by the stethoscope. This is the systolic value. As the cuff pressure is reduced further, the sound suddenly becomes faint. This is the diastolic value.

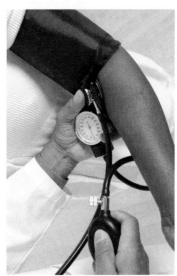

Hypertension is defined as a systolic pressure at rest that averages 140 mm Hg or higher, a diastolic pressure at rest that averages 90 mm Hg or higher, or both. As shown in Table 8.1, the higher the blood pressure, the greater the risks. In most people with hypertension, both systolic and diastolic pressures are high. Although hypertension can be successfully controlled, in most cases (over 90 percent of the time) its actual cause remains a medical mystery. This condition is formally known as *essential* or *primary hypertension.*

Hypertension is widespread in the U.S. population, affecting nearly one in three adults. Of those with hypertension, about 20 percent don't know they have it. A popular myth is that one can "sense or feel" when blood pressure is high. This is not true. Some folks believe that if they don't feel ill, they must be OK. In reality, hypertension has no symptoms for many years. This is why hypertension is known as the "silent killer."

A clinician measuring blood pressure using a sphygmomanometer and stethoscope.

© Comstock Images/Jupiterimages

High blood pressure, or **hypertension,** is a chronic elevation of blood pressure, defined as a systolic pressure of 140 mm Hg or higher and/or a diastolic pressure of 90 mm Hg or higher.

TABLE 8.1 CLASSIFICATION OF BLOOD PRESSURE

CATEGORY	SYSTOLIC (mm Hg)		DIASTOLIC (mm Hg)
Normal	<120	and	<80
Prehypertension	120–139	or	80–89
Hypertension			
Stage 1	140–159	or	90–99
Stage 2	≥160	or	≥100

Note: High blood pressure is not diagnosed based on a single reading. If an initial reading is high, a second reading should be taken a few minutes later. Elevated readings should then be confirmed in the other arm.

Source: *Seventh Report of the Joint National Committee on Prevention, Detection, Evaluation and Treatment of High Blood Pressure*, 2003.

Compared to people with normal blood pressure, those with uncontrolled hypertension have a two- to threefold greater risk of heart attack and a three- to fourfold greater risk of stroke. Other prominent risks include kidney damage and heart failure. Hypertension is more common in people who are obese and African Americans.

If you don't know your blood pressure or if it's been more than a year since it was checked, get a reading and record it. Everyone should know their numbers. Surprisingly, only about 50 percent of those with hypertension are effectively managing it. So, if you have hypertension, work out a personalized plan with your doctor to control it. There are a variety of approaches combining weight reduction, dietary changes, aerobic exercise, stress management, and drug therapy.

HIGH BLOOD CHOLESTEROL

A **high blood cholesterol** is another important modifiable risk factor. A total cholesterol value equal to or greater than 240 mg/dL (milligrams per deciliter of blood) is defined as high, putting a person at increased risk of atherosclerosis and thus heart attack, stroke, and peripheral arterial disease. Elevated cholesterol values can be due to many factors: a diet high in saturated fats, smoking, obesity, physical inactivity, and diabetes. Like hypertension, high cholesterol has no symptoms, and many people are unaware that they have the risk factor. About one out of four American adults has high blood cholesterol.

Cholesterol is transported through the circulatory system by combining with lipoprotein carriers that vary in size and weight. Low-density lipoprotein (LDL) cholesterol is readily deposited on arterial walls and is a major constituent of plaque. LDL cholesterol—the "bad" cholesterol—is the largest component of total cholesterol and the primary target for cholesterol-lowering treatment. Conversely, high-density lipoprotein (HDL) cholesterol functions in the opposite manner and prevents plaque buildup. Thus, HDL cholesterol is dubbed the "good" cholesterol. It is the only blood lipid in which higher levels are better.

High blood cholesterol, or hypercholesterolemia, is an abnormally elevated total cholesterol level (≥240 mg/dL) as measured from a blood sample.

The preferred blood test is a fasting lipoprotein profile that measures total blood cholesterol and its components: LDL cholesterol, HDL cholesterol, and triglycerides. Blood lipid values and associated risks are presented in Table 8.2. Notice the target values: total cholesterol less than 200 mg/dL, LDL cholesterol under 100, and HDL cholesterol 60 or greater.

One index of cardiovascular risk is determined from the ratio of total cholesterol to HDL cholesterol. Ratios range from 3 or less (e.g., 180/60), which would be low risk, to 10 or higher (e.g., 250/25), which would be high risk. An ideal target is to keep the total cholesterol well below 200, with the HDL cholesterol accounting for 30 percent or more.

Average ratios (total cholesterol/HDL cholesterol) are 3.3 to 3.8 for young men and 3.0 to 3.5 for young women. The more favorable ratio in women is due to their higher levels of HDL cholesterol, which is associated with the female hormone estrogen. This is one reason why women are at lower risk for heart disease and stroke through midlife. After menopause (as estrogen levels diminish), women lose this HDL cholesterol advantage, and the incidence of atherosclerotic diseases increases.

How do we decrease LDL cholesterol and increase HDL cholesterol? For those with borderline values, a prudent diet and aerobic exercise, respectively, are the first lines of action. If your LDL cholesterol is very high (>190 mg/dL), your doctor may prescribe drug therapy—using a class of drugs known as statins—to significantly lower the "bad" cholesterol.

Recent findings show one in five teenagers has abnormal lipid levels. Since 2011, the American Academy of Pediatrics has recommended all children be screened for high cholesterol between the ages of 9 and 11 years, and again between ages 17 and 21 years. If you have not had a lipid profile done within the past several years, get one. Know your numbers.

TABLE 8.2 CLASSIFICATION OF BLOOD LIPIDS

TOTAL CHOLESTEROL (mg/dL)	
<200	Desirable
200–239	Borderline high
≥240	High risk
LDL CHOLESTEROL (mg/dL)—PRIMARY TARGET OF THERAPY	
<100	Optimal
100–129	Near optimal
130–159	Borderline high
160–189	High risk
≥190	**Very high risk**
HDL CHOLESTEROL (mg/dL)	
<40	High risk
≥60	Cardioprotective

Source: *Third Report of the Expert Panel on Detection, Evaluation, and Treatment of High Blood Cholesterol in Adults,* 2004.

Health & the Media Health Messages That Inspire Action…Are You Ready?

Communicating health messages has broadened from awareness campaigns of risk factors and consequences of various conditions to motivating individuals to act in emergency situations. This advertisement delivers a simple, powerful narrative. Professional British footballer Fabrice Muamba, 26, suffered a sudden cardiac arrest during a routine football match in 2012. Thankfully, measures were in place to ensure he had the best chance of survival: not only was CPR administered on the scene, but an AED was on hand. When coupled with basic revival techniques, these measures increase the chance of survival tenfold, from 5% to 50%. We have a responsibility to ourselves—and others—when faced with a situation such as Fabrice's. Be ready to act, and act fast. Now is The Time.

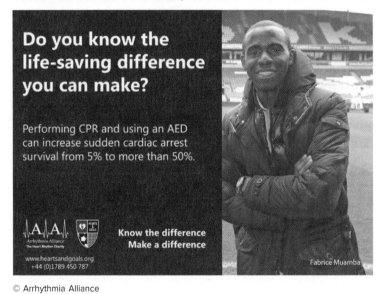

© Arrhythmia Alliance

INACTIVITY, OBESITY, AND DIABETES

Until the 1990s, the American Heart Association identified only three *major* risk factors that could be changed: cigarette smoking, high blood pressure, and high blood cholesterol. Other modifiable risk factors were described as *secondary* or *contributing* risk factors. However, as research evidence continued to mount, it became clear that several of the secondary risk factors were of similar importance as the first three. Accordingly, physical inactivity in 1992 and then obesity and diabetes in 1998 were upgraded to *major* risk factors.

Physical Inactivity

Article 8.2

Physical inactivity is an independent risk for heart attack and stroke. When inactivity is combined with overeating, obesity and diabetes can result. All contribute to

the development of atherosclerosis. Conversely, regular moderate-to-vigorous physical activity reduces the risk of heart and blood vessel diseases. Yet, only about 2
in 10 adults are active enough to achieve these health benefits. Or put another way,
8 in 10 are not engaging in sufficient levels of physical activity. Although any
increase in physical activity imparts some benefit, regularly engaging in moderate
activities (e.g., 30 minutes of brisk walking five days a week) is known to improve
cardiorespiratory function and lower the risk of cardiovascular disease. Physical
activity follows a dose-response curve—the more active you are, the better. Refer
to Chapter 3 for more information on exercise guidelines.

Obesity

People with excess body fat—particularly if the fat is in the waist/trunk area
(abdominal obesity)—are at higher risk of cardiovascular disease. Obesity also contributes to the development of other risk factors for atherosclerosis: high blood
pressure, high blood cholesterol, and diabetes. However, obesity puts people at
higher risk of cardiovascular disease even if they don't have other risk factors. One
in three American adults is obese (BMI $\geq$ 30). Losing excess body fat reduces a
person's risk for atherosclerosis as well as associated disorders. Even modest weight
loss (5 to 10 percent of body weight) can help significantly. Refer to the section on
healthy weight in Chapter 2 for information on safe and effective weight loss.

Diabetes

Persons with diabetes have a two- to sixfold higher risk for developing atherosclerosis than those without diabetes. Diabetes—a fasting blood glucose level of
126 mg/dL or higher—is a disease in which the body does not produce or respond
properly to insulin. The most common form—type 2 diabetes—develops during
middle age, although recent findings show onset is occurring at younger ages. Nine
percent of Americans aged 20 and older have diabetes and another 25 percent have
pre-diabetes (100–125 mg/dL). Most diabetics die from cardiovascular disease. Diabetes damages the blood vessels and is linked with low HDL cholesterol, high triglycerides, and high blood pressure. Women with diabetes are not protected from
atherosclerosis before menopause. Also, physical inactivity and weight (fat) gain
contribute to the development of diabetes. This dangerous combination of risk
factors—elevated blood sugar, abnormal blood lipids, high blood pressure, and
obesity—is called the *metabolic syndrome* (discussed in Chapter 10). Diabetes is
largely a preventable disease, but it is not reversible. Refer to Chapter 10 for an
expanded discussion on diabetes.

OTHER RISK FACTORS

Although not considered major risk factors, other factors are known to compromise
heart health. For example, some individuals have particularly intense cardiovascular responses (e.g., sharp spikes in heart rate and blood pressure) to stressful conditions. Under conditions of continual stress, this high "physiological reactivity"
can contribute to the development of atherosclerosis. People who score high on
personality traits of anger and hostility are also at higher risk. Such individuals,
primarily men, typically display an explosive temper or expect the worst from
people. This is damaging to their own health as well as unpleasant for those around
them. Third, drinking too much alcohol can raise blood pressure and triglycerides
and cause other cardiac problems as well as contributing to obesity, alcoholism,

suicide, and accidents. As a side note, moderate alcohol consumption has been shown to reduce cardiovascular risk by elevating HDL cholesterol. However, the evidence is not strong enough to recommend that teetotalers should begin drinking to improve their cardiovascular health!

Scientists continue to search for clues to early diagnosis of cardiovascular disease. Two promising blood tests include homocysteine, an amino acid associated with blood vessel damage, and lipoprotein(a), a subclass of LDL cholesterol. Two scanning tests include coronary artery calcification and carotid intima-media thickness. Research also continues on the role viruses and other infectious agents may play in the instigation and early stages of atherosclerosis. Specific biochemical markers may eventually lead to additional or better methods for predicting cardiovascular disease.

Self Assessments 8.1 & 8.2

To estimate your risk for heart disease and stroke, take the Self-Assessments. It may be eye opening to calculate risk profiles for a few relatives too—like a brother, sister, parent, or grandparent. To get a sense of what your cardiovascular health might be like in another 25 to 30 years, take a hard look at your parents. If you are concerned with what lies ahead, be proactive.

> ✓ **NEED TO KNOW**
>
> Major risk factors for heart disease and stroke are categorized as non-modifiable and modifiable. The three nonmodifiable risk factors are age, gender, and family history. The six modifiable risk factors are cigarette smoking, high blood pressure, high blood cholesterol, physical inactivity, obesity, and diabetes. Heart disease and stroke are largely preventable diseases.

➤ Interventions

The aim of this section is to provide a brief overview of the most common behavioral, pharmacological, and surgical approaches to reduce risk of heart attack and stroke and to treat atherosclerosis.

BEHAVIORAL APPROACH

If you have one or more of the six modifiable risk factors, the first step should be to consider lifestyle modification to reduce risk. Your primary care doctor will be glad to hear of your willingness to make healthful changes and will support you in developing an appropriate plan. Practical, science-based, online resources are cited throughout *iHealth* to help you break the smoking habit, improve eating and exercise patterns, and reach and maintain a healthy weight. If you plan these risk-lowering behavior changes on your own, it would be smart to consult with your physician before starting. It's important to have your doctor's support. Depending on your overall health status and risk profile, your doctor may feel it necessary to prescribe medications in conjunction with your steps to improve lifestyle behaviors.

Occasionally a doctor may not support a person's desire to improve health habits and may recommend relying solely on medications to control risk factors. This approach is not common, but it does occur. If the doctor's rationale is unclear, then get a second opinion. A time-honored principle in the practice of medicine is to do the patient no harm. This reminds us that—even in the 21st century, when drugs are available for nearly every known malady—medications should be used only as needed. If nondrug lifestyle changes are available and feasible, they should be tried first.

PHARMACOLOGICAL APPROACH

This overview focuses on the use of medicines and the importance of patient–doctor communication to break tobacco dependence or treat and control high blood pressure and abnormal blood lipids. Dozens of other cardiovascular drugs are available to treat a multitude of related conditions. While discussion of these is beyond the scope of *iHealth,* an excellent resource to learn about specific prescription and over-the-counter drugs is the *Physicians' Desk Reference* website (**www.pdrhealth.com/drug**).

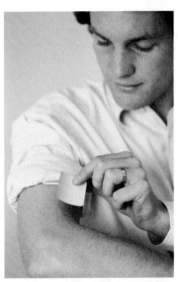

Nicotine replacement treatments via gum, inhaler, nasal spray, or patch are often prescribed for tobacco users who want to stop smoking, chewing, or dipping. Consult with your doctor about using nicotine or other drugs to help break the habit of tobacco dependence. He or she will gladly discuss drug treatment as well as counseling and behavioral options. Some doctors record history of tobacco use (i.e., current, former, never) as a vital sign along with their patients' pulse, blood pressure, temperature, and respiratory rate. If you use tobacco, talk to your doctor about stopping.

Drugs to treat and control high blood pressure and high blood cholesterol are two of the most common types of drugs prescribed in the United States. There are a variety of both antihypertensive drugs and LDL-cholesterol-lowering drugs available. Doctors have many choices regarding specific drugs and dosages. Yet, a major challenge to doctors is noncompliance; that is, patients not taking their medications. During

A nicotine patch can help a smoker quit by easing withdrawal symptoms.

© Stockdisc/PunchStock

initial drug treatment, many people abruptly stop taking medication due to unpleasant side effects and *do not follow up* with their doctor. It's critical for individuals to report side effects to their doctor so that adjustments can be made. Successful treatment depends on the patient and doctor working in partnership, with the patient taking an active role in his or her own health.

To be fair, noncompliance is understandable. Most patients with high blood pressure or high cholesterol feel fine. Yet, they are told that their condition must be treated. In turn, the prescribed medicines may make them feel odd or ill or disrupt their normal patterns—for example, they begin experiencing sluggishness, achiness, frequent trips to the toilet, difficulty sleeping, or a host of other side effects.

What is the solution? First, realize that, if left untreated, high blood pressure and abnormal blood lipids will cause significant health problems down the road. The damage caused by either of these conditions is cumulative and permanent. Second, be aware that if your doctor recommends drug therapy, side effects may occur. It may take several office visits over many months to find the right drug–dose combination. Work with your doctor to find a solution. If you know others who are having difficulty staying on their medicines, strongly encourage them to go back to their doctors.

SURGICAL APPROACH

Since the 1960s, coronary angiography, also known as *cardiac catherization,* has been the gold standard for determining the degree of blockage in the coronary arteries. After a series of initial diagnostic tests, angiography is typically performed when CHD is suspected. In this procedure, a tiny hollow tube or catheter is inserted into an artery in the arm or leg and guided to the heart, where a contrast dye is released and X-rays are taken. From the resulting images, the degree of atherosclerosis—the narrowing of the coronary arteries—can be measured. If severe blockage is present in one or more coronary arteries, the options are usually coronary angioplasty with stent placement or coronary artery bypass surgery.

Both types of surgery are amazingly common, remarkably safe, and, in the vast majority of cases, successful in restoring functional capacity and relieving symptoms such as chest pain (angina). However, if patients don't follow prescribed lifestyle changes and drug treatments after surgery, the benefits may be relatively short term. Some people find themselves back on the operating table a few years later for a second surgery. About 500,000 angioplasty procedures and 220,000 bypass surgeries are performed annually in the United States. That's about 1,400 angioplasties and 600 bypass surgeries per day, every day throughout the year, year after year!

Coronary Angioplasty

Coronary angioplasty, or balloon angioplasty, is technically known as *percutaneous coronary intervention (PCI)* (*percutaneous* means "through the skin"). This catheter-based procedure is performed to open up a blocked coronary artery and restore blood flow to the heart muscle. Angioplasty is preferred to bypass surgery as it is less invasive and faster. In fact, in most cases the patient remains awake and conscious during the entire procedure. Coronary angioplasty involves guiding a catheter (thin tube) through a large peripheral artery in the arm or leg into the aorta and eventually into the narrowed part of the artery (Figure 8.4).

A very thin wire tipped with an expandable balloon and stent is threaded across the blocked area (A). The balloon is inflated and deflated several times to compress the surrounding plaque and open the artery (B). The balloon is then deflated and the catheter removed, leaving the stent in place. The stent—a tiny, metal mesh tube—acts as a scaffold to keep the artery from closing again. The artery is now wider and blood can flow more easily (C). The patient usually returns home from the hospital within one to two days. During the next several weeks, the artery heals around the stent.

> **Coronary angioplasty** is a surgical procedure in which a balloon-tipped catheter is inserted into a diseased, narrowed coronary artery; inflation of the balloon stretches the vessel opening, improving blood flow through it. Also called *balloon angioplasty,* and technically known as *percutaneous coronary intervention.*

FIGURE 8.4 CORONARY ANGIOPLASTY WITH STENT

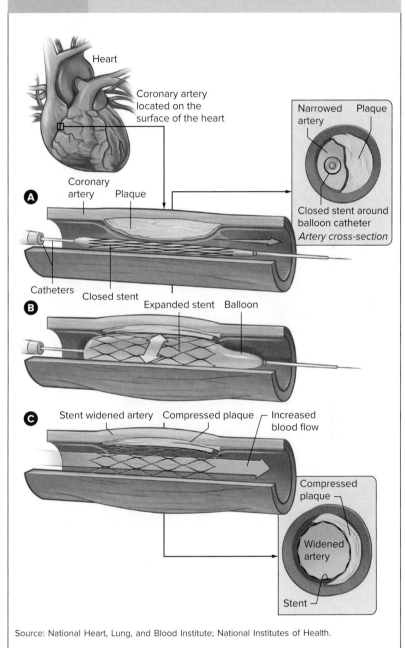

Source: National Heart, Lung, and Blood Institute; National Institutes of Health.

Coronary Artery Bypass Graft

Coronary artery bypass graft, commonly called *bypass surgery,* consists of grafting vessels taken from another part of the body (e.g., vein from leg or artery from chest wall) to a coronary artery and the aorta. Blood flow is thus rerouted, skipping over (bypassing) the narrowed or blocked area. In the traditional surgery, an incision is made down the center of the chest from the neck to the top of the stomach, and the breastbone is parted.

The patient is on a heart-lung machine, which adds oxygen to the blood and circulates blood to other parts of the body during the surgery. This open-heart surgery can take four to six hours depending on the number of blood vessels to be grafted. The modifier before *bypass*—for example, *triple* or *quadruple*—refers to the number of arteries that are bypassed. The hospital recovery stay is typically five to seven days (Figure 8.5).

FIGURE 8.5   CORONARY ARTERY BYPASS GRAFT

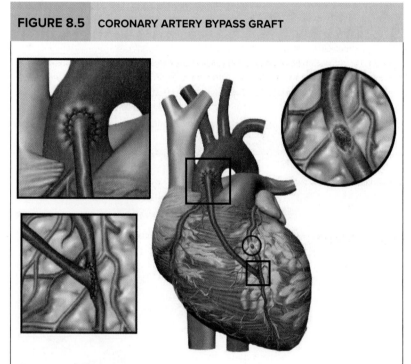

The cardiac surgeon uses a vein removed from the leg or an artery from inside the chest wall to provide a new path for blood flow from the aorta to the heart muscle.

Source: Blausen Images.

Coronary artery bypass graft, or bypass surgery, creates a new route around a significantly narrowed coronary artery or multiple diseased arteries using a vein from the leg or an inner chest-wall artery, permitting increased blood flow to deliver oxygen and nutrients to the heart muscle. Bypass surgery is one of the most commonly performed major operations.

Other surgical techniques and technologies are being used more frequently. One increasingly popular method, called *off-pump coronary artery bypass,* avoids use of the heart-lung machine. This operation allows the bypass to be created while the heart is still beating. Another less-invasive alternative is the use of smaller incisions that avoid splitting the breastbone. Last, some bypass procedures are being performed using surgeon-directed robotics.

Carotid Endarterectomy

Carotid endarterectomy is a related vascular surgery done to prevent strokes by removing plaque from the carotid arteries. The carotid arteries are located on each side of the neck and extend from the aorta to the base of the skull. Narrowed carotid arteries are diagnosed using medical imaging techniques. Although less well known and less frequently performed than angioplasty or bypass surgery, carotid endarterectomy is a common operation (over 100,000 per year) and a safe and long-lasting treatment.

The patient may be given a general anesthesia or, alternately, only the neck area may be numbed to allow the patient to communicate with the surgeon during the operation. The surgery involves making an incision to expose the narrowed carotid artery. The artery is temporarily clamped or bypassed, and another incision is made directly into the blocked section of the artery (Figure 8.6). The surgeon removes the plaque deposits, stitches the artery, removes the clamps or the bypass, and closes the neck incision. The procedure lasts about two hours. Following surgery, the average hospital stay is one or two days.

We have reviewed three of the most common cardiovascular surgeries. Surgical techniques are continually being modified and improved. Moreover, applications of new technologies are providing new options for removing arterial plaque—for example, miniaturized devices and tools using the latest laser, mechanical, and chemical technology.

Heart Transplants

As an endnote to this section on surgical approaches, let's consider the ultimate cardiovascular surgery—heart transplantation. For a few patients with advanced heart disease, it may represent the only option left. The first heart transplant was performed in 1967 in Groote Schuur Hospital, Cape Town, South Africa, by Professor Christiaan Barnard and his surgical team. It was a milestone in medicine. While the patient lived only 18 days, dying due to pneumonia, his new heart beat strongly to the end. Dr. Barnard showed the world that a human heart transplant was possible.

Half a century later, the science of organ transplantation is highly sophisticated and recipient outcomes are remarkably successful. Heart transplantation is performed at over 150 medical centers in the United States. Since 1990, there have been more than 2,100 heart transplants per year. Survival rates are about 90 percent for one year and 75 percent for five years. As expected, the costs are enormous—surgery and treatments for the first year are estimated to be about one million dollars.

Carotid endarterectomy is a surgical procedure in which a narrowed carotid artery is opened and the plaque is removed to restore adequate blood flow to the brain.

FIGURE 8.6 CAROTID ENDARTERECTOMY

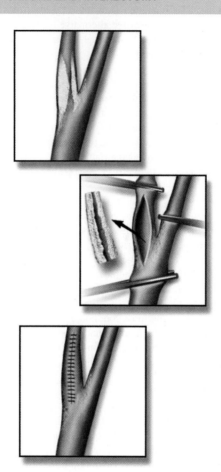

The sequence illustrates the surgical removal of plaque from a carotid artery.

Source: Blausen Images.

✓ NEED TO KNOW

Interventions to treat risk factors for heart disease and stroke can be categorized as behavioral, pharmacological, and surgical. Modifying lifestyle habits—the behavioral approach—is arguably the best. Motivation and perseverance are necessary, but the cost and side effects are minimal. Drugs are available to help people stop smoking and to control high blood pressure and abnormal blood lipids. Standard surgeries include angioplasty and bypass procedures to treat CHD and carotid endarterectomy to prevent stroke. Effective interventions may use combinations of behavioral, pharmacological, and surgical approaches.

➤ Prevention

Humans are intrigued with scientific and medical achievements. We are particularly dazzled by medical advances. The discovery of new drugs and the refinement of surgical techniques to treat cardiovascular disease are shining examples. With the constant highlighting of medical breakthroughs, we tend to minimize or overlook the enormous human pain and financial costs that come with heart disease and stroke—that is, until it strikes close to home.

No one purposely chooses a path that leads to disease and surgery, with the emotional and physical toll of the incisions, the tubes, and the pills. But by default, this is the path many follow. And more often than not, it leads to a life with limitations and loss of independence. In retrospect, many heart disease survivors encourage young people to pay attention to their health *now*. Don't wait until you're 40 or have a heart attack before you take stock of your lifestyle.

To gain insight into the emotional dimension and impact on quality of life, you should discuss the process of heart surgery with someone who has gone through it. A family member or a neighbor may be willing to share a firsthand account of the disease progression, surgery, and rehabilitation. Surgical options can indeed be lifesaving treatments. Yet, if one can prevent the need for surgery by following a healthy lifestyle, then the choice seems clear.

Article
8.3

Over 90 percent of those who develop atherosclerosis or experience a heart attack or stroke have one or more of the major risk factors. Science-based guidelines are available for all six of the modifiable risk factors. To keep your risk low, focus on these four behaviors: don't smoke, eat a prudent diet, exercise regularly, and maintain a healthy weight. And monitor your blood pressure, blood lipid profile, and blood glucose level and intervene as necessary to keep them in a healthy range. These goals are captured in the American Heart Association's campaign titled Life's Simple 7.

LIFE'S SIMPLE 7

1. Stop Smoking	5. Manage Blood Pressure
2. Eat Better	6. Control Cholesterol
3. Get Active	7. Reduce Blood Sugar
4. Lose Weight	

Note: Program developed by the American Heart Association.

Notable scientists assert that cardiovascular disease need not influence one's quality of life until the age of 80 or later. Esteemed cardiologist Dr. Paul Dudley White stated that "dying from cardiovascular disease nor sudden death itself are to be regretted, provided they take place at an advanced age after a healthy, happy, and useful life right up to the last minute."

✓ NEED TO KNOW

The big-picture message is clear: cardiovascular disease is largely preventable through our own actions. The lifestyle habits you establish now will have a bearing on whether or when you will face drug therapy and surgery in the years ahead. If the public were to adopt preventive measures, premature death and disability would decline markedly.

≡ connect Resources

ARTICLES

8.1 "Paul Dudley White, MD, Preventive Cardiologist and Exercise Advocate." Author Phil Sparling writes a profile on the father of American cardiology.

8.2 "Sedentary Behavior: Emerging Evidence for a New Health Risk." *Mayo Clinic Proceedings.* Prolonged sitting may have dire long-term health consequences distinct from those due to lack of regular exercise.

8.3 "Fewer Americans Than Ever Sticking to Heart-Healthy Lifestyle, Study Finds." *HealthDay.* The dilemma is many of us simply don't take care of ourselves.

SELF-ASSESSMENTS

8.1 Disease Risk Questionnaire for Heart Disease
8.2 Disease Risk Questionnaire for Stroke

Website Resources

American Heart Association **www.heart.org**
American Red Cross: CPR & AED Courses **www.redcross.org/take-a-class**
American Stroke Association **www.strokeassociation.org**
Heart Disease & Stroke Prevention (CDC) **www.cdc.gov/dhdsp**
Physicians' Desk Reference **www.pdrhealth.com/drugs**
Quit Smoking Today! **smokefree.gov**

Knowing the Language

Understanding the Content

1. Define *atherosclerosis, coronary heart disease,* and *stroke.*
2. How do the signs of a heart attack differ from those of a stroke?
3. What is the difference between a modifiable and a nonmodifiable risk factor? Provide examples of each.
4. Give an example of a behavioral, a pharmacological, and a surgical intervention to reduce risk for cardiovascular disease.

1. Assume you are walking across campus early one morning, and you see a person lying on the ground who appears to have passed out. What would you do?
2. Prescription drugs are available to control high blood pressure and abnormal blood lipids, yet many people stop taking their medicines. What are possible explanations? What are possible solutions?
3. What lifestyle behaviors will lower the likelihood that we develop atherosclerosis? Considering the modifiable risk factors, describe the key cardioprotective behaviors.

Selected References

American Academy of Pediatrics. 2014 recommendations for pediatric preventive health care. *Pediatrics* 133: 568–570, 2014.

American Heart Association. Cardiac Procedures and Surgeries. **www.heart.org/Procedures-and-Surgeries**

American Heart Association. Warning Signs of Heart Attack, Stroke and Cardiac Arrest. **www.heart.org/warning_signs**

Centers for Disease Control and Prevention. Heart Disease Fact Sheet. Atlanta, GA: CDC. **www.cdc.gov/dhdsp/data**

Centers for Disease Control and Prevention. Prevalence of abnormal lipid levels among youths—United States, 1999–2006. *MMWR* 59 (2): 29–33, 2010.

Centers for Disease Control and Prevention. Smoking and Tobacco Use. **www.cdc.gov/tobacco**

Eckel RH, Jakicic JM, Ard JD, et al. 2013 AHA/ACC guideline on lifestyle management to reduce cardiovascular risk. *Circulation* 129: S76–S99, 2014.

Framingham Heart Study: A Project of the National Heart, Lung and Blood Institute and Boston University. **www.framinghamheartstudy.org**

Go AS, Bauman MA, Coleman King SM, et al. An effective approach to high blood pressure control. *Hypertension* 63: 878–885, 2014.

Havranek EP, Mujahid MS, Barr DA, et al. Social determinants of risk and outcomes for cardiovascular disease. *Circulation* 132: 873–898, 2015.

Hurst JW. Meaningful quotations from Paul Dudley White. *Clinical Cardiology* 21: 617–618, 1998.

James PA, Oparil S, Carter BL, et al. 2014 evidence-based guideline for the management of high blood pressure in adults: Report from the panel members appointed to the Eighth Joint National Committee (JNC 8). *JAMA* 311: 507–520, 2014.

Kraus WE, Bittner V, Appel L, et al. The National Physical Activity Plan: A call to action from the American Heart Association. *Circulation* 131: 1932–1940, 2015.

Lear MW. *Heartsounds.* Pp. 11–12. New York: Simon & Schuster, 1980.

Meschia JF, Bushnell C, Boden-Albala B, et al. Guidelines for the primary prevention of stroke. *Stroke* 45: 3754–3832, 2014.

Mosca L, Benjamin EJ, Berra K, et al. Effectiveness-based guidelines for the prevention of cardiovascular disease in women—2011 update: A guideline from the American Heart Association. *Circulation* 123: 1243–1262, 2011.

Mozaffarian D, Benjamin EJ, Go AS, et al. Heart disease and stroke statistics—2015 update: A report from the American Heart Association. *Circulation* 131: e29–e322, 2015.

Neumar RW, Shuster M, Callaway CW, et al. 2015 AHA guidelines update for cardiopulmonary resuscitation and emergency cardiovascular care. *Circulation* 132: S315–S367, 2015.

Piscatella JC, Franklin BA. *Prevent, Halt, and Reverse Heart Disease: 109 Things You Can Do*. New York: Workman, 2011.

Seventh Report of the Joint National Committee on Prevention, Detection, Evaluation and Treatment of High Blood Pressure. *Hypertension* 42: 1206–1252, 2003.

Spring B, Ockene JK, Gidding SS, et al. Better population health through behavior change in adults. *Circulation* 128: 2169–2176, 2013.

Stone NJ, Robinson JG, Lichtenstein AH, et al. 2013 ACC/AHA guideline on the treatment of blood cholesterol to reduce atherosclerotic cardiovascular risk in adults. *Journal of the American College of Cardiology* 63: 2889–2934, 2014.

Third Report of the Expert Panel on Detection, Evaluation, and Treatment of High Blood Cholesterol in Adults. *Circulation* 106: 3143–3421, 2002.

World Health Organization and the Centers for Disease Control and Prevention. *The Atlas of Heart Disease and Stroke.* **www.who.int/cardiovascular_diseases**

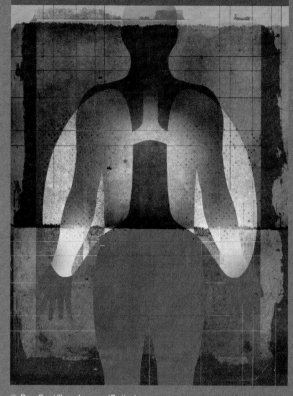

I know how scary cancer diagnosis can be—it was for me. But I beat cancer and I know we can turn tears of sorrow into tears of joy if we support this movement (Stand Up to Cancer).

—Sophia Vergara

© Roy Scot/Ikon Images/Getty Images

Chapter 9

CANCERS

In Chapter 9 we try to defuse the perception that cancer is synonymous with death. While people do die from cancer, there have been phenomenal advances in diagnosis and treatment. There is now hope where there was once none. This chapter discusses the basic disease process of cancer and also explains risks, prevention-oriented behaviors, early detection strategies, and treatment options.

Chapter 9 | CANCERS

Cancer
WHAT IS CANCER?

CANCER TERMINOLOGY

Causes of Cancer
HEREDITY

ENVIRONMENT

VIRUSES

LIFESTYLE

Diagnosing Cancer
EXAMINATIONS AND BIOPSIES

STAGING OF CANCER

Common Cancer Sites
BREAST CANCER

LUNG CANCER

COLON CANCER

PROSTATE CANCER

CERVICAL CANCER

TESTICULAR CANCER

LEUKEMIA

SKIN CANCER

Cancer Treatment
EARLY DETECTION AND PREVENTION

BATTLE* AND *LOST are two words often used by the media to describe people who have been diagnosed with cancer. In recent years, celebrities including Patrick Swayze, Farrah Fawcett, and Dennis Hopper all lost their battles with cancer: Patrick Swayze of pancreatic cancer at age 57; Farrah Fawcett of anal cancer at age 62; and Dennis Hopper of prostate cancer at age 74.

The word *win* is not usually used in describing surviving cancer; instead, the words *cancer-free* or *cancer survivor* are favored. The reason for this can be summarized by another well-known saying: You don't know you're cured until you die of something else. That's because there is always a chance for recurrence with cancer. So while celebrities such as Sheryl Crow, Melissa Etheridge, Kylie Minogue, Lance Armstrong, Ann Romney, Rod Stewart, Sofia Vergara, Christina Applegate, and Robert DeNiro have not necessarily "won" their battles with cancer yet, they have remained cancer-free and healthy since their treatments.

Reducing the impact of cancer is difficult because it requires proactive efforts on two fronts. People need to engage in healthy diet and behaviors throughout life to limit risk of developing cancer in the first place. Additionally, people should have regular screenings so in the event cancer does occur, it can be detected early and treated effectively. There are still many unknowns about why cancer strikes certain people and not others, and why some people respond better to treatment than others. But science continues to unravel these puzzles over time. Although the disease in Patrick Swayze, Farrah Fawcett, and Dennis Hopper followed the "traditional" pattern of late detection and a subsequently quick death, the good news is that more and more people are diagnosed with cancer early and respond favorably to treatments. Many become cancer-free after initial therapies and stay that way for the rest of their lives. And for others, cancer is not cured outright but is managed like a chronic disease, so that many people with cancer continue living productive lives despite being ill.

➤ Cancer

This year approximately 1,658,370 new cases of cancer will be diagnosed, and over 589,430 Americans will die from the disease. One in four deaths in the United States is attributable to cancer. The good news is that, according to the American Cancer Society, the five-year survival rate for all cancers increased from 49 percent in 1975–1977 to 68 percent in 2010. More people are surviving cancer because of education, early detection methods, and sophisticated treatment.

WHAT IS CANCER?

Cancer is a broad term that refers to the growth and spread of abnormal cells in the body. The cell is the basic unit of life. Cells that are alike group together and form tissue. Tissue makes organs, and organs make up body systems. There are nine major body systems: cardiovascular, respiratory, digestive, endocrine, skeletal, muscular, nervous, reproductive, and excretory.

Human cells have two major characteristics. They "survive" by dividing into new cells, and each type of cell has a specific function. For example, cells in the digestive system may secrete digestive enzymes, while those on the tongue may allow you to taste.

Cancer is the growth and spread of abnormal cells.

FIGURE 9.1 BODY STRUCTURE AND CANCER GROWTH

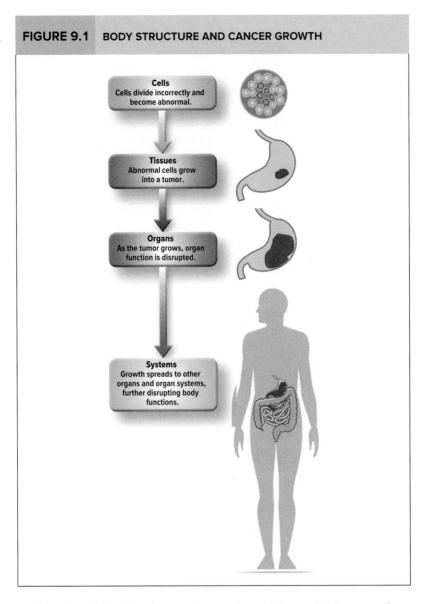

Normally cells divide and create the same types of tissues that they came from. But sometimes, something goes wrong in the division process. Two unhealthy cells derive from a normal one, and then those two cells continue creating more abnormal cells. The abnormal tissue created can make an organ unhealthy. Unhealthy organs will make a body system malfunction. Figure 9.1 represents the progression of cancer. If the process goes on unchecked, death can result.

CANCER TERMINOLOGY

A multitude of terms describe cancer and the disease process. The most basic ones are fairly simple. When a healthy cell becomes abnormal, it is said to mutate. Some

FIGURE 9.2 LOSS OF CONTROL OF NORMAL CELL GROWTH

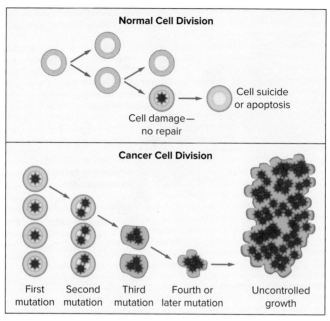

Source: National Cancer Institute "Understanding Cancer Series."

mutations lead to cancers, but not all do. An abnormal cell that is not cancerous is referred to as **dysplasia.**

Chemicals from outside the body that influence cells to grow in abnormal ways are known as *carcinogens.* On the other hand, within the body, some people have genes in their DNA that are known to be correlated with increased chance for certain types of cancers. These are referred to as **oncogenes.**

Finally, when cancer spreads from its point of origin to another area, the process is known as **metastasis.** For example, one might hear that the cancer has metastasized from the lungs to the bone, meaning that the cancer has spread from the lungs to the skeleton. Figures 9.2 and 9.3 show diagrammatic representations of all of these terms.

Mutation is the process by which a normal cell becomes abnormal.

Dysplasia is an abnormal cell that is not cancer.

An **oncogene** is a gene that increases the risk of cancer in a person who carries it.

Metastasis is the spread of cancer from its place of origin to somewhere else in the body.

FIGURE 9.3   METASTASIS

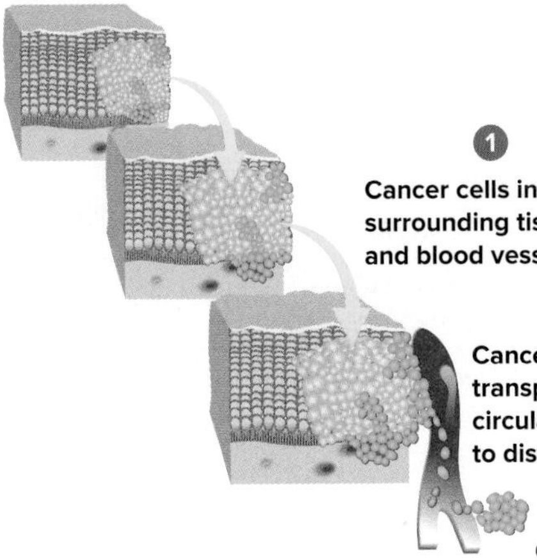

1 Cancer cells invade surrounding tissues and blood vessels

2 Cancer cells are transported by the circulatory system to distant sites

3 Cancer cells reinvade and grow at new location

Source: National Cancer Institute "Understanding Cancer Series."

When abnormal cells divide, they normally form a structure referred to as a *tumor*. A tumor is a stacking of cells, sometimes also called a *growth*. Tumors do not have to contain cancer cells—a benign tumor is a growth of normal cells, and a malignant tumor is a growth of cancer cells. It should be noted that just because something is referred to as *benign* doesn't necessarily mean it is not dangerous. Some benign tumors can significantly interfere with the function of an organ and body system and, as a result, can be life-threatening.

Often the terms *tumor* and *cyst* are used interchangeably, but this is incorrect. Cysts are a mass of cells with fluid in the center. Tumors have solid centers. Both, however, are growths. Another difference is that cysts are usually benign.

Tumors normally arise from certain types of body tissues and are named in a way that defines their origin. Tumor names also end with the suffix *-oma*. **Sarcomas** are tumors that arise from bone, cartilage, or muscle. **Lymphomas** originate in lymphatic tissue, and **carcinomas** arise from epithelial tissue, such as that in the skin, nose, and mouth. From a clinical perspective, the specific location of the tumor is often referred to when discussing the tumor. For example, the term *basal cell carcinoma* describes a tumor that is made up of basal cells found in skin.

A **sarcoma** is a tumor that arises in bone, cartilage, or muscle.

A **lymphoma** is a tumor that originates in lymphatic tissue.

A **carcinoma** is a tumor that arises from epithelial tissue.

➤ Causes of Cancer

Many factors influence cellular change over time. Like many diseases, cancer generally has more than one cause.

HEREDITY

There are 23 pairs of chromosomes in the nucleus of every cell in our body (except for red blood cells, sperm, and ova). **Deoxyribonucleic acid (DNA)** is the cellular molecule containing the genetic code that organisms need to function, and genes are made of DNA. Genes lie on the chromosomes and influence all sorts of body traits, from height and eye color to the propensity to develop certain types of cancers. If a person has a gene sequence that is linked with cancer, it usually means that at a certain point in a person's life, specific cells are more likely to grow abnormally than they would in a person without that oncogene.

In recent years health researchers have focused on decoding human DNA by mapping what different gene expressions do. Mapping the human genome is not a small task, because there are an estimated 20,000–25,000 genes in human DNA, with 3 billion chemical base pairs involved.

The alignment of the chemical base pairs spells out the genetic code, including disease. The Human Genome Project has estimated that there are about 1.4 million locations where single-base DNA differences occur in humans that seem to correlate with cancer and other diseases. The genetic sequences that are linked to a disease are sometimes referred to as "markers." In the case of cancer, having a marker does not mean the person will inevitably develop cancer. But it indicates that the person is at a much higher risk for developing a form of the disease if certain environmental variables are present. For example, people who have a marker for lung cancer but do not smoke have a low risk of lung cancer. If they do smoke, then their risk of lung cancer is very high—bigger than the risk of a smoker who doesn't have the lung cancer marker. Again, it is the marker combined with the unfavorable environment (via smoking) that greatly increases the overall chance for cancer.

Although it sounds like science fiction, someday we may be able to alter a problematic line of code in a person's DNA and eradicate hereditary-linked cancers. Until then, the best way to deal with what we may be genetically predisposed to is

Deoxyribonucleic acid (DNA) is the genetic code inside nearly all cells that gives instructions on how the cells will divide, grow, and function.

to be aware of the kinds of cancer that run in our family, to try to live a healthy lifestyle, and to get early and regular screenings to minimize risks.

ENVIRONMENT

Some chemicals in our environment can cause cancer. These substances are called **carcinogens.** Some of the more common ones include sulfur dioxide, arsenic, asbestos, benzene, chromium, radon, soot, tar, vinyl chloride, wood dust, and ultraviolet light.

Sulfur dioxide is a product of combustion engines and is a component in air pollution. Exposure to sulfur dioxide over time can cause cell mutations that contribute to the development of lung cancer. Arsenic is found in pesticides and has been linked to lung, skin, and liver cancer. Asbestos, a risk factor for lung cancer, was once a key chemical in glues, home insulation, and tile products. As a result, many construction workers who worked before asbestos was outlawed in the late 20th century were put at risk for cancer. Similarly, petroleum workers are often exposed to benzene, which has been linked to leukemia, and metal workers must deal with exposure to chromium, a chemical that increases the risk of lung cancer.

Radon is an underground gas found in geological pockets in many parts of the United States. It can leak through the foundation of homes unnoticed because it has no odor. Prolonged exposure to radon can increase the risk of lung cancer. Excessive soot and tar exposure, such as that experienced by industrial workers, has been linked to lung, skin, and liver cancers. Frequent exposure to wood dust has been associated with nasal cancer. Finally, exposure to ultraviolet light from the sun is strongly related to the development of skin cancer.

Again, it is important to note that exposure doesn't automatically mean disease. But people who have high levels of exposure to carcinogens run greater than average risks for developing certain cancers, and the longer the duration of exposure, the higher the probability of getting cancer. Environmental health specialists are very skilled at implementing ways to reduce exposure, so although an occupation may be risky, certain precautions like protective masks, sunscreen, or special clothing can help minimize harmful exposures.

VIRUSES

Viruses are microorganisms that invade other organisms and use their cellular materials to replicate itself. (A more detailed explanation of viruses is in Chapter 11.) Since cancer involves abnormal replication of body cells, it makes sense that if viruses are capable of disrupting the genetic mechanisms in cells, their process might be a contributing factor to cancer. Fortunately, only a few viruses are thought to actually cause cancer.

Herpes virus 2, the most common form of genital herpes, can affect cervical cells and increase a woman's risk of cervical cancer. The same holds true for women infected with human papillomavirus (HPV). Hepatitis B affects liver cells and may increase the risk of liver cancer. Epstein-Barr virus (EBV), the cause of mononucleosis, increases the risk of lymphoma, and human T-cell lymphotrophic virus is related to leukemia.

A **carcinogen** is a chemical or substance in the environment that can cause cancer in someone who is exposed to it.

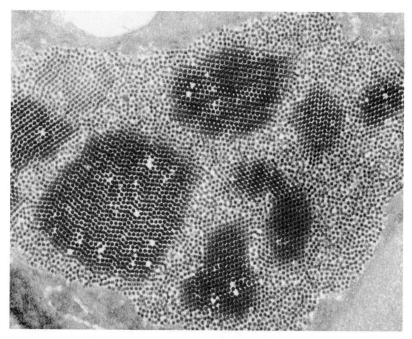

The human papillomavirus (HPV) is a leading cause of cervical cancer in women. Pap smear tests are important screening tools in finding abnormal cells early.
© Steve Gschmeissner & Carol Upton/Science Source

People who have been infected with cancer-linked viruses should be monitored closely. For example, a woman with a herpes 2 infection should have Pap smears more frequently than a woman who isn't infected with herpes 2. Understanding the early signs of related cancers is important so people can seek medical help early, if necessary. A more thorough discussion about herpes and HPV, including the issues surrounding Gardasil, the vaccine for HPV, can be found in Chapter 11.

LIFESTYLE

As with so many diseases, the everyday choices we make can influence our risk for cancer. Lifestyles are a key factor in the etiology of many common cancers. Tobacco use is strongly implicated in the development of lung cancer. People who smoke 30 cigarettes or more each day have a 15 times greater risk of developing lung cancer than nonsmokers. Even smoke that nonsmokers inhale—secondhand smoke—can increase the risk of lung cancer. Additionally, combining cigarettes and alcohol increases the risk of cancer of the esophagus. People who drink more than four drinks a day and smoke have a 40 times greater chance of developing cancer of the esophagus than people who don't combine heavy alcohol consumption with smoking.

Self Assessment 9.1

Meat consumption and colon cancer are also related. The higher the consumption of red meat, the greater the risk of colon cancer. The population of the United States consumes large amounts of red meat and has one of the highest incidences of cancer of the colon. Specific information regarding reducing one's risk will be discussed later in the chapter.

➤ Diagnosing Cancer

Diagnosing cancer requires an examination of cells to determine if they are normal or malignant (cancerous). The protocol for diagnosis involves the same steps used for identifying any disease. It begins when people explain their medical history, describe their symptoms, and are examined by a medical professional.

EXAMINATIONS AND BIOPSIES

When people have physical symptoms that are of concern, they usually visit a physician who asks about the severity of symptoms and the length of time they have been occurring. The physician performs physical examinations to determine health status, such as listening to the heart and lungs and measuring blood pressure. This examination may reveal suspicious findings that require further testing.

In the case of cancer, further testing can include examinations with imaging technologies such as X-rays, CT scans, or MRIs (see Chapter 12 for more explanation of some of these technologies). Some cancers leave traces in the blood, so tests may also be conducted on blood samples. For example, if a man has prostate cancer, his blood might have high levels of prostate specific antigen (PSA).

If something looks abnormal in blood work or a scan image, a biopsy is performed. A **biopsy** is the removal and examination of a segment of the abnormal tissue or tumor. The cells are examined to determine if they are benign or malignant. Biopsies can be performed in a range of ways. The least invasive type is with a needle inserted into the tumor, which draws out cells for study. Other times, surgery may be needed to obtain a tissue sample. Most biopsies are uncomfortable but not usually highly painful.

STAGING OF CANCER

Once cells are determined to be malignant, the next step is to determine how serious and advanced the malignancy is. In other words, how deep is the cancer and

Biopsy is the removal and testing of a sample of cells or tissue to look for abnormalities.

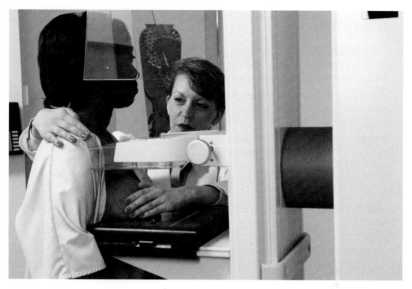

Mammograms are X-rays used to detect breast cancer.
© Keith Brofsky/Getty Images

has it metastasized? **Staging** is the term used to determine how invasive the cancer is. There are three types of staging: tumors (*T*), nodes (*N*), and metastasis (*M*). *T, N,* and *M* values are assigned after the diagnosis of cancer.

If a tumor cannot be measured or found, then it is called *TX*. When there is no evidence of a primary tumor, a *T0* is noted, which means that cancer has been diagnosed, but the tumor has not been found. If the tumor has not started to grow into the surrounding tissues, then it is staged as *Tis*. Finally, *T1–T4* are used to describe the size and invasiveness of the tumor, with *T4* being the largest and most invasive.

N staging is also important because if the cancer has spread from the tumor to the lymph nodes, it very possibly has spread to other parts of the body, too. The notations in *N* staging include *NX, N0, N1, N2,* and *N3. NX* means that nearby lymph nodes cannot be measured. When the nearby lymph nodes don't contain cancer, an *N0* is assigned. *N1, N2,* and *N3* refer to the size, location, and number of lymph nodes involved. The higher the *N* value, the more lymph nodes involved and the more dangerous the cancer is.

M staging is used to describe the extent of metastasis of the cancer. Only three stages are used: *MX, M0,* and *M1. MX* means metastasis cannot be measured or found. *M0* means that there is no known distant metastases, and *M1* means metastases are present.

The evaluation of *TNM* will determine the course of treatment. As a general rule, the worse the *TNM* staging, the more intense the treatment. For people who are diagnosed with cancer, the staging they want to hear or see on their medical chart is *TX, NX, MX.*

Staging is a description of the size and spread of a cancer.

NEED TO KNOW

Diagnosing cancer is a complex and sophisticated process. Depending on the type of suspected cancer, a diagnosis may involve physical exams, X-rays, blood evaluation, and biopsy. Cancer must be staged, or rated, for an effective treatment plan to be devised. Staging describes three factors: whether a tumor has been found, if the original cancer has been discovered in lymph nodes as well, and if metastasized cancer can be found outside the original cancer site. Cancer tumors that are small and have not spread are the easiest to treat successfully.

➤ Common Cancer Sites

Any cell in the body has the potential to become cancerous. Figures 9.4 and 9.5 show the estimated cancer incidences and deaths by gender for 2015. It will be quickly noticed that the more common sites for cancer to develop include the breast, lung, colon, prostate, cervix, testicles, blood, and skin. We will examine these kinds of cancers with respect to signs and symptoms, risk factors, early detection, and treatment.

FIGURE 9.4   ESTIMATED CANCER CASES BY GENDER

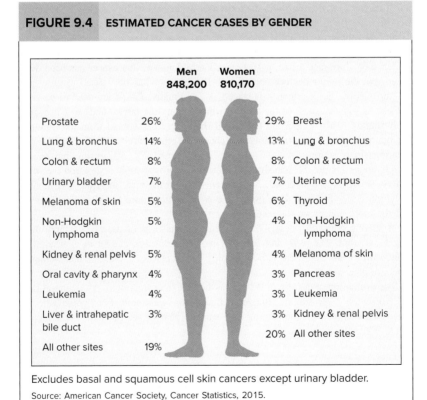

	Men 848,200	Women 810,170	
Prostate	26%	29%	Breast
Lung & bronchus	14%	13%	Lung & bronchus
Colon & rectum	8%	8%	Colon & rectum
Urinary bladder	7%	7%	Uterine corpus
Melanoma of skin	5%	6%	Thyroid
Non-Hodgkin lymphoma	5%	4%	Non-Hodgkin lymphoma
Kidney & renal pelvis	5%	4%	Melanoma of skin
Oral cavity & pharynx	4%	3%	Pancreas
Leukemia	4%	3%	Leukemia
Liver & intrahepatic bile duct	3%	3%	Kidney & renal pelvis
		20%	All other sites
All other sites	19%		

Excludes basal and squamous cell skin cancers except urinary bladder.

Source: American Cancer Society, Cancer Statistics, 2015.

FIGURE 9.5   ESTIMATED CANCER DEATHS BY GENDER

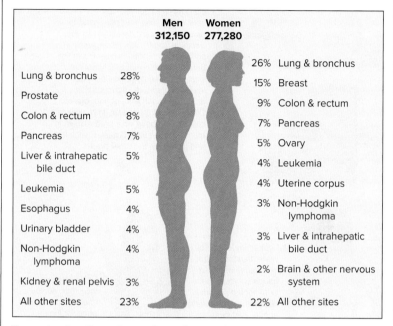

	Men 312,150	Women 277,280	
Lung & bronchus	28%	26%	Lung & bronchus
Prostate	9%	15%	Breast
Colon & rectum	8%	9%	Colon & rectum
Pancreas	7%	7%	Pancreas
Liver & intrahepatic bile duct	5%	5%	Ovary
Leukemia	5%	4%	Leukemia
Esophagus	4%	4%	Uterine corpus
Urinary bladder	4%	3%	Non-Hodgkin lymphoma
Non-Hodgkin lymphoma	4%	3%	Liver & intrahepatic bile duct
Kidney & renal pelvis	3%	2%	Brain & other nervous system
All other sites	23%	22%	All other sites

Source: American Cancer Society, Cancer Statistics, 2015.

BREAST CANCER

Of the estimated 230,000 new cases of breast cancer each year, 99 percent are found in women and less than 1 percent are in men. Breast cancer is the most common form of cancer diagnosed among women and the second most common site for cancer deaths in women. The most common symptoms of breast cancer are a lump in the breast or changes in the nipple. Although most lumps are benign, lumps still remain the most common symptom of breast cancer. Other symptoms include breast swelling, tenderness, nipple pain and/or dimpling, and nipple discharge. Any of these symptoms warrant immediate medical evaluation.

Like most cancers, the causes are unknown. Risk factors include a family history, a long menstrual history including periods that started early and ended late in life, obesity after menopause, postmenopausal hormone therapy, never bearing children, and having a first child after age 30. None of these events are strongly enough correlated with cancer to conclude cause and effect, but they are factors that increase one's relative risk.

Early detection of breast cancer is key to survival. The simplest early detection method is breast self-examination performed once a month. Women who properly practice self-examinations have a higher probability of identifying a lump or tumor so that less invasive procedures can be used to remove the lump. Figure 9.6 shows the proper procedures for examinations.

Mammography is a type of X-ray examination of the breast. If a lump or mass is seen in the X-ray image, it will be biopsied. Unless directed by a physician, the

FIGURE 9.6   BREAST SELF-EXAMINATION

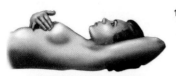

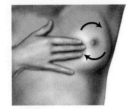

1. Lie down and put your left arm under your head. Use your right hand to examine your left breast. With your 3 middle fingers flat, move gently in small circular motions over the entire breast, checking for any lump, hard knot, or thickening. Use different levels of pressure - light, medium, and firm - over each area of your breast. Check the whole breast, from your collarbone above your breast down to the ribs below your breast. Switch arms and repeat on the other breast.

2. Look at your breasts while standing in front of a mirror with your hands on your hips. Look for lumps, new differences in size and shape, and swelling or dimpling of the skin.

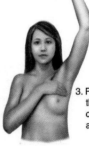

3. Raise one arm, then the other, so you can check under your arms for lumps.

4. Squeeze the nipple of each breast gently between your thumb and index finger. Report to your healthcare provider right away any discharge or fluid from the nipples or any lumps or changes in your breast.

general medical consensus is that all women should begin yearly mammograms at age 40. The earlier the breast cancer is detected, the less intense the treatment. If the cancer hasn't invaded other tissue or the lymph nodes, then all that may be necessary is a lumpectomy (removal of the growth). If the cancer is more advanced, then removal of the affected breast, called *mastectomy,* might be necessary. In addition to surgery, there may be a need for follow-up chemotherapy and/or radiation, both of which will be discussed in the section on cancer treatment.

LUNG CANCER

Lung cancer accounts for approximately 14 percent of the new cases of cancer, or about 221,200 cases annually. It is the second most commonly diagnosed cancer among both men and women, and it is also the most typical site for cancer deaths among both genders. The most frequent symptoms for lung cancer include persistent cough, sputum streaked with blood, chest pain, and recurring bouts with respiratory infections, such as pneumonia and bronchitis.

Lung cancer tumors can grow and spread without symptoms. Unfortunately, lung cancer has a lower rate of survival than other cancers, mostly because it is usually discovered late. By the time a tumor is visible on an X-ray, it is well advanced.

The most important risk factor for lung cancer is cigarette smoking. Other risk factors include exposure to secondhand smoke and to carcinogenic environmental chemicals. Although family history is always an important variable in the development of cancer, lung cancer is clearly more related to environmental exposure.

Chest X-rays, analysis of cells in sputum, and fiber-optic examination of the bronchial passages are detection methods. Unfortunately, they are not very effective for early detection. Treatment options include surgery, chemotherapy, and radiation.

Article 9.1

COLON CANCER

Approximately 93,090 cases of colon cancer are diagnosed each year in the United States. It is the third most common cancer, in both incidence and mortality, for both men and women. The most typical symptoms are rectal bleeding, blood in the stool, change in bowel habits, and cramping pain in the lower abdomen. Unfortunately, there are no early signs of the disease.

The major risk factors for colon cancer include family history, colon polyps, inflammatory bowel disease, low-fiber diet, obesity, and a diet high in saturated fat and red meats.

Because there are no early signs of colon cancer, the emphasis is on early detection. Early detection can be done through a number of procedures. The simplest is a noninvasive procedure to determine if there is blood in the stool. Another procedure is an endoscopic exam called a *colonoscopy*; the person is given a sedative, and a scope is inserted deep into the bowel so that the bowel wall can be examined for cancer. An endoscopic exam is recommended for all adults over 50 years of age.

Treatment for colon cancer can range from removal of the tumor to removal of sections of the colon. It depends on how advanced the cancer is. Follow-up with chemotherapy and radiation may also be necessary.

PROSTATE CANCER

Prostate cancer is the most commonly diagnosed cancer among men and typically affects men over 50 years of age. Many experts say that, like women's risk of breast cancer, if men live long enough, they will eventually develop prostate cancer. Approximately 220,800 new cases of prostate cancer are diagnosed each year.

Like many other of the cancers discussed, symptoms usually occur in the advanced stages. The common symptoms include weak or interrupted urine flow, inability to urinate, need to urinate frequently, blood in the urine, pain or burning with urination, and pain in the lower back, pelvis, or upper thighs. Symptoms usually mean the cancer has spread.

Risk factors for prostate cancer are age, ethnicity, and family history. The older a man is, the greater the risk. More than 70 percent of all prostate cancer cases are diagnosed in men older than 65. African American men have the highest prostate cancer rates in the United States.

Treatment options for prostate cancer usually include surgery, chemotherapy, and radiation. In early stage prostate cancer, radioactive seed implants can be inserted into the prostate to shrink the tumor. However, some prostate cancers are slow growing, and if a man is quite old, the cancer may be monitored and not removed because it might not present a threat to life and health.

CERVICAL CANCER

The cells of the cervix are susceptible to mutation especially with the presence of certain viruses such as HPV. Cervical cells can change and over time mutate into cancer cells without a woman experiencing other symptoms. Approximately 12,900 new cases of cervical cancer are diagnosed each year.

Symptoms of cervical cancer don't usually occur until the abnormal cervical cells invade surrounding vaginal and cervical tissue. Then, the symptoms are usually abnormal vaginal bleeding and vaginal discharge. The main risk factor for cervical cancer is infection with HPV. Also, women who had sexual intercourse at an early age or who have had multiple partners are also at higher risk.

The Pap test is the most common early detection measure used to determine the health of the cervical cells and the first indication of cancer. A Pap test consists of a swab of cervical cells that are examined under a microscope. A trained lab technician can distinguish between healthy cells and cancer cells. Sometimes a Pap test will be reported as dysplasia. This term describes cells that aren't normal, yet aren't cancer either. Women with dysplasia are monitored more closely and have Pap tests more often. If cervical cancer is diagnosed, then surgery, chemotherapy, and radiation are most likely to follow.

TESTICULAR CANCER

Testicular cancer is called a young man's cancer because the majority of the almost 8,430 diagnosed cases each year occur in men 20–40 years of age. Like other cancers, testicular cancer in the early stages has no specific symptoms. A common symptom is a lump in the testicle. The lump may or may not be painful. Testicular swelling, hardness, and a feeling of heaviness or aching in the scrotum or lower abdomen are other possible symptoms of testicular cancer.

Article
9.2

Risk factors for testicular cancer are not clearly understood. Undescended testicles are the major risk factor. In the absence of risk factor information, the key is early detection. The American Cancer Society recommends that men, especially between the ages of 20 and 40, practice testicular self-examination (TSE) once each month. Figure 9.7 highlights the simple TSE procedures.

Treatment for testicular cancer can range from chemotherapy to removal of the testicular lump to removal of the testicle or both testes.

LEUKEMIA

When blood cells mutate and become cancerous, **leukemia** can result. Approximately 54,270 new cases of all forms of leukemia are diagnosed each year. Acute

Leukemia is a type of cancer that occurs when blood cells mutate and become cancerous.

FIGURE 9.7   TESTICULAR SELF-EXAMINATION

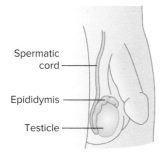
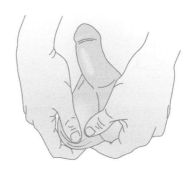

Spermatic cord

Epididymis

Testicle

Self-Exam

It's best to do a TSE during or right after a hot shower or bath. The scrotum (skin that covers the testicles) is most relaxed then, which makes it easier to examine the testicles.

1. Use both hands to gently roll each testicle (with slight pressure) between your fingers. Place your thumbs over the top of the testicle, with the index and middle fingers of each hand behind the testicle, and then roll it between your fingers.
2. You should be able to feel the epididymis (the sperm-carrying tube), which feels soft and ropelike and is slightly tender to pressure; it is located at the top of the back part of each testicle. This is a normal lump.
3. Remember that one testicle (usually the right one) is slightly larger than the other for most men—this is also normal.
4. When examining each testicle, feel for any lumps or bumps along the front or sides. Lumps may be as small as a grain of rice or a pea.
5. If you notice any swelling, lumps, or changes in the size or color of a testicle, or if you have any pain or achy areas in your groin, let your doctor know right away.

Lumps or swelling may not be cancer, but they should be checked by your doctor as soon as possible. Testicular cancer is almost always curable if it is caught and treated early.

Source: "How to Perform a Testicular Self-Exam" from TeensHealth.org. This information was reprinted with permission from KidsHealth, one of the largest resources online for medically reviewed health information written for parents, kids, and teens. For more articles like this one, visit **www.KidsHealth.org** or **www.TeensHealth.org**. Copyright: 1995–2011. The Nemours Foundation/KidsHealth.

leukemia is the major form affecting children, and its symptoms appear quickly. Chronic leukemia is the major form affecting adults and is characterized by a slow progression of symptoms.

The major signs of leukemia are fatigue, paleness, weight loss, repeated infections, fever, bruising easily, nosebleeds, and other hemorrhages. Some of these symptoms are common to other conditions as well, making the diagnosing of leukemia difficult. The major risk factors for leukemia include exposure to environmental carcinogens, radiation, and specific types of viruses.

Other than paying close attention to ongoing fatigue, weight loss, and other symptoms with a follow-up diagnosis, there is no early detection method. Blood tests in suspect patients can indicate leukemia, and sometimes a bone marrow biopsy might be needed to examine bone marrow for cancer cells.

SKIN CANCER

Skin cancer is an epidemic. There are over 5 million cases of skin cancer diagnosed in the United States each year. The good news is that most skin cancer is curable if detected early. Symptoms of skin cancer are more ambiguous than other forms of cancer discussed because the symptoms are mostly changes on the skin, so one has to notice those changes.

There are three major types of skin cancer. **Basal cell carcinoma** usually appears as flat, firm, pale areas of the skin or as small, raised, pink or red shiny areas. **Squamous cell carcinoma** appears as growing lumps with a rough surface or as flat, red patches that grow slowly. **Malignant melanoma** represents approximately 2 percent of all skin cancers diagnosed but the majority of deaths due to skin cancer, so it is considered the most dangerous of the skin cancers.

Article
9.3

Malignant melanoma, the fifth and seventh most common form of cancer diagnosed in males and females, respectively, is very aggressive, and the incidence is rising faster than any other cancer in the United States. Malignant melanoma appears as an unusual mole, and if untreated it will grow deep into the body and metastasize. Melanomas appear asymmetrical—that is, one side doesn't match the other. They also tend to have irregular borders and wide variation in colors including yellow, green, and red tinges. Finally, the size of melanomas tends to be more than 6 mm (¼ in.), or about the size of a pencil eraser.

Self
Assessment
9.2

The chief risk factor for malignant melanoma is exposure to the sun. It is estimated that 86 percent of melanomas are related to ultraviolet (UV) exposure. There are three major forms of UV rays, called UV-A, UV-B, and UV-C. All forms of ultraviolet light are found in the sun's rays, and when the rays reach the skin, they traumatize it. The skin responds by secreting pigment, which is what causes a suntan. So a suntan is not a sign of health but rather a sign of the skin trying to protect itself from damage. Tanning booths are also a source of UV rays (see "Breaking It Down" on the safety of tanning booths).

Early detection for malignant melanoma uses an A, B, C, D, and E screening. A stands for "asymmetrical." Symmetrical moles are usually not melanoma, which have irregular edges. Likewise, the borders (B) of the moles observed should be round, not irregular. The color (C) of a malignant melanoma is not brown, but might be brownish, red, yellow, or green. It does not look like a typical, common brown mole. A malignant melanoma will have a diameter (D) more than 6 mm or the size of a pencil eraser. Finally, E refers to evolving, meaning that a mole is starting to

Basal cell carcinoma is a flat, firm, pale area of the skin or a small, raised, pink or red shiny area.

Squamous cell carcinoma appears as a growing lump with a rough surface or as a flat, red patch that grows slowly.

Malignant melanoma is the most dangerous form of skin cancer because it is fast growing and can metastasize quickly.

FIGURE 9.8   IDENTIFYING MALIGNANT MELANOMA

Normal		Cancerous
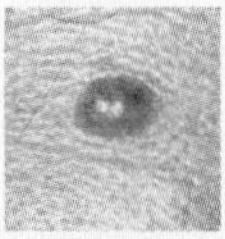	**"A" is for Asymmetry** • If you draw a line through the middle of the mole, the halves of a melanoma won't match in size.	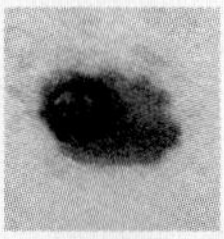
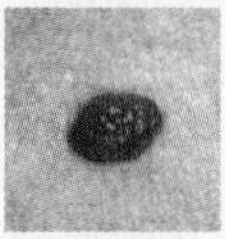	**"B" is for Border** • The edges of an early melanoma tend to be uneven, crusty, or notched.	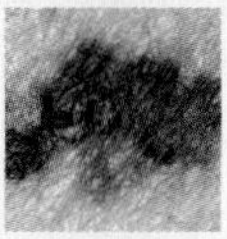
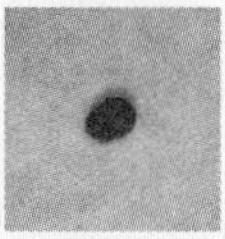	**"C" is for Color** • Healthy moles are uniform in color. A variety of colors, especially white and/or blue, is bad.	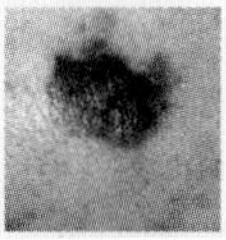
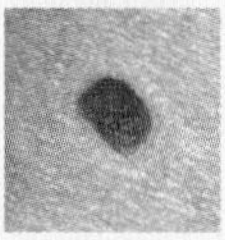	**"D" is for Diameter** • Melanomas are usually larger in diameter than a pencil eraser, although they can be smaller.	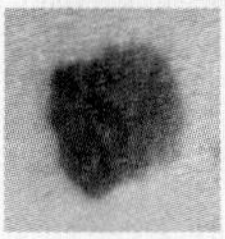
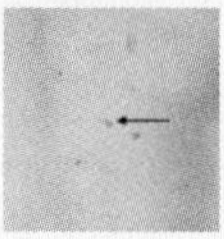	**"E" is for Evolving** • When a mole changes in size, shape, or color, or begins to bleed or scab, this points to danger.	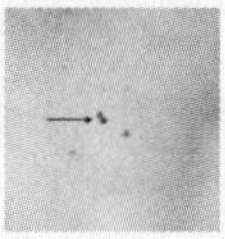

© The Skin Cancer Foundation.

change. If any mole on the body has abnormal characteristics of *A, B, C, D,* or *E,* a follow-up evaluation is necessary. Figure 9.8 shows the *A, B, C, D, E* of identifying malignant melanoma.

Treatment for malignant melanoma is like that for other cancers: surgery, chemotherapy, and radiation. Generally speaking, the earlier a melanoma is diagnosed, the better the outcome. If found in the early stages, then all that may be necessary for treatment is the removal of the mole.

In spring–summer 2012 the Food and Drug Administration (FDA) implemented new sunscreen regulations. The aim of the new regulations is to educate the consumer on the benefits or lack of benefits in using a particular sunscreen. The following are among the new regulations:

• Broad-spectrum-labeled sunscreens must provide protection from both UV-A and UV-B radiation.
• Those products with an SPF (sun protection factor) of 15 or higher can make the claim that they protect against skin cancer if used as directed with other sun protection measures.
• Sunscreens with an SPF of 2–14 are required to have a warning stating that the product has not been shown to help prevent skin cancer or early aging.

Breaking It Down Are Tanning Booths Safe?

Studies show that more than 2 million new cases of skin cancer will be diagnosed in the United States this year and that over 10,000 deaths will be traced to skin cancer in the same time period. Exposure to the sun is the major risk factor associated with the development of skin cancer, especially the deadliest skin cancer, melanoma. Approximately 28 million Americans visit tanning booths each year, and many assume that tanning booths are safer than regular sun exposure. Is this a correct assumption?

In fact, tanning booths are not safer than the sun. Booth equipment doesn't emit much UV-B light, which is what causes surface damage and sunburns. Instead, booths emit mostly UV-A light, which penetrates deeper into the skin and can damage internal organs or a person's DNA. UV-A exposure can increase the risk of melanoma.

A case in point. Anna Tremblay was a student at James Madison University in Virginia. She used tanning booths frequently, feeling it was a "social thing to do." Just before her senior year, she noticed a mole on her lower hip. After a trip to the dermatologist and a biopsy, she was diagnosed with melanoma.

Anna then had surgery to remove a large section of tissue from the area around the melanoma as well as other suspicious areas on the waist. According to Anna, her whole midsection "was just completely cut up. It was horrible." In the next four years she had two other melanomas diagnosed and treated. The good news is that Anna is a cancer survivor—however, because of her overuse of tanning booths, she now has to visit a dermatologist every six months for the rest of her life.

According to the Skin Cancer Foundation,

- UV light is a proven human carcinogen.
- Exposure to tanning beds before age 35 increases melanoma risk by 75 percent.
- People who use tanning beds are 2.5 times more likely to develop squamous cell carcinoma.
- Occasional use of tanning beds almost triples the chances of developing melanoma.

Yes, tanning booths can be found anywhere—spas, shopping malls, hotels. Just because they are abundant doesn't mean they are safe. For years the American Cancer Society and other groups have been very vocal regarding the dangers of tanning booths. Finally, there has been a response. President Bush signed the Tanning Accountability and Notification Act (TAN Act), which gives the Food and Drug Administration the authority to regulate tanning equipment including language used on warning labels. Expect to see the public's view of the safety of tanning booths change to regarding them as a high-risk behavior in the next few years.

- The terms *sunblock, sweatproof,* and *waterproof* can no longer be included on sunscreen labels.
- A sunscreen can claim to be water resistant, but the product must specify it offers 40 or 80 minutes of protection while swimming or sweating. Sunscreens that are not water resistant must include a direction instructing consumers to use a water-resistant sunscreen if swimming or sweating.
- Sunscreens cannot claim to provide sun protection for more than two hours without reapplication.

- The FDA emphasized that sunscreen alone is not enough and should be used in conjunction with a complete sun protection regimen, including finding shade and wearing long pants, long-sleeved shirts, hats, and sunglasses.
- Limit exposure to the sun between 10 a.m. and 2 p.m.
- Do not burn.
- Avoid tanning and UV tanning booths.
- Cover up with clothing, including a broad-brimmed hat and UV-blocking sunglasses.

Protecting against skin cancer is simple. In addition to consistently using a broad-spectrum, water-resistant sunscreen (SPF of 15 or higher) and applying 1 ounce to your entire body 30 minutes before going outside and reapplying every two hours or immediately after swimming or excessive sweating, the following should be observed:

- Examine your skin head-to-toe every month to check for suspicious moles (A, B, C, D evaluation).
- See your physician for a professional skin exam each year.

✔ NEED TO KNOW

There are signs and symptoms for the common sites for cancer. Through an understanding of the signs and symptoms and the early detection methods, you can reduce your risk of being a cancer-mortality number and increase the probability of a successful outcome with the cancer. Many cancers are a result of choices people make—diet, smoking, sun exposure, and use of certain medications. Knowing the long-term effect of your health choices and acting appropriately can significantly reduce your risk.

➤ Cancer Treatment

Cancerous tissue must be removed in some manner. Surgery is the chief option for excising both the cancer and surrounding tissue. Once the cancer is removed, then a radiation and/or chemotherapy regime is instituted to prevent it from growing back.

Article 9.4

Chemotherapy simply means "chemical therapy," or the use of a variety of anticancer drugs. Some cancers do not require surgery and can be cured with just chemotherapy, whereas other cancers require both surgery and "chemo." There are many categories of anticancer drugs, some of which are quite toxic and have a very narrow margin of safety. The whole emphasis of chemotherapy is to kill new cancer cells before the cancer reoccurs.

Chemotherapy is hard on the body. Although drugs are becoming more precisely targeted, they often kill all fast-growing cells in a body, not just the cancerous ones. (People on chemotherapy sometimes lose their hair because scalp cells are fast growing.) Chemotherapy also can suppress the immune system and leave a person open to infection. Further, it can cause nausea and weakness.

Radiation therapy is the last component of cancer treatment. Similar to chemo, the goal of radiation treatment is to destroy both cancer cells and cells that divide

Chemotherapy is the use of numerous drugs to kill cancer cells.

Radiation therapy exposes cancer-ridden body areas to radiation doses to kill cancerous cells.

Health & the Media Quack Cancer Treatments

Amigdalina (amygdalin) has often been referred to as vitamin B_{17}. However, it is not really a vitamin but a chemical found in the pits of apricots and other fruits. *Laetrile* is the common term for the drug form of the chemical. Because laetrile produces cyanide, which is a poison that kills cells, it has been marketed (particularly in Mexico) as a cancer cure. Amygdalin was first used as a cancer treatment in Russia in the 1840s. But modern studies show no scientific or clinical evidence that laetrile cures cancer. Nonetheless, some people diagnosed with cancer are tempted to try laetrile despite the numerous studies indicating it won't work.

Why are people susceptible to this quack drug? Some people do not research treatments before embracing them, so they remain ignorant of the science and evidence. This makes them easy prey for those who continue to market laetrile therapy. Others may have tried traditional cancer therapies but remain uncured. People who are desperate to extend their life may try almost any treatment if they think it gives them even the tiniest chance for improvement. Still others are drawn to the idea that "natural" or "simple" cures like laetrile, a drug derived from plants, must be better than invasive surgery or the arduous regimens of radiation or chemotherapy. So for a variety of reasons, quack drugs like laetrile continue as cancer treatments.

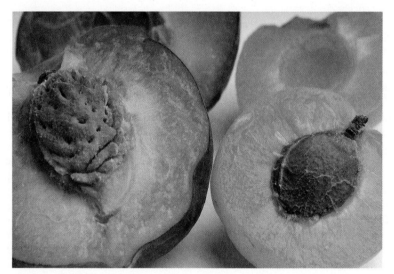

© McGraw-Hill Education/Jill Braaten, photographer

rapidly, which could be cancer cells. This treatment increases the likelihood that cancer cells remaining after surgery will be destroyed along with any cells that might become cancerous. In addition to killing cancer cells, radiation can help reduce symptoms if a cancer cure is not possible.

Although there have been many remarkable advances in cancer treatment, there is no guarantee that surgery, chemotherapy, and radiation will be effective with everyone. What has been described is the conventional approach, and the implementation of this treatment protocol requires the clinical judgment of physicians and the decision of the patient. Cancer is such a serious condition that there is wisdom in getting a second opinion—not just about the diagnosis but also before committing to an aggressive treatment protocol. Finally, and most importantly, early detection is critical to increase the options for less intense treatment and survival.

NEED TO KNOW

More people are surviving cancer. Effective treatment modalities are the key to survival—surgery, chemotherapy, and radiation. Although these therapies are not pleasant, they are effective. There is much more hope for surviving cancer today than there was just a few years ago.

EARLY DETECTION AND PREVENTION

Each type of cancer discussed has implications for early detection. Unfortunately, some kinds of cancer do not have symptoms until the cancer is advanced. Further, pain is a symptom of advanced cancer, so pain is not an early warning sign and should not be considered one. Figure 9.9 shows the array of cancer screenings available, when they should be done, and the appropriate age group.

To make cancer symptoms easy to remember, the American Cancer Society created the acronym CAUTION. If any of the symptoms below are noticed for at least two weeks, then a follow-up medical evaluation should be undertaken. CAUTION stands for:

Changes in bowel or bladder habits, like bloody stool/urine, or painful elimination.
A sore that doesn't heal—a sign of skin cancer.
Unusual bleeding or discharge—possibly a symptom of cervical or bladder cancer.
Thickening or lump in the breast or elsewhere.
Indigestion or difficulty in swallowing—digestive-tract cancer symptoms.
Obvious change in color of a wart or mole—a key sign of skin cancer.
Nagging cough or hoarseness—symptoms of lung or throat cancer.

Increasing the options to prevent cancer focuses mainly on the choices people make that affect risk. These choices are related to tobacco use, diet, and exposure to environmental carcinogens.

Tobacco is related to most cases of lung, mouth, and throat cancer, so abstaining from tobacco would be a significant effort in reducing the risk of respiratory cancers. Diets high in saturated fat and red meat increase the risk of cancer of the colon, so moderation in intake of saturated fats and red meat will reduce one's risk of cancer of the colon. Environmental carcinogens range from ultraviolet light to industrial chemicals, and reducing exposure will reduce risk.

NEED TO KNOW

There is not always a clear way to prevent cancer because we do not know with confidence what is related to the development of certain cancers. Just as important as prevention is early detection. CAUTION provides a simple framework for a basic set of symptoms that might indicate cancer. Learn and apply them. They may save your life.

FIGURE 9.9 RECOMMENDED CANCER SCREENINGS

Cancer-Related Checkup

Physicians should conduct appropriate cancer screenings based on factors such as age, gender, family history, and risk factors. Further, the screenings are in accordance with guidelines for early cancer detection promoted by the American Cancer Society. The American Cancer Society routinely evaluates cancer screening guidelines and, if necessary, revises the guidelines based on expert judgment and medical/scientific evidence.

Colon & Rectum

For both men and women, screenings for cancer of the colon and rectum are recommended beginning at age 50 and should include one (or more) of the following:

- A fecal occult blood test (FOBT) or fecal immunochemical test (FIT) every year

- A double-contrast barium enema every 5 years

- A flexible sigmoidoscopy (FSIG) every 5 years

- A colonoscopy every 10 years

Prostate

Beginning at age 50, men should have an annual PSA test and a digital rectal examination. Those men at high risk, such as African American men and those with a strong family history of first-degree relatives diagnosed with prostate cancer at an early age, should begin PSA and digital rectal examinations at age 45.

Breast

- Women should be familiar with how their breasts feel normally and be sensitive to changes. Starting in their 20s, women should practice breast self-exam at least once a month and seek medical assistance if changes are noted.

- Women in their 20s and 30s should have a periodic health exam every 3 years and the evaluation should include a clinical breast exam. Women in their 40s should have a yearly clinical breast exam.

- Mammograms should be done yearly starting at age 40.

- For women with a strong family history of breast or ovarian cancer or who were treated for Hodgkins diseases, screening MRIs may be recommended.

FIGURE 9.9 RECOMMENDED CANCER SCREENINGS *(concluded)*

Uterus

Cervix: Between age 21 and 29, women should be screened for cervical cancer every 3 years. Between age 30 and 65, screenings should be done every 5 years when combining the HPV screening and the Pap test or screenings every 3 years if being screened with the Pap test alone. Women 65 and older could stop cervical cancer screening if they have had either 3 or more consecutive negative Pap tests or 2 or more consecutive negative HPV and Pap tests within the previous 10 years.

Endometrium: For women with or at risk for hereditary nonpolyposis colon cancer, a yearly screening for endometrial cancer including endometrial biopsy should begin at age 35. Women at the time of menopause should be informed about signs and symptoms of cancer of the endometrium and should be encouraged to seek medical assistance if they notice any of the signs or symptoms.

Source: American Cancer Society, *Cancer Facts and Figures, 2015.* Atlanta: American Cancer Society, Inc.

Knowing the Language

 connect Resources

ARTICLES

9.1 "The Deadliest Cancer." *Newsweek.* This article highlights why lung cancer is considered the deadliest cancer.

9.2 "Getting to the Root of Testicular Cancer." *ED Insider.* Epididymitis and testicular torsion are two conditions affecting young males. This article highlights the diagnosis and treatment of both.

9.3 "The Sunscreen Myth: How Sunscreen Products Actually Promote Cancer." *NaturalNews.com.* This controversial article's premise is that sunscreens might not protect one from skin cancer.

9.4 "Conquering Cancer in the 21st Century: Leading a Movement to Save More Lives Worldwide." *Health Education and Behavior.* The executive director of the American Cancer Society writes about the current state of the global fight against cancer.

SELF-ASSESSMENTS

9.1 Cancer Risk Factors
9.2 Skin Cancer Prevention

Website Resources

American Cancer Society **www.cancer.org**
American Institute for Cancer Research **www.aicr.org**
American Medical Association **www.ama-assn.org**
American Public Health Association **www.apha.org**
Centers for Disease Control and Prevention **www.cdc.gov**
Harvard Center for Cancer Prevention **www.diseaseriskindex.harvard.edu**
MedlinePlus Cancer Information **www.nlm.nih.gov/medlineplus/cancers.html**
National Comprehensive Cancer Network **www.nccn.org**
Skin Cancer Organization **www.skincancer.org**

Knowing the Language

1. What is meant by *cancer* and *metastasis*?
2. Where are the most common sites where cancer occurs, and what are the major risk factors for each site?
3. What are the major methods used to treat cancer? Are they successful?
4. How can cancer be prevented?
5. What does the acronym CAUTION mean?

Exploring Ideas

1. Why is it that when people hear the word *cancer,* they think immediately of death?
2. At which sites are college-age students at risk for cancer? What can be done to reduce risk?
3. What steps should be taken after a person is diagnosed with cancer?
4. Is there a role for complementary and alternative medicine in cancer treatment, and if so when?
5. Do you think the statement is true that if a person lives long enough he or she will most likely develop cancer? If so, why would this be true?

Selected References

American Cancer Society. *Cancer Facts and Figures.* Atlanta, GA: American Cancer Society, 2015.

American Cancer Society. *Cancer: What Causes It. What Doesn't.* Atlanta, GA: American Cancer Society, 2006.

Calle EE, Rodriquez C, Walker-Thurmond K, et al. Overweight, obesity, and mortality from cancer in a prospectively studied cohort of U.S. adults. *New England Journal of Medicine* 348: 1625–1638, 2003.

Chao A, Thun MJ, Connell CJ, et al. Meat consumption and risk of colorectal cancer. *JAMA* 293 (2): 172–182, 2005.

Christenson LJ, Borrowman TA, Vachon CM, et al. Incidence of basal cell and squamous cell carcinomas in a population younger than 40 years. *JAMA* 294 (6): 681–690, 2005.

Curry SJ, Byers T, Hewitt M, eds. *Fulfilling the Potential of Cancer Prevention and Early Detection.* Washington, DC: National Academic Press, 2003.

Elmore JG, Armstrong K, Lehman CD, et al. Screening for breast cancer. *JAMA* 293 (10): 1245–1256, 2005.

Fung T, Hu FB, Fuchs C, et al. Major dietary patterns and the risk of colorectal cancer in women. *Archives of Internal Medicine* 163 (3): 309–314, 2005.

Kapp J, Yankaskas BC, LeFevre ML. Are mammography recommendations in women younger than 40 related to increased risk? *Breast Cancer Research and Treatment* 119: 485–490, January 2009.

Paules RS, Aubrecht J, Corvi R, et al. *Moving Forward in Human Cancer Assessment.* Bethesda, MD: National Institutes of Environmental Health Sciences, December 2010.

Raloff J. Sun struck: Data suggest skin cancer epidemic looms. *Science News Online* 168 (7), August 13, 2005.

Ruckington C, Straus JJ. *The Encyclopedia of Cancer.* New York: Facts on File, 2005.

Samaniego FS, Matias KP. Studies of the viral origins of some cancers lead to new prevention, treatment strategies. *OncoLog* 39 (1), 2004.

Skin Cancer Foundation. Skin Cancer Facts. **www.skincancer.org/skin-cancer-information/skin-cancer-facts.** February 9, 2015.

U.S. Food and Drug Administration. FDA Sheds Light on Sunscreens, June 2011. **www.fda.gov/ForConsumers/ConsumerUpdates/ucm258416.htm**

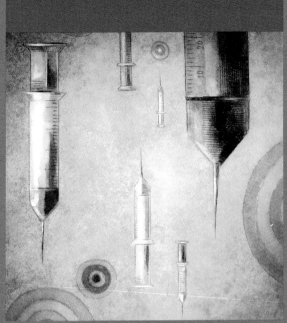

Good health is a serious business. Like life itself, it has to be worked at and it takes on added meaning with effort.

—Norman Cousins

Chapter 10

DIABETES

In this chapter, we focus on what public health experts describe as the fastest-growing chronic disease among Americans today—diabetes. Metabolic syndrome (associated with diabetes, heart disease, and obesity) is also discussed. The interrelatedness of these chronic conditions underscores the importance of establishing a balanced lifestyle at an early age.

DIABETES IS DISABLING, deadly, and on the rise. New evidence indicates that one in three Americans born in 2000 will develop diabetes. Due to the rapid rise in prevalence—a tripling over the past three decades—and the dire prediction for further increases, an expanded look at this disease called *diabetes* is warranted. An understanding of diabetes is important because it may well affect our personal health or the health of those close to us. Moreover, facing the challenges of diabetes provides a striking example of how lifestyle, medicine, and technology converge in 21st-century American society.

The Greeks described the disease as a "melting down of the flesh and limbs into urine." Indeed, the symptoms of diabetes have been recognized for centuries. Early records describe a puzzling and deadly condition that caused intense thirst, excessive urine production, and a wasting away of the body. And, oddly, the urine of those afflicted was sweet. Thus, the full medical term, *diabetes mellitus,* comes from the Latin words meaning "siphon" (in reference to excessive urine output) and "sweet like honey," respectively.

Little was understood about the cause of diabetes until the late 19th century, when the pancreas, a little-known organ, was discovered to play a central role. Experiments involving the removal of the pancreas from dogs resulted in diabetes, confirming the relationship between the organ and the disease. The focus then shifted toward identifying a substance in the pancreas that could be the key to solving the diabetes puzzle. This led to the discovery of insulin in 1921. For this remarkable scientific achievement, Canadian researchers Frederick G. Banting and John Macleod were awarded the 1923 Nobel Prize in Medicine.

Subsequent events continued to advance our understanding and treatment of diabetes. Soon after the discovery of insulin, Eli Lilly and Company started commercial production of insulin from the pancreases of animals. Concurrently, home testing kits for sugar (glucose) in the urine were developed. Yet, it would be the 1950s before it was realized that diabetes could be caused in two ways. This finding spurred the discovery of (noninsulin) drugs to lower blood glucose levels. In the 1970s, treatment innovations included blood glucose meters and insulin pumps. They were followed in the early 1980s by the commercial production of bioengineered "human" insulin.

Despite major advances in treatment, diabetes among Americans continues to rise. Researchers agree the primary cause is a combination of too much eating and too little exercise among a large proportion of the population. This "fattening of America" is clearly triggering the onset of diabetes along with increasing risk for heart disease and stroke. Related to these changes, a clustering of chronic disease risk factors has been recognized and named the *metabolic syndrome.*

Article 10.1

In large part, diabetes, like atherosclerosis, is an unintended consequence of our technologically advanced, affluent society where food is plentiful, and physical demands are nearly nonexistent. For those with diabetes, the disease is not reversible or curable. Thankfully though, it is highly treatable. And for those without diabetes, the key is prevention. Let's learn about diabetes and see what we can do to turn the tide, for ourselves and society.

➤ Diabetes

Diabetes is the seventh leading cause of death in the United States behind heart disease, cancer, stroke, chronic lower respiratory disease, unintentional accidents, and Alzheimer's disease. Over 9 percent of the population has diabetes—nearly 30 million children and adults—with about the same number of males and females being affected. Of these, about 3 out of 10 are undiagnosed; that is, these individuals have the disease but are unaware of it. The risk for early death among people with diabetes is at least two times that of people without diabetes.

Among all American adults (aged 20 or older), 12.3 percent or about one in eight have diabetes. As shown in Figure 10.1, the prevalence of diabetes increases with age. About one in six midlife adults has diabetes and the rate increases to one in four among older adults. Risk of diabetes is also associated with race/ethnicity, as illustrated in Figure 10.2. Native Americans, Blacks, and Hispanics are about one and a half to two times more likely to have diabetes than Whites of similar age.

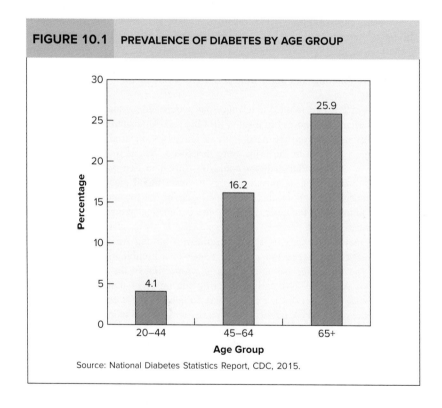

FIGURE 10.1 PREVALENCE OF DIABETES BY AGE GROUP

Source: National Diabetes Statistics Report, CDC, 2015.

Diabetes (or technically *diabetes mellitus*) is a group of disorders characterized by hyperglycemia resulting from defects in insulin production, insulin action, or both.

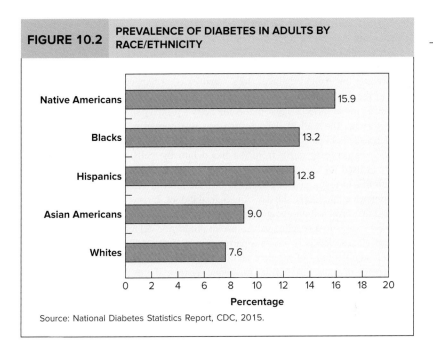

FIGURE 10.2 PREVALENCE OF DIABETES IN ADULTS BY RACE/ETHNICITY

Source: National Diabetes Statistics Report, CDC, 2015.

PANCREAS, METABOLISM, AND DIABETES

Just what is diabetes? Diabetes is a group of disorders in which there is a defect in the transfer of glucose (sugar) from the bloodstream into cells. This leads to abnormally high levels of blood glucose, which is known as **hyperglycemia** (*hyper-* means "high" or "elevated"; *-glycemia* refers to glucose in the blood). Blood glucose levels are controlled by **insulin,** a hormone produced by the pancreas that helps move glucose from the blood into the cells of muscles and other tissues.

The pancreas, sandwiched between the stomach and the spine, is an oblong gland about the size and shape of a flattened banana. Part of it lies behind the stomach, and the other part is nestled in the curve of the small intestine (duodenum). The pancreas makes hormones and enzymes that help the body digest and use food. Throughout the pancreas are clusters of cells called the *islets of Langerhans.* These islets are made up of two types of cells: alpha cells, which make glucagon, a hormone that raises the level of glucose in the blood, and beta cells, which make the hormone insulin.

Balancing the release of glucagon and the release of insulin into the bloodstream to regulate glucose needs of the body is normally an efficient physiological system.

Hyperglycemia is high blood glucose levels and is the hallmark of uncontrolled diabetes.

Insulin is a hormone produced in the pancreas that helps glucose pass into the cells where it can be used for energy.

However, if the beta cells do not produce enough insulin, diabetes will develop. Diabetes can also result if the body does not respond properly to the insulin that is made. Last, diabetes can occur by a combination of both defects—insulin deficiency and insulin resistance.

To better understand diabetes, let's consider what happens when a person eats. Once in the gastrointestinal tract, food is broken down into constituents including glucose, a simple form of sugar that is the body's primary source of energy. Glucose passes through the wall of the intestine and is absorbed into the bloodstream and stimulates the beta cells in the pancreas to produce and release insulin. Insulin then allows the glucose to move from the blood into the cells. Once inside the cells, glucose is used for energy or stored until it's needed.

With this in mind, you might expect that the level of glucose in the blood would vary somewhat throughout the day. And indeed it does. It rises after a meal and returns to a baseline level within about two hours after eating. Once the level of glucose in the blood returns to a baseline value, insulin production decreases. Standard variation in blood glucose levels is within a narrow range of about 70 to 110 milligrams per deciliter (mg/dL) most of the time and up to 140 mg/dL following meals.

Diabetes disrupts this normal metabolic system. If the body does not produce enough insulin to move the glucose into the cells or if there is a defect in the action of the insulin that limits its effect, the resulting high level of glucose in the blood and the inadequate amount of glucose in the cells together produce the symptoms and complications of diabetes. There are three main types of diabetes: type 1, type 2, and gestational diabetes.

TYPE 1 DIABETES

Type 1 diabetes is diagnosed in children, teenagers, and young adults. The incidence of type 1 diabetes peaks at puberty. In this form of diabetes, the beta cells, the insulin-producing cells of the pancreas, are destroyed by the body's immune system. This abnormal autoimmune response—a targeted attack and destruction of the body's own cells—is linked to genetic predisposition, but it may also be associated with environmental factors. Although pieces of the puzzle are coming together, the actual causes are still not well understood. The eventual permanent destruction of all or nearly all of the beta cells typically leads to absolute insulin deficiency—that is, a complete inability to produce insulin. Most people who have type 1 diabetes develop it before age 25 and must take insulin for the rest of their lives. Due to the acute onset of symptoms (e.g., increased urination, increased thirst, unexplained weight loss), type 1 diabetes is nearly always diagnosed soon after symptoms appear. Although the preferred term is *type 1 diabetes,* this condition is also referred to as *insulin-dependent diabetes* or *juvenile diabetes.* From a public health perspective, it's important to note that only 5 to 10 percent of people with diabetes have this form of the disease.

Type 1 diabetes develops during childhood or young adulthood due to pancreatic beta cell destruction. This form includes cases of diabetes caused by an autoimmune process and those with unknown etiology.

Type 2 diabetes usually develops in people older than 40 and becomes more common with age. It is by far the most prevalent type of diabetes—over 90 percent of all people with diabetes have type 2. In this type of diabetes, the pancreas continues to produce insulin, but the body develops what is known as *insulin resistance.* This is a condition in which the body's cells do not use insulin properly. Initially, the pancreas compensates by producing more insulin at higher-than-normal levels. Over time, however, the pancreas cannot supply enough insulin in response to meals. Excess body fat (adipose tissue) is the primary cause of insulin resistance and the chief risk factor for type 2 diabetes. It's estimated that 80–90 percent of people with type 2 diabetes are obese. This type of diabetes, like type 1, is also associated with a genetic predisposition and tends to run in families. In contrast to type 1, though, type 2 develops gradually. People can have high blood glucose levels for years— with ongoing damage to tissues—yet have no symptoms. The only way to tell is with regular screening for diabetes. Type 2 is also referred to as *noninsulin-dependent diabetes* because insulin is usually not needed to treat the condition, at least initially.

For many decades, type 2 diabetes was considered solely a disease of middle age and commonly referred to as *adult-onset diabetes.* From the 1930s until the 1990s, if a child or young adult had diabetes, it was known that they had type 1 (juvenile diabetes). Type 2 diabetes was simply not seen in children or young adults. But then in the 1990s, a few unusual cases were reported. Physicians began to diagnose type 2 diabetes in individuals in their 30s, 20s, and even occasionally in their teens. This was surprising and puzzling. What could cause premature development of type 2 diabetes? Were these cases rare occurrences, or were they early indications of a troubling trend?

Twenty years later, we know the answer: Development of type 2 diabetes in children and young people is primarily a consequence of excess body weight (an obesity epidemic), which in turn is largely ascribed to unhealthy eating and sedentary lifestyle. The prevalence of American children and adolescents who are overweight has tripled over the past three decades. Since about 90 percent of type 2 diabetes is attributed to weight gain, it's easy to see why type 2 diabetes is rising among our youth. There is also evidence that exposure to diabetes *in utero* (gestational diabetes) may be a major contributor. Although the epidemiology of type 2 diabetes in children and teenagers is limited, clinical reports and regional studies indicate type 2 diabetes is being diagnosed more frequently, particularly in Native Americans, Mexican Americans, and African Americans. The International Diabetes Federation states that type 2 diabetes in young people is a global phenomenon affecting children in both developed and developing countries.

Article
10.2

Type 2 diabetes, the most common form of diabetes, encompasses cases that range from an inability to make enough insulin (secretory defect) to an inability to use the insulin that is made (insulin resistance).

GESTATIONAL DIABETES

Gestational diabetes develops in about 1 out of 20 women during the late stages of pregnancy. It is more common among obese women, certain ethnic/racial groups (African American, Hispanic, Native American), and those with a family history. This form of diabetes is typically caused by the development of insulin resistance late in pregnancy. Gestational diabetes requires treatment to normalize the maternal blood glucose levels to avoid complications in the infant. Treatment usually consists of dietary changes and avoiding excess weight gain. Although gestational diabetes usually resolves after the baby is born, women who develop it are more likely to develop type 2 diabetes later in life. Following pregnancy, a small proportion of women with gestational diabetes (5–10 percent) are found to have type 2 diabetes, and a larger proportion (40–60 percent) are at risk for developing type 2 diabetes within the next 5 to 10 years. For additional information, go to: **www.diabetes.org/gestational.**

PRE-DIABETES

Pre-diabetes is a condition that causes blood glucose levels to be higher than normal but not high enough for a diagnosis of diabetes. People with pre-diabetes are at increased risk for developing diabetes. This borderline condition is similar to the pre-hypertension category for blood pressure. There are three times as many Americans with pre-diabetes as those with diabetes. Before people develop type 2 diabetes, they almost always have pre-diabetes. Recent evidence indicates initial damage to the body, especially the heart and circulatory system, starts during pre-diabetes. However, not all individuals with pre-diabetes inevitably progress to diabetes. Interventions work. Improving diet, increasing physical activity, and losing weight can reverse pre-diabetes and delay or prevent diabetes. Being diagnosed with pre-diabetes represents an important crossroad. It is a last window of opportunity for true prevention, because once diabetes is developed, it doesn't go away.

✓ NEED TO KNOW

Diabetes is a group of metabolic diseases characterized by hyperglycemia resulting from defects in insulin secretion, insulin action, or both. Type 1 diabetes develops during childhood due to destruction of the beta cells of the pancreas. Lifelong insulin therapy is required. Type 1 accounts for 5–10 percent of all cases of diabetes. Type 2 diabetes generally appears during adulthood and is associated with weight gain and insulin resistance. It is by far the most common (over 90 percent of all cases). Pre-diabetes is a transitional condition in which blood glucose is in a borderline range. People with pre-diabetes are at high risk for developing type 2 diabetes. For these people, lifestyle strategies are available to prevent or delay the onset of the disease.

Gestational diabetes is diabetes that first appears during pregnancy; it affects about 5 percent of pregnant women.

Pre-diabetes is a borderline condition in which the blood glucose level is between normal and diabetic levels.

We all know individuals with diabetes. Yet, unless we actually live with a person who has diabetes or have it ourselves, it's difficult to fully appreciate the disease. People with diabetes may experience serious, long-term complications. Although some complications may begin within months of the onset of diabetes, most develop over a period of years. Nearly all complications are progressive. If not managed, diabetes can be extremely disabling in a number of ways.

DAMAGE TO BLOOD VESSELS

Uncontrolled diabetes damages both the small blood vessels (such as arterioles, capillaries, and venules) and the large ones (arteries and veins). Compounds accumulate within the tiny vessels that compromise the microvascular systems, causing them to thicken and leak. Blood flow is restricted, especially to the skin and nerves. High glucose levels also cause the levels of fats in the blood to rise, hastening atherosclerosis in the larger blood vessels. As a result, atherosclerosis occurs at younger ages and is at least twice as common in people with diabetes as in those without diabetes.

HEART ATTACK AND STROKE

Over time, elevated blood glucose levels and compromised circulation harm multiple organs, including the heart and brain. Angina, heart attack, stroke, and heart failure can result. Heart disease and stroke cause about two out of three deaths among people with diabetes.

EYE DISEASE AND BLINDNESS

Diabetic eye disease is the leading cause of blindness in adults. Complications from diabetes primarily result in damage to the retina (retinopathy) but also include cataracts and glaucoma. Diabetic retinopathy is caused by a breakdown of the small blood vessels in the retina. All three diabetic complications of the eye can result in loss of vision and eventual blindness.

KIDNEY DISEASE

Over 40 percent of all new cases of kidney disease (nephropathy) are in people with diabetes. Diabetic kidney disease develops as the tiny blood vessels in the kidney are damaged, and the system to filter the blood is slowly degraded. Eventually, this can lead to kidney failure requiring dialysis or kidney transplantation.

NERVE DAMAGE

In 60–70 percent of people with diabetes, high blood sugar and related metabolic factors lead to nerve damage (neuropathy). Although nerve problems can occur in every organ system, the most common is peripheral neuropathy, which causes pain, tingling, or numbness (loss of feeling) in the toes, feet, legs, hands, and arms.

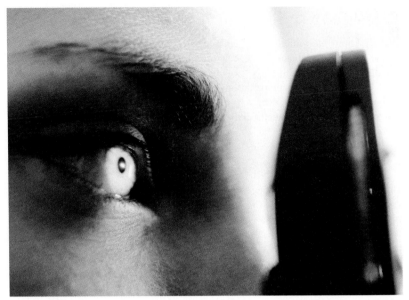

Diabetes is a leading cause of blindness in the United States.
© image100/Getty Images

Blisters and sores may appear on numb areas of the foot because pressure or injury goes unnoticed. Peripheral neuropathy may also cause muscle weakness and loss of balance and coordination.

AMPUTATIONS

Poor circulation and nerve damage can lead to ulcers, infections, and poor wound healing. People with diabetes are especially likely to have skin breakdown and infections of the feet and legs. Such wounds typically heal slowly or not at all. More than half of all lower-limb amputations in the United States occur in people with diabetes.

The complications just highlighted are only the major ones. There are other outcomes, less vivid but still debilitating. Diabetes can also compromise immune function; flu- and pneumonia-related deaths are three times more likely among people with diabetes than those without diabetes. And there are gender-specific concerns such as pregnancy complications affecting women and their babies and the risk of impotence among men.

Although diabetes-related complications can be severe, they don't have to be. The more tightly a person with diabetes controls his or her blood glucose level (glycemic control), the less likely complications will develop or worsen. Early detection, comprehensive medical care, and vigilant self-management are proven strategies in preventing or minimizing complications. Regular medical exams should include careful screening for heart disease and stroke, eye disease, kidney disease, skin and foot infections, and nerve damage.

✓ **NEED TO KNOW**

Early diagnosis of diabetes is extremely important because complications from untreated diabetes are extensive. Over time high glucose levels in the bloodstream and insufficient levels in the cells cause irreversible damage. Both microvascular and macrovascular systems are affected. Serious complications include heart disease, stroke, blindness, kidney damage, nerve damage, and lower-limb amputations. The key to preventing or minimizing complications is to control blood glucose levels and associated risk factors such as hypertension, abnormal blood lipids, and overweight/obesity. Moreover, people with diabetes should follow preventive care practices for their eyes, kidneys, and feet.

➤ Diagnosis and Control

As previously mentioned, undiagnosed diabetes is common; nearly 30 percent of those with type 2 diabetes are unaware of their condition. Similar to high blood pressure or abnormal lipid levels, type 2 diabetes can be present for years before symptoms arise. When symptoms do develop, they may be subtle. Increased urination and thirst are mild initially, then gradually worsen over months. Eventually, the person experiences extreme fatigue, is likely to develop blurred vision, and may become chronically dehydrated. Even during the early stages of type 2 diabetes— before the symptoms—uncontrolled high blood glucose (hyperglycemia) causes microvascular disease (e.g., damage to the retinas and kidneys) and may cause or contribute to macrovascular disease (e.g., heart disease, stroke, peripheral vascular disease). Undiagnosed diabetes is a serious condition.

For apparently healthy adults, testing for diabetes is recommended beginning at age 40, particularly if overweight (i.e., BMI $\geq$ 25). If results are normal, testing should be repeated every three years. Screening should begin earlier for individuals with other known risk factors for diabetes. Targeted testing is suggested for children and adults who are overweight and have one or more of the following risk factors:

- Parent or sibling with diabetes.
- Previous diagnosis of pre-diabetes.
- Member of high-risk ethnic/racial group—Black, Hispanic, Native American, Pacific Islander.
- History of gestational diabetes.
- High blood pressure.
- Abnormal blood fats.
- Habitual physical inactivity.

Awareness and appropriate action are critical. In a study from Oregon, two out of three adults at high risk for developing diabetes reported being unconcerned about their risk for developing the disease, and only one out of five had discussed their risk of diabetes with their doctor. These surprising findings indicate a need for individuals at high-risk *and* health care professionals to recognize and discuss the looming threat of diabetes.

Diabetes and pre-diabetes can be diagnosed by measuring blood glucose in one of four ways: a fasting plasma glucose test, an A1c test, an oral glucose tolerance test, or a random plasma glucose test. Each test has advantages and disadvantages. Figure 10.3 summarizes the diagnostic values for the first three methods.

The *fasting plasma glucose (FPG)* test is the most common measure. (Plasma is the fluid portion of blood after the cells are removed.) Fasting is defined as no caloric intake for at least eight hours. Typically a blood sample is drawn in the morning after an overnight fast. Normal fasting glucose levels range from about 70–99 mg/dL. Pre-diabetes is defined as 100–125 mg/dL, while diabetes is diagnosed as a value of 126 mg/dL or above.

A second approach is the *A1c* test. No fasting is required for this blood test. The A1c test indicates a person's average blood sugar level for the past two to three months. An A1c level between 5.7 and 6.4 percent indicates pre-diabetes, while a level of 6.5 percent or higher indicates diabetes. This test is not for everyone, though, and should not be used for pregnant women, people who have had recent severe bleeding or blood transfusions, those with kidney or liver disease, and people with blood disorders. (More on the A1c test in the upcoming section on managing diabetes.)

A third method is the *oral glucose tolerance test (OGTT)*. The OGTT requires a fasting plasma glucose test, followed by drinking a standard glucose solution (75 grams dissolved in water) to "challenge" one's system, and then two hours later another blood draw. Pre-diabetes is indicated if the 2-hour value is between 140 and 199 mg/dL, and diabetes is indicated if the value is 200 mg/dL or higher. The OGTT is not widely used, as it's more burdensome on patients (requires fasting, multiple blood draws), more time-consuming, and more costly. In certain cases, though, it may be the best choice.

The fourth and least common approach is to measure the *random plasma glucose.* In this test, the blood sample can be taken at any time of day without regard to when the last meal was eaten. A diagnosis of diabetes is indicated if the glucose level is 200 mg/dL or above *and* the person has the classic symptoms of diabetes (i.e., increased urination, increased thirst, unexplained weight loss).

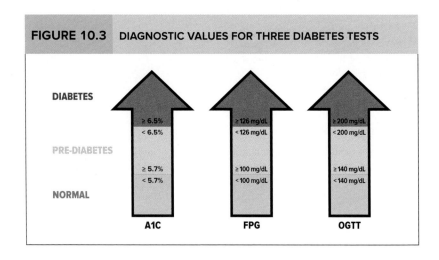

FIGURE 10.3   DIAGNOSTIC VALUES FOR THREE DIABETES TESTS

DIABETES

PRE-DIABETES

NORMAL

	A1C	FPG	OGTT
Diabetes	≥ 6.5%	≥ 126 mg/dL	≥ 200 mg/dL
	< 6.5%	< 126 mg/dL	< 200 mg/dL
Pre-diabetes	≥ 5.7%	≥ 100 mg/dL	≥ 140 mg/dL
	< 5.7%	< 100 mg/dL	< 140 mg/dL

Health & the Media Ratcheting Up PSAs from Risk Awareness to Disease Management

Diabetes is now so widespread in the United States that public service announcements (PSAs) such as this are designed for a broad audience—not just for people with diabetes but also their families and friends. Perhaps more than any other chronic disease, diabetes requires daily vigilance and appropriate actions to manage the disease. Using cartoon-like characters to catch the eye, this PSA is an example of how an information-dense message can be conveyed in a creative and engaging manner. The highlighted A, B, Cs combine the diabetes-specific measurement of A1c with measurements of blood pressure and cholesterol (discussed in Chapter 8), reinforcing the interrelatedness of the major cardiovascular and metabolic diseases.

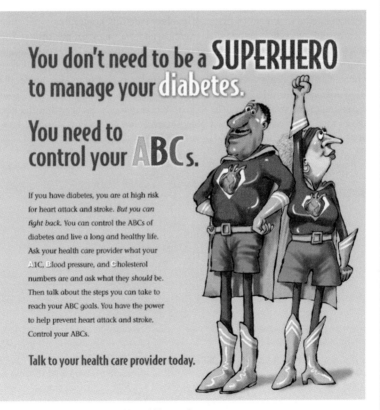

Source: U.S. Department of Health and Human Resources

Regardless of the method used, if diabetes is diagnosed, it must be confirmed with a subsequent test on a separate day. Any one of the four tests can be used to confirm an initial positive diagnosis. Of the four, the fasting plasma glucose test (FPG) is the preferred method and most widely accepted. It's a routine measurement made on blood samples during annual physical exams. The test is easy to perform, relatively convenient for patients, and low cost.

CHALLENGE OF TREATMENT

The goal for successfully treating diabetes is to do what the body does naturally for most people—to maintain the proper balance between glucose and insulin. In diabetes the glucose–insulin synergy is impaired, due to either a lack of insulin being produced (insulin deficiency), an inability to effectively use the insulin (insulin resistance), or a combination of the two. Even with these limitations, the overall physiological processes remain operational. Food still makes the blood glucose level rise. Insulin and exercise make it fall. But the normal responsiveness and sensitivity to these variables are lacking.

Consequently, treatment of diabetes involves carefully controlling type, amount, sequence, and interaction among diet, exercise, and, for many people, drugs. Among adults with diagnosed diabetes, 14 percent take insulin only, 15 percent take both insulin and oral medication, 57 percent take oral medication only, and 14 percent are treated without drugs (Figure 10.4). With multiple factors to coordinate, diabetes self-management education is an integral part of medical care. The goal of diabetes treatment never stops. It is to keep blood glucose levels within the normal range as much as possible. If blood glucose levels are carefully controlled, complications are less likely to develop.

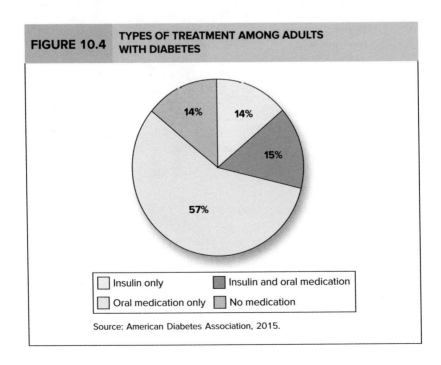

FIGURE 10.4 **TYPES OF TREATMENT AMONG ADULTS WITH DIABETES**

14%   14%

15%

57%

Insulin only
Oral medication only
Insulin and oral medication
No medication

Source: American Diabetes Association, 2015.

Keeping blood glucose levels from getting too high—hyperglycemia—is the primary challenge. But the problem with tightly controlling levels to prevent high blood glucose is that low blood glucose, or **hypoglycemia,** may occur. Most cases of low blood glucose—lower than 70 mg/dL—are caused by an "overshoot" or excessive effect of the insulin or oral medications taken to lower glucose levels. Hypoglycemia is uncommon among people without diabetes. Symptoms of hypoglycemia vary. They can progress from mild discomfort to severe confusion to fainting or coma. They can begin slowly or come on suddenly. Hypoglycemia should be treated immediately because prolonged hypoglycemia can cause brain damage.

Symptoms are relieved within minutes of consuming sugar in any form such as a few ounces of fruit juice or a regular (not diet) soft drink or a few pieces of candy. Many people with diabetes carry these quick-fix foods, glucose tablets, or foil packets of a glucose-containing liquid. Milk is actually better than juice or glucose because it has lactose, fat, and protein, and this combination not only raises blood sugar but also keeps it more stable over time. However, milk is not easily carried or always readily available. A doctor may prescribe a glucagon kit for those prone to hypoglycemia, as an injection will quickly raise one's blood glucose. Family, friends, and coworkers can be taught how to inject glucagon in an emergency.

Less frequent but even more dangerous is a condition called **ketoacidosis.** If glucose is not readily available to the body's tissues, fat is broken down as a source of energy, and ketones are produced as a byproduct. If the body burns too much fat too quickly, ketones will accumulate in the bloodstream and make the body too acidic, upsetting normal chemical balance and leading to ketoacidosis. Untreated, this condition can lead to coma and death. Symptoms include excessive thirst and urination; nausea; vomiting; rapid, shallow breathing; stomach and chest pain; and fatigue. Hospital treatment involves intravenous administration of large amounts of fluids with electrolytes to replace those lost through excessive urination. Insulin is also generally given intravenously so that it works quickly and the dose can be adjusted frequently. Controlling blood glucose levels and replacing fluid and electrolytes usually allow the body to restore the normal acid–base balance.

MANAGING DIABETES

Diabetes is a complex disease and best treated with a team approach. Two key elements for optimally managing diabetes are patient education and a specialized medical team. People with diabetes benefit greatly from learning as much as possible about the disease—particularly, the practical, everyday steps that must be taken to control it. For example, self-testing of blood glucose is a daily routine. People with diabetes check their blood glucose level several times throughout the day using a drop of blood from a finger prick and a small, easy-to-use glucose monitor. Each test indicates the blood glucose level at that particular time and can guide the person's subsequent actions regarding eating, exercise, and medications.

Hypoglycemia is low blood glucose levels and can occur as a side effect of diabetes treatment.

Ketoacidosis is a life-threatening condition requiring immediate treatment; it is associated with uncontrolled diabetes and characterized by accumulation of ketones in the blood and increased acidity of the blood.

A specialized medical team provides patient education along with medical care. If the person's primary care doctor does not have expertise and experience in treating diabetes, the person is typically referred to an endocrinologist, a physician specializing in the treatment of hormonal and metabolic diseases. Other members of a diabetes-care medical team often include a nurse practitioner or a physician assistant, a dietitian, an exercise specialist, a pharmacist, and a mental health professional such as a social worker, a psychologist, or a counselor. Many are certified as diabetes educators by the American Association of Diabetes Educators (**www.diabeteseducator.org**), a multidisciplinary professional organization that ensures the delivery of quality self-management training to diabetic patients.

An important marker of blood glucose management (glycemic control) is the A1c test because it indicates how well blood glucose has been controlled over the past several months. As glucose circulates in the blood, some of it spontaneously binds to hemoglobin A (the primary form of hemoglobin). Hemoglobin is the protein that carries oxygen in the red blood cells. Once the glucose is bound to the hemoglobin A, it remains there for the life of the red blood cell (about 120 days). The more glucose there is in the blood, the more it binds to hemoglobin A. This combination of glucose and hemoglobin A is called *A1c* or *hemoglobin A1c* (see the earlier discussion of the A1c test). Measuring this compound reflects the overall blood glucose level over the previous two to three months. The A1c test helps the patient and doctor know if the treatment plan is working or needs to be adjusted. A1c should be measured two to four times a year, and the goal is to have a reading that is less than 7 percent.

People with diabetes should let friends and coworkers know about their diabetes so that they are aware of the needs associated with diabetes management—such as dietary control, medications, and, for some people, injections. Those with diabetes should carry or wear a medical identification bracelet or tag to alert paramedics and other health care professionals to the presence of diabetes. This allows medical professionals to respond appropriately, whether treating a diabetes-related emergency or an injury or accident unrelated to the disease.

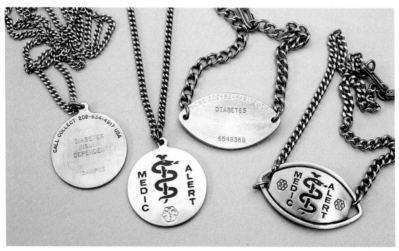

Individuals with diabetes may wear a medical alert tag or bracelet to ensure quick medical intervention in an emergency.

© McGraw-Hill Education/Rick Brady, photographer

To deal with the complexities of diabetes, treatment and management should be individualized and address medical, psychosocial, and lifestyle issues. Acceptance of the disease and compliance with a management plan are not trivial issues. A team approach works only if the patient takes an *active role* in his or her care. The actions a person chooses will determine how full a life he or she leads and to what degree disability is prevented.

Management of Type 1 Diabetes

Due to the lack of insulin production, type 1 diabetes is the most difficult form of diabetes to control. Type 1 is treated with insulin replacement along with a structured diet and physical activity regimen. Eating times, types and amounts of foods and beverages, and physical activity patterns should be consistent from day to day. Blood glucose is measured several times a day, and multiple insulin injections are necessary. Insulin can't be taken by mouth because the digestive juices destroy it. Most people find giving the injections to be simple and relatively painless because the needle is very small. Insulin is given at regular intervals, usually two to four times a day. Each injection may contain one type or a combination of different types of insulin—short-acting, intermediate-acting, or long-acting. As an alternative to injections, insulin pumps are increasingly being used. These pumps are small, computerized devices—about the size of a small cell phone—worn outside the body (in a pocket, pouch, or on a belt). They provide continuous insulin delivery through a small, soft tube. Future prospects for treatment include the possibility of delivering insulin through an inhaler.

Article
10.3

Breaking It Down "Human" Insulin— A First in Genetic Engineering

Since the discovery of insulin in 1921, a variety of insulins have been developed for people with diabetes. Harvesting human pancreases from corpses was not practical commercially, so the pancreases of cows and pigs were used. Both have "insulin activity" in humans because they are nearly identical to human insulin. However, even a slight difference is enough to elicit an allergic response in some people.

To overcome this problem, researchers looked for ways to make better insulin. Since the early 1980s, two methods have been used to make human insulin from nonhuman sources. One method involves the use of enzymes to convert insulin from pigs into human insulin by altering the one amino acid that is different. The second and more widely used method comes from genetic engineering, or recombinant DNA technology. Eli Lilly and Company marketed the first biogenetically engineered synthetic human insulin in 1982.

Genetic engineering is the manipulation of genetic material of cells in the lab to change hereditary traits or produce biological products. In this instance, bacteria are genetically altered to produce human insulin in large amounts. To provide a reliable source of human insulin, researchers obtain from human cells the DNA carrying the gene with the information to make insulin. They then make a copy of this DNA and move it into a bacterium. As the bacterium grows, the microbe splits from one cell into two, and both cells get a copy of the insulin gene. As these two grow, they divide into four, those four into eight, and so forth. All the cells have a copy of the genetic "recipe card" for insulin and, thus, produce insulin.

(continued)

This synthesized human insulin is identical to the insulin naturally produced in healthy humans. Recombinant DNA technology put to rest the fear that insulin production from animals would not be able to meet the need of the ever-increasing diabetic population. It had been forecast as early as 1976 that by the early 1990s demand would outstrip supply. Today, insulin from cows is no longer available, and insulin from pigs is being phased out. The cost of "human" insulin has remained similar to that of animal-derived insulin.

Genetic engineering is controversial—and it should be. After all, genetic engineering provides the means to alter the normal biology of living organisms by increasing the yield of a crop species, introducing a novel trait, or producing a new protein. As such, it brings on a host of legal, regulatory, and ethical challenges. In the case of "human" insulin, there has been little debate. A major medical need was met, and no major side effects or long-lasting adverse events have been identified.

Biotechnology products are regulated by the U.S. Department of Agriculture, the Environmental Protection Agency, and the Food and Drug Administration. Together, these agencies apply three criteria when assessing new products: safety, efficacy, and quality. Is the product sufficiently safe for humans and the environment? Does the product work as intended? Can the quality of the product be ensured? Other considerations include potential or probable social and economic impacts. The more we know about biotechnology, the better prepared we are to make personal choices and provide input on policies about the use of new technologies and their products.

Management of Type 2 Diabetes

In the past, type 2 diabetes was considered the milder form of diabetes. This is no longer the case. Although most people with type 2 do not require insulin, the consequences of not controlling high blood glucose can lead to the same serious

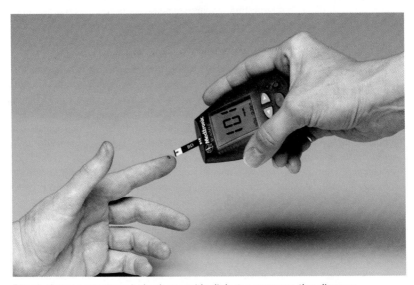

Blood glucose monitors help those with diabetes manage the disease.
© McGraw-Hill Education/Kevin May, photographer

metabolic and tissue damage complications as type 1. Generally, type 2 can be controlled with diet and exercise, especially if detected early. When lifestyle measures don't provide adequate blood glucose control, then medication in tablet form is used. The different types of medicine work in one of several ways: helping the beta cells of the pancreas make more insulin, increasing the use of glucose and decreasing glucose production, slowing the absorption of glucose from the intestine, or stimulating insulin release from the pancreas. Over time, even a careful diabetes management plan (i.e., optimal diet, exercise, oral medication therapies) may not be sufficient to keep type 2 diabetes under control. If this occurs, then insulin injections may become necessary.

✓ NEED TO KNOW

The most widely used criterion measure for diagnosing diabetes is a fasting blood glucose level equal to or greater than 126 mg/dL. Pre-diabetes is indicated when the fasting blood glucose level is in the borderline range of 100–125 mg/dL. Since 3 out of 10 people with type 2 diabetes are undiagnosed, it's important to know the risk factors and be screened as appropriate. The goal of treatment is to keep glucose levels within the normal range. Hypoglycemia and ketoacidosis are conditions that may occur with poor glycemic control. With the help of a diabetes health care team, a management plan addressing lifestyle, medical, and psychosocial issues is tailored to each individual. The key then becomes careful implementation and maintenance. In the final analysis, success depends on vigilant self-care.

➤ Prevention of Type 2 Diabetes

To date, there is no known method to prevent type 1 diabetes, although pancreatic islet transplantation shows promise and may become a viable option for selected patients within the next decade. In marked contrast to type 1, type 2 diabetes is largely a preventable disease. Yet, unless lifestyle changes are widely adopted, public health experts forecast the rise in type 2 diabetes will continue—and one out of three people born in the year 2000 will develop diabetes.

Responsibility to take action rests squarely on the shoulders of individuals and families. We need to avoid health-compromising habits and take the initiative to establish health-promoting practices. Once a person has diabetes, the decision to make smart choices seems so clear *in retrospect*. Humans, unlike other animals, have the capacity to plan and then follow a course of action. We should apply this capacity to our health and the prevention of disease just as we do in other aspects of our lives.

Be aware of the risk factors for diabetes and pre-diabetes, and be screened as appropriate. Remember that a significant proportion of people with diabetes are undiagnosed and that diabetes is occurring at earlier ages. Being overweight and having a family history of diabetes are the two most obvious risk factors.

Self Assessment 10.1

For those diagnosed with pre-diabetes, the potential to prevent the onset of diabetes with diet and exercise is excellent. In a major three-year clinical trial known as the Diabetes Prevention Program, high-risk participants randomly assigned to a lifestyle intervention group reduced their risk of getting diabetes by 58 percent. This intervention focused on healthful changes in diet and physical activity. Participants increased intake of whole-grain foods and reduced intake of saturated fats. They also built up to 30 minutes of exercise per day—engaging in brisk walking or similar moderate-intensity activity.

In a second group, participants were treated with standard diabetes oral medication (metformin). They reduced their risk of getting diabetes by 31 percent—a nice reduction, but not as great as the reduction for those in the lifestyle intervention. Those in the lifestyle intervention group lost about 6 percent of their body weight compared to no weight loss among those in the medication group.

This landmark study was conducted at 25 centers nationwide and involved over 3,000 people with pre-diabetes. Participants ranged in age from 25 to 85 with an average age of 51, and nearly half were from minority groups that disproportionately develop type 2 diabetes. All were overweight. The structured lifestyle intervention worked as well in men as women, in all ethnic groups, and across the age range.

The study ended a year early because the data clearly answered the main research question within the first three years. Ending a clinical trial study early due to excellent results is highly unusual. While both the lifestyle and oral medication treatments were found to be effective, lifestyle intervention was found to be better. NIH Director Francis S. Collins stated: "If you're tipping over into diabetes, you're better off with diet and exercise than you are with medication" (Diabetes Prevention Program).

✓ NEED TO KNOW

Type 2 diabetes is a preventable disease, yet its prevalence among Americans has been climbing steadily since 1990. Prevention depends on awareness and proactive steps by individuals and families. If you know someone with advanced diabetes, your incentive to take action may be particularly strong. Research has convincingly shown that the best strategy is to eat properly, exercise regularly, and maintain a healthy weight.

➤ Metabolic Syndrome

Metabolic syndrome is a cluster of risk factors for cardiovascular disease and type 2 diabetes, which occur together more often than by chance alone. Leading health organizations—including the American Heart Association; the National Heart, Lung, and Blood Institute (NHLBI); and the International Diabetes Association—have issued consensus statements to define and describe metabolic syndrome and to provide guidance on diagnosis and treatment.

TABLE 10.1   DEFINITION OF METABOLIC SYNDROME

Metabolic syndrome is defined as having at least 3 of 5 criteria:

RISK FACTORS	CRITERIA
Abdominal obesity (waist circumference)	$\geq$ 40 inches for men, $\geq$ 35 inches for women
Triglycerides	$\geq$ 150 mg/dL
HDL cholesterol	< 40 mg/dL for men, < 50 mg/dL for women
Blood pressure	$\geq$ 130/85 mm Hg
Fasting blood glucose	$\geq$ 100 mg/dL

Source: Alberti et al. *Circulation* 120: 1640–1645, 2009.

WHAT IS METABOLIC SYNDROME?

Metabolic syndrome appears to be precipitated by multiple underlying risk factors. The most important of these are abdominal obesity and insulin resistance. Other risk factors include poor diet, physical inactivity, aging, and genetic or ethnic predisposition. People with metabolic syndrome are three times as likely to have a heart attack or stroke and five times as likely to develop type 2 diabetes, compared with people without the syndrome.

First described in 1988, multiple definitions of metabolic syndrome have been proposed. The criteria most widely accepted are those adopted in 2009 (Table 10.1). These criteria are based on five common clinical measurements: waist circumference, triglycerides, HDL cholesterol, blood pressure, and fasting blood glucose. The presence of abnormalities in any three of these five measures constitutes a diagnosis of the syndrome.

A brief comment on abdominal obesity is warranted. Substantial research has shown that accumulation of upper body fat (on the trunk)—also known as abdominal or visceral fat—is more highly associated with both type 2 diabetes and atherosclerosis than lower body fat (on the hips and thighs). For this reason, a large waist circumference ($\geq$35 inches for women and $\geq$40 inches for men) is used in lieu of a high BMI as a criterion for metabolic syndrome.

The schematic in Figure 10.5 presents a simple depiction of a complex web of interactions and likely causal links among lifestyle factors, human physiology, and metabolic syndrome. The middle box reflects a biological "mixing pot"—still a scientific black box in many respects—where multiple physiological systems attempt to adapt to health-compromising factors as well as to one another. Behaviors can be viewed as input; the biological "pot" is where compensatory interplay among systems and disease processes occurs; and the resulting related diseases that constitute metabolic syndrome are presented as output. Over time, cascading and wide-ranging effects toward disease (or health) can result from lifestyle behaviors.

Metabolic syndrome is a cluster of conditions—excess abdominal fat, abnormal lipid levels, high blood pressure, and elevated blood glucose—that occur together and increase risk for coronary heart disease, stroke, and type 2 diabetes.

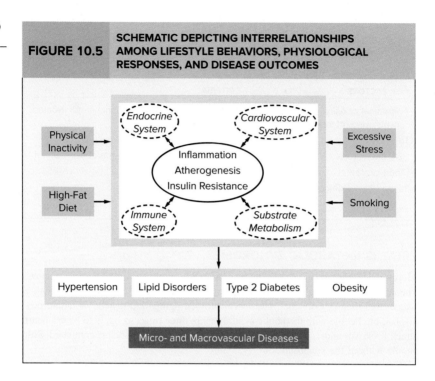

FIGURE 10.5 SCHEMATIC DEPICTING INTERRELATIONSHIPS AMONG LIFESTYLE BEHAVIORS, PHYSIOLOGICAL RESPONSES, AND DISEASE OUTCOMES

TREATMENT GOALS AND STRATEGIES

The primary goal in treating metabolic syndrome is to reduce risk for atherosclerosis—namely, heart disease and stroke—and to decrease the risk for type 2 diabetes in people who do not yet have the disease. As in managing the diseases separately, the first-line approach is to reduce the major risk factors: that is, strive to normalize blood pressure, blood lipids, blood glucose, and body weight to recommended goals. And, if a smoker, negotiate a program to stop.

At age 27, Mike acknowledged that he was overweight but gave little thought to his overall health. After all, he was simply a big person, still relatively young, and busy with work and home activities. Then he volunteered to give blood during a blood drive at work and was turned away because of high blood pressure. Surprised by this, he saw his doctor, who confirmed his hypertension and told him his blood lipids were off the chart, too. His doctor was direct and to the point: "You need to lose 70 pounds. It's time to get serious about your health." Mike suddenly realized his poor eating habits and his sedentary lifestyle had caught up with him, and he was at risk for heart disease, stroke, and diabetes.

Whenever possible, initial treatments for metabolic syndrome begin with life-style interventions—weight loss in overweight and obese people, a change in dietary patterns toward a prudent diet (low in saturated fats and refined sugars; high in whole grains, fruits, vegetables), and an increase in regular physical activity. Such changes will produce a reduction in all metabolic syndrome risk factors simultaneously. The greatest benefit will be derived from consistent and lasting lifestyle intervention. As a second tier of treatment, an array of drug therapies are

Mike decided to do something about his deteriorating medical condition and the inattention he had shown to his health. He made a promise to himself to turn around his situation. He started going to the gym regularly and made consistent adjustments in his diet, eating fewer processed foods and more fruits and vegetables. He relates, "I didn't cut out all the fun stuff; rather I just began to make better choices." These days, Mike feels healthier than he has in a long time. He is glad he finally recognized the need to take action and now would not have it any other way.

In closing, the term *metabolic syndrome* describes a condition in which risk factors for metabolic and atherogenic diseases cluster in the same people more often than would be expected by chance. This provides a practical means for early detection of individuals at high risk for type 2 diabetes and cardiovascular disease and indicates an interaction among diseases once thought to be separate conditions.

The American Diabetes Association, and American Heart Association have joined together to promote clinical and public health interventions to reduce tobacco use, poor diet, and sedentary living—the major risk factors for diabetes and cardiovascular disease. These leading scientific organizations are committed to ongoing collaboration in the prevention and early detection of interrelated chronic diseases.

✓ NEED TO KNOW

Metabolic syndrome is a clustering of risk factors associated with diabetes and cardiovascular disease. Metabolic syndrome provides a striking example of the continuous interaction among circulatory, metabolic, endocrine, and immune systems in their adaptations to lifestyle behaviors. Our body's physiological systems do not operate separately. Rather, complex interactions and compensatory influences are at work among them. Likewise, our health behaviors affect more than a single system or disease. Indeed, lifestyle habits have overall effects—for better or worse.

connect Resources

ARTICLES

10.1 "A Sweet and Sticky End." *The Lancet.* Movie review of *That Sugar Film,* an entertaining documentary on the effects of sugar in the diet.

10.2 "Type 2 Diabetes Surges in People Younger Than 20." *Washington Post.* A disease formerly associated with adults is now occurring in children and teens.

10.3 "Creating a Family Culture of Healthy Eating One Step at a Time." *Diabetes Health.* A mother provides insights and practical tips on making dietary changes for the whole family when her son is diagnosed with type 1 diabetes.

SELF-ASSESSMENT

10.1 Disease Risk Questionnaire for Type 2 Diabetes

Website Resources

DIABETES

American Association of Diabetes Educators **diabeteseducator.org**
American Diabetes Association **www.diabetes.org**
Diabetes Prevention Program **https://dppos.bsc.gwu.edu/**
International Diabetes Federation **www.idf.org**
Joslin Diabetes Center **www.joslin.harvard.edu**
National Diabetes Education Program **http://ndep.nih.gov**

METABOLIC SYNDROME

American Heart Association **www.heart.org/MetabolicSyndrome**

Knowing the Language

diabetes, 292
gestational diabetes, 296
hyperglycemia, 293
hypoglycemia, 293
insulin, 293

ketoacidosis, 303
metabolic syndrome, 309
pre-diabetes, 296
type 1 diabetes, 294
type 2 diabetes, 295

Understanding the Content

1. Where is insulin produced, and what is its role in the body?
2. Explain the differences among type 1 diabetes, type 2 diabetes, and pre-diabetes.
3. What are the risk factors for diabetes?
4. Define metabolic syndrome and the criteria for diagnosis.

1. Type 2 diabetes is by far the most common form of the disease, yet it's largely preventable. Its prevalence in the population is at an all-time high and projected to rise even higher. Why is this happening, and what needs to be done to turn the tide?

2. Just as with high blood pressure and abnormal blood lipids, we should know the numbers that define the condition. What fasting blood glucose levels define pre-diabetes and diabetes? What is the A1c measurement, and when is it used?

3. Explain how eating a healthy diet and exercising regularly lowers a person's risk for developing type 2 diabetes and metabolic syndrome.

Selected References

Alberti KG, Eckel RH, Grundy SM, et al. Harmonizing the metabolic syndrome: A joint interim statement of the International Diabetes Federation; National Heart, Lung, and Blood Institute; American Heart Association; World Heart Federation; International Atherosclerosis Society; and International Association for the Study of Obesity. *Circulation* 120: 1640–1645, 2009.

American Diabetes Association. Mike's Story. Posted at blog about diabetes in 2010. **http://diabetesstopshere.org/**

American Diabetes Association. Standards of medical care in diabetes—2015. *Diabetes Care* 38: S1–S94, 2015.

American Diabetes Association. Statistics. **www.diabetes.org/statistics**

Blaha M, Elasy TA. Clinical use of the metabolic syndrome: Why the confusion? *Clinical Diabetes* 24: 125–131, 2006.

Centers for Disease Control and Prevention. Childhood Overweight and Obesity. **www.cdc.gov/obesity/childhood/**

Centers for Disease Control and Prevention. Diabetes Report Card. **www.cdc.gov/diabetes**

Danaei G, Finucane MM, Lu Y, et al. National, regional, and global trends in fasting plasma glucose and diabetes prevalence since 1980: Systematic analysis of health examination surveys and epidemiological studies with 370 country-years and 2.7 million participants. *Lancet* 378: 31–40, 2011.

Diabetes Prevention Program Research Group. Reduction in the incidence of type 2 diabetes with lifestyle intervention or metformin. *New England Journal of Medicine* 346: 393–403, 2002.

Eckel RH, Alberti KG, Grundy SM, et al. The metabolic syndrome. *Lancet* 375: 181–183, 2010.

Eckel RH, Kahn R, Robertson RM, et al. Preventing cardiovascular disease and diabetes: A call to action from the American Diabetes Association and the American Heart Association. *Diabetes Care* 29: 1697–1699, 2006.

Grundy SM, Cleeman JI, Daniels SR, et al. AHA/NHLBI scientific statement: Diagnosis and management of the metabolic syndrome. *Circulation* 112: 2735–2752, 2005.

Hu FB. Globalization of diabetes: The role of diet, lifestyle, and genes. *Diabetes Care* 34: 1249–1257, 2011.

International Diabetes Federation. *Diabetes Atlas.* **www.idf.org/atlas**

Kemple AM, Zlot AI, Leman RF. Perceived likelihood of developing diabetes among high-risk Oregonians. *Preventing Chronic Disease*, November 2005.

Nobel Prize in Physiology or Medicine, 1923. **nobelprize.org/med1923**

Reaven GM. Role of insulin resistance in human disease. *Diabetes* 37: 1595–1607, 1988.

Sanders LJ. *The philatelic history of diabetes: In search of a cure.* Alexandria, VA: American Diabetes Association, 2001.

Steinberger J, Daniels SR., Eckel RH, et al. AHA scientific statement: Progress and challenges in metabolic syndrome in children and adolescents. *Circulation* 119: 628–647, 2009.

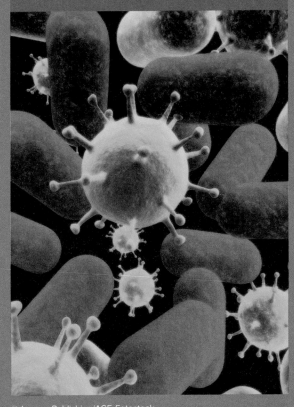

Epidemics have often been more influential than statesmen and soldiers in shaping the course of political history, and diseases may also color the moods of civilizations.

—René Dubos

© Ingram Publishing/AGE Fotostock

Chapter 11

INFECTIONS

The relationship between people and microbes has in part defined our world. In 2014, Americans were riveted to media sources trying to make sense of the Ebola pandemic and, in particular, how it might affect them. Yet, if people were aware of the processes involved in the spread of communicable diseases, they would have known that they were at minimal if any risk of Ebola. In Chapter 11 we examine all facets of the infectious disease process including signs, symptoms, treatment, risk factors, and risk reduction. At the end of the chapter we explore emerging issues, from new diseases to bioterrorism.

Chapter 11 | INFECTIONS

> The fate of most microbes that invade us is quick death. Sometimes, though, a
> microbe finds in humans an ideal environment, with plenty of nourishment and
> mere Maginot resistance. And it has its own weapon; it can attack or elude white
> blood cells, produce toxins, and kill and feed on tissues anywhere from the toes to
> the depths of the brain. If it multiplies unhindered, it may kill the host. But should
> that happen before the germ finds transport to another home, the meeting becomes
> a dead end for host and parasite alike.

As the quote from Karlen's book describes, the world is filled with microbes that
infect and sicken humans. Some cause illnesses that are easy to transmit but prove
more annoying than serious. Others are life-threatening but hard to catch. A few are
unfortunately both deadly and easy to spread. An example of the last type of infection
is the one that was responsible for the influenza pandemic of 1918, which is estimated to have killed tens of millions of people—more than died in World War I.

In the second half of the 20th century, the development of antibiotics greatly
reduced the number of deaths from bacteria infections. But microbes have mutated
and adapted defenses against many antibiotics in the past few decades. Each year
approximately 18,000 Americans die from MRSA (methicillin-resistant *Staphylococcus
aureus*), a common bacterium that has become resistant to antibiotics. Because of this
resistance, the bacterium can multiply unhindered and may kill the host.

In this chapter we will discuss the communicable disease process and the human
immune response that protects us. We will also describe some of the more common
infections that affect people today.

➤ Communicable Disease Process

The common link shared by all communicable diseases is that they are caused by
microorganisms called **pathogens,** *germs,* or *microbes.* Thousands of communicable
diseases have been identified. The American Public Health Association publishes
the *Control of Communicable Diseases in Man,* the definitive resource that describes
all communicable diseases and all facets of the communicable disease process
including transmission, prevention, and treatment.

Any communicable disease is defined by not only the pathogen responsible for
the disease but also the process by which the pathogen can infect people. The communicable disease process involves pathogens, reservoir, modes of transmission,
hosts, and stages of response (incubation, prodromal, acute, and recovery). Communicable diseases follow the process shown in Figure 11.1.

PATHOGENS

Six major groups of pathogens cause communicable diseases. These include bacteria, viruses, fungi, rickettsia, metazoa, and protozoa. Most common diseases are
caused by bacteria, viruses, and fungi. Pathogens are living organisms and, as such,
must have a place where they can live and reproduce in their natural environment.
This place is termed a *reservoir.* Not surprisingly, the reservoir for the most common
diseases that affect people is the human body.

Pathogens are microorganisms that cause communicable diseases.

FIGURE 11.1   CHAIN OF INFECTION

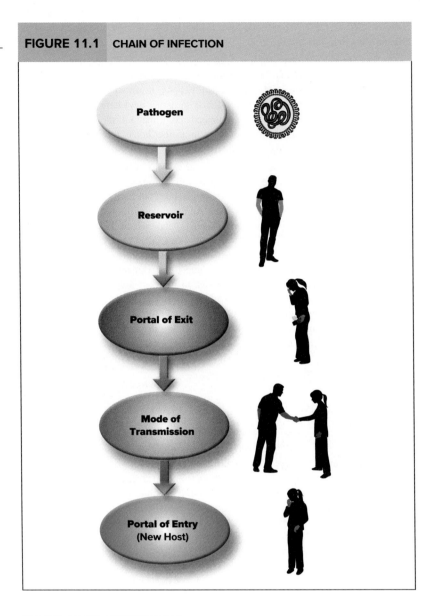

MODE OF TRANSMISSION

Infection occurs when a pathogen leaves the reservoir (that is, an infected person) and enters another person. This process is referred to as the *mode of transmission.* **Direct modes of transmission** are person to person via coughing, sneezing, or

> **Direct mode of transmission** is disease transmission through person-to-person contact.

sexual contact. **Indirect modes of transmission** include vectors and vehicles.
Vectors can be insects, such as mosquitoes or ticks, that carry a pathogen. An insect
that carries a pathogen bites a person in order to feed and as a result gives the
person the pathogen that causes disease. Vehicles are substances like water and food.
If a pathogen exists in the vehicle, it is consumed. Inanimate objects such as drinking glasses and eating utensils are also considered vehicles, since people can pick
up pathogens from their contaminated surfaces.

PORTALS OF ENTRY AND EXIT

Pathogens require portals of entry and exit in order to infect a person and for that
person to pass the infection to others. Portals include the nose, mouth, and reproductive system. The skin normally protects against infection, but when its surface is
broken by a cut, scrape, or insect bite, then it too becomes a possible portal of entry.
Finally, during sexual activity, pathogens can be transmitted from mucous membrane to mucous membrane.

STAGES OF RESPONSE

Once inside the body, pathogens have specific mechanisms of action on body cells.
There are many variations within pathogen groups that result in differences in infec-
tion mechanisms. Some of these will be noted when discussing selected diseases.
Regardless of the variations, there are four stages of response to any pathogen.

The first stage is called **incubation,** which is defined as the time between exposure to the pathogen and the onset of clinical symptoms. It is the time when the
pathogen is reproducing in the system and doing whatever it uniquely does to take
over the body.

After incubation, the infected person begins to experience early symptoms of
the disease, called *prodrome* or the **prodromal stage.** During the prodromal stage,
most people don't realize they are sick, and they tend to attribute the symptoms to
something else—lack of sleep, allergies, or general tiredness. As the symptoms get
more intense and the person begins to feel sick, the infection enters the **acute,** or
peak **stage.**

One of three things can happen after the acute stage: death (the pathogen wins),
recovery (the person's immune response system wins), or relapse (the person begins
to recover and then goes back into another acute stage). Relapse normally occurs if
a person doesn't get the right amount of rest or stops taking prescribed medication
too soon, allowing the pathogen to once again gain the upper hand.

Indirect mode of transmission is disease transmission via food or insects.

Incubation is the time between exposure to a pathogen and the onset of the
infection's symptoms.

In the **prodromal stage** the person experiences the early symptoms of a
disease.

The **acute stage** is the period when a person is the sickest with an infection.

Recovery is overcoming the infection and getting better.

Most common infectious diseases are caused by bacteria, viruses, and fungi. Direct modes of transmission are person to person via coughing, sneezing, or sexual contact. Indirect modes of transmission include vectors (such as insects) and vehicles (such as food, utensils, or other objects). Stages of infection are incubation, when symptoms have not yet appeared; prodromal, when symptoms first begin to emerge; and acute, when the full-blown infection is obvious. The acute stage is followed by recovery if the host successfully conquers the infection, or by death if the pathogen completely overwhelms the host. In long-term infectious diseases, the acute stage may sometimes be followed by a series of partial recoveries and relapses to the acute stage.

➤ Fighting Disease

Our body interprets infection with a pathogen as an invasion and tries to fight. A war of sorts ensues, with the pathogen trying to multiply on one side, and the body trying to kill off the pathogens on the other. The most effective method of fighting infections is our own immune system. Other methods include drugs such as vaccines, antibiotics, and antivirals.

IMMUNE SYSTEM

The immune system continually guards against foreign substances called **antigens.** Pathogens are considered antigens. White blood cells called **leukocytes** are the most basic unit of the immune system. Phagocytes and lymphocytes are the two main types of leukocytes. **Phagocytes** will surround, engulf, and digest pathogens or other material that is recognized as being foreign to the body. Phagocytes can also be specialized. For example, neutrophils are a type of phagocyte that primarily targets bacteria. A clinical application of this knowledge about different kinds of white blood cells is a blood test ordered by a physician to determine neutrophil count. If the count is higher than normal, it indicates a bacterial infection, which then has implications for the physician's recommendations about treatment.

 Lymphocytes originate in the bone marrow, and they can stay in the bone marrow and develop into B lymphocytes, often referred to as **B cells.** T lymphocytes, or **T cells,** are those that leave the bone marrow and mature in the thymus

An **antigen** is a foreign substance in the body that triggers the production of antibodies.

Leukocytes are white blood cells.

Phagocytes are white blood cells that surround and destroy foreign substances in the body.

Lymphocytes are a type of white blood cell and are the most basic unit of immunity. **B cells** are lymphocytes that produce antibodies. **T cells** are small circulating lymphocytes that mediate immune response.

gland. T cells and B cells work in partnership. If a pathogen invades the body, it is detected by the B cells, which produce antigen-specific **antibodies,** specialized proteins capable of destroying antigens. The T cells then destroy the pathogens.

The process of immunity is defined by lymphocytes and antibodies, but the broader types of immunity include active immunity and passive immunity. In active immunity, the protection develops after direct exposure to the pathogen. Cells in our immune response recognize the pathogen if we are subsequently exposed, and that increases our body's capability to fight that particular type of infection. Passive immunity is a process by which people get antibodies from another source, such as when infants ingest them in breast milk. Passive immunity is short-lived.

VACCINES

Vaccines can be an effective way to prevent an infection. When people are vaccinated, they are given a weakened or dead form of the pathogen, and they develop an immunity to it through their body's formation of antibodies. Figure 11.2 shows the diseases for which vaccinations are available.

ANTIBIOTICS

As their name implies, **antibiotics** fight bacterial infections. They are antibodies that, once administered, either destroy the bacteria directly or block bacterial biological processes, causing the pathogens to self-destruct. Antibiotics are specific to certain types of bacteria, so a diagnosis must be made in order to prescribe the correct drug. It is also important that once an antibiotic is prescribed, the person takes the whole prescription in the course of treatment. If not, resistant strains of the bacteria can result. Resistance to antibiotics is becoming a serious problem because the altered bacteria cause infections that can become very virulent, difficult to treat, and deadly.

Some individuals are allergic to antibiotics, and their reaction to them can be life-threatening. Physicians should ask any patient about known antibiotic allergies before prescribing an appropriate drug.

ANTIVIRALS

Antivirals are drugs that block the reproductive ability of viruses; they can be effective in treating certain viral conditions such as influenza. Tamiflu is an example of an antiviral. Use of antiviral drugs is tricky because in many instances there is

Antibodies are proteins that are produced to destroy antigens, including pathogens.

Vaccines are a treatment made from weakened or dead pathogens that allow the body to build up immunity against specific diseases.

Antibiotics are antibodies given as a drug that disrupt bacterial processes and stop an infection from growing.

Antivirals are drugs that treat viral infections.

FIGURE 11.2 ADULT IMMUNIZATION SCHEDULE

VACCINE ▼ / AGE GROUP ▶	19–49 Years	50–64 Years	≥65 Years
Tetanus, Diphtheria, Pertussis (Td/Tdap)[1],*	1 dose Td booster every 10 yrs; Substitute 1 dose of Tdap for Td		
Human papillomavirus (HPV)[2],*	3 doses females (0, 2, 6 mos)		
Measles, Mumps, Rubella (MMR)[3],*	1 or 2 doses	1 dose	
Varicella[4],*	2 doses (0, 4–8 wks)		
Influenza[5],*	1 dose annually		
Pneumococcal (polysaccharide)[6,7]	1–2 doses		1 dose
Hepatitis A[8],*	2 doses (0, 6–12 mos or 0, 6–18 mos)		
Hepatitis B[9],*	3 doses (0, 1–2, 4–6 mos)		
Meningococcal[10],*	1 or more doses		
Zoster[11]		1 dose	

For all persons in this category who meet the age requirements and who lack evidence of immunity (e.g., lack documentation of vaccination or have no evidence of prior infection).

Recommended if some other risk factor is present (e.g., on the basis of medical, occupational, lifestyle, or other indications).

*Covered by the Vaccine Injury Compensation Program.

Adult immunization schedule by vaccine and medical and other indications

VACCINE ▼ / INDICATION ▶	Pregnancy	Immuno-compromising conditions (excluding human immunodeficiency virus [HIV]), medications, radiation[13]	HIV infection[3,12,13] CD4+ T lymphocyte count <200 cells/μL	HIV infection[3,12,13] CD4+ T lymphocyte count ≥200 cells/μL	Diabetes, heart disease, chronic pulmonary disease, chronic alcoholism	Asplenia[12] (including elective splenectomy and terminal complement deficiencies)	Chronic liver disease	Kidney failure, end-stage renal disease, receipt of hemodialysis	Health care personnel
Tetanus, Diphtheria, Pertussis (Td/Tdap)[1,*]	Substitute 1 dose of Tdap for Td	1 dose Td booster every 10 yrs							
Human papillomavirus (HPV)[2,*]		3 doses for females through age 26 yrs (0, 2, 6 mos)							
Measles, Mumps, Rubella (MMR)[3,*]	Contraindicated	Contraindicated	Contraindicated	1 or 2 doses					
Varicella[4,*]	Contraindicated	Contraindicated	Contraindicated	2 doses (0, 4–8 wks)					
Influenza[5,*]	1 dose TIV annually								1 dose TIV or LAIV annually
Pneumococcal (polysaccharide)[6,7]	1–2 doses								
Hepatitis A[8,*]	2 doses (0, 6–12 mos or 0, 6–18 mos)								
Hepatitis B[9,*]	3 doses (0, 1–2, 4–6 mos)								
Meningococcal[10,*]	1 or more doses								
Zoster[11]	Contraindicated	Contraindicated	Contraindicated	1 dose					

For all persons in this category who meet the age requirements and who lack evidence of immunity (e.g. lack documentation of vaccination or have no evidence of prior infection).

Recommended if some other risk factor is present (e.g. on the basis of medical, occupational, lifestyle, or other indications).

*Covered by the Vaccine Injury Compensation Program.

Report all clinically significant postvaccination reactions to the Vaccine Adverse Event Reporting System (VAERS). Reporting forms and instructions on filing a VAERS report are available at www.vaers.hhs.gov. Additional information about the vaccines in this schedule is available at www.cdc.gov/vaccines.

Source: CDC.

a narrow therapeutic window for effectiveness at the very beginning of the infection. Most people don't visit their physician until they are very ill, when the use of antivirals is less effective, if not contraindicated.

Health & the Media Hand Sanitizer Dangers

Can the alcohol in hand sanitizers cause poisoning? You may have heard a story about a little girl who was rushed to the emergency room after becoming lethargic and unable to focus her eyes. Tests failed to discover the problem until a preschool teacher reported that children witnessed the child licking hand sanitizer before falling ill. Blood alcohol tests then showed the girl had dangerously high levels of alcohol in her system. The story ends with strict cautions about how deadly hand sanitizer can be.

Although this tale was widely distributed via e-mail with enough factual errors (such as an impossibly high blood alcohol level) that led it to be classified as an urban myth, the basic premise behind the story is true. Hand sanitizers contain up to 65 percent alcohol, and if ingested in sufficient amounts, they can cause alcohol poisoning. Although this isn't an issue for adults, who understand that sanitizer is for washing and not drinking, accidental poisoning could occur with small children.

Although nonalcoholic versions of hand sanitizers are available, some doctors and health policy administrators caution strongly against using this type. In this case, the worry is that widespread use of these alternative sanitizers may help build drug-resistant "superbugs." (See "Breaking It Down" for more information on drug-resistant infections.) Alcohol-based sanitizers are believed to kill more types of bacteria than other types, and the mechanism by which they work does not create drug-resistant pathogens.

Given their ability to reduce the spread of gastrointestinal and respiratory illness and the fact their use doesn't increase drug-resistant microbes, getting rid of alcohol-based hand sanitizers entirely is probably too strong a reaction. They have their place in the fight against infections. However, keeping them out of reach of children and allowing children to use them only with adult supervision are wise practices.

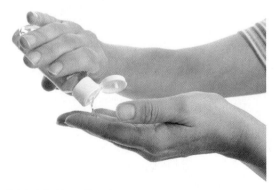

© Ashok Rodrigues/Getty Images

Vaccines, antibiotics, and antivirals are all valuable ways to prevent infections or lessen their intensity and duration. Good hygiene is also important in the prevention of infections. Perhaps the most important behavior one can perform to prevent disease is to wash hands frequently. Many of the more common pathogens are found on hands and thus are capable of being transmitted to other people. Additionally, maintaining a good lifestyle (such as exercising regularly, eating healthy foods, and getting enough sleep routinely) also helps keep the immune system in good shape, which in turn helps the body fight off infections.

✓ **NEED TO KNOW**

The human immune system is by far the most effective tool for fighting off infections. White blood cells, called B cells, target antigens by creating antibodies, while other white blood cells (T cells) then destroy the pathogens. Vaccines are drugs that are administered to prevent infections. Antibiotics are drugs that kill bacteria, and antiviral drugs fight viruses. People who maintain good health habits and are well rested will usually have a better immune response against infections than people who are stressed or have unhealthy habits. All people can decrease the chance of infections by frequently washing their hands.

Self
Assessment
11.1

➤ Bacterial Infections

Bacteria are very simple pathogens. It should be noted that many bacteria do not cause disease and can even be beneficial to human health. Bacteria are single-celled plants that, after entering a body, divide until they reach sufficient numbers to cause symptoms. One cell becomes two, two cells become four, four cells become eight, and so on until they reach billions and trillions. It is only after huge numbers of bacteria are present that a person becomes aware of the infection, because that is the point at which symptoms arise.

There are many common bacterial infections. Some will be covered in this section and some will be covered in the section "Sexually Transmitted Infections." Because most foodborne diseases (food poisoning) are bacterial, those diseases are discussed in Chapter 2.

STAPH INFECTIONS

Staph (staphylococcal) bacteria are common bacteria found on the skin and the membranes that line the nose and throat. In most instances the bacteria are harmless, but if conditions are right, the bacteria can invade the body, secrete a toxin, and result in disease. Common **staph infections** include impetigo, boils, and cellulitis.

Staphylococcal infections include cellulitis, impetigo, skin boils, and the much-feared, drug-resistant MRSA.

Impetigo is a contagious skin infection that can result when the staph bacteria invade the skin through a crack or broken area. During an impetigo infection, blisters can appear, and the affected skin can become red. When the blisters burst, the infection can spread, and the area where the blister fluid dries can have a crusty appearance. Antibiotics can clear up the infection quickly.

Boils are inflamed, pus-filled lumps on the skin that are also caused by staph bacteria. Normally these lumps are infected hair follicles. To avoid spreading the infection, it is important that the boil not be burst. A hot compress can shrink the boil and facilitate drainage. In some instances antibiotics are prescribed to facilitate ending the infection.

Cellulitis is a staph infection of the skin and the tissues beneath. Usually the infection results from a wound. Cellulitis normally affects the neck, face, and legs. In addition to redness of the affected skin, fever and chills can result. Again, antibiotics are used to treat the infection.

Toxic shock syndrome is an uncommon staph infection, but because it is largely preventable and the people with the highest risk are young menstruating women, it warrants discussion. In rare instances, toxic shock syndrome results when a woman inserts a tampon without first washing her hands. Staph bacteria on the hands are transmitted to the vagina via the tampon. If the staph grow in sufficient numbers, they can secrete a toxin that causes a sudden drop in blood pressure, high fever, skin rash, dizziness, disorientation, and possibly shock. The mortality rate is about 3 percent. Treatment is the same antibiotics used for other staph infections.

STREP INFECTIONS

Streptococcal (strep) infections are common, with the most common being strep throat. One of the least common yet most highly publicized is flesh-eating bacteria. Strep throat usually starts one to five days after exposure, and its chief symptoms include fever, sore throat, and swollen neck glands. A simple throat culture can confirm the diagnosis, and antibiotics can be effective in treating the condition. In extreme or untreated cases, the initial strep infection can develop into a body rash known as scarlet fever, or turn into rheumatic fever, which causes heart problems.

Breaking It Down   Superbugs

Pathogens capable of surviving antibiotics and other medications designed to kill them are called *superbugs*. Such pathogens, the most common of which is methicillin-resistant *Staphylococcus aureus* (MRSA), have the potential to become a significant medical and public health problem.

MRSA is colonized in approximately 1 percent of the population. The bacterium itself is not harmful unless it invades the skin or body organs and causes infection.

Streptococcal infections include strep throat and flesh-eating bacteria.

There are about 90,000 reported infections each year. These bacteria are a real danger because infection has a 20 percent mortality rate.

Until recently MRSA was a problem mostly found in hospitals and nursing homes, where approximately 85 percent of the reported cases originate. These settings are ideal for transmission because elderly and/or sick people tend to be more susceptible to infections. In the case of hospitals, invasive procedures such as surgery also provide an easy way for these bacteria to find their way into the body.

Although medical facilities are the riskiest locations for coming into contact with MRSA, infection can occur in any setting, especially where towels, soap, or equipment are shared by many. This is why we have seen outbreaks of MRSA in students at the same school, among U.S. soldiers returning from Afghanistan and Iraq, and even within the ranks of the St. Louis Rams football team.

MRSA is not the only superbug. Other strains of *Staphylococcus aureus* are becoming antibiotic resistant. *Enterococcus,* which is responsible for infections that range from the urinary tract to heart valves, and *Streptococcus pneumonia,* which can cause pneumonia and meningitis, are also developing tolerance to drugs that formerly killed them easily. There is also some evidence that the pathogens responsible for gonorrhea, salmonella, and *Escherichia coli (E. coli)* disease are also becoming antibiotic resistant.

If more superbugs emerge, we could potentially see a new era where the leading causes of death will be communicable diseases, much as it was during the centuries before modern advances in medical care. In that event, medical efforts would shift to emphasizing the prevention of communicable diseases instead of chronic illnesses such as diabetes and heart disease. Further, if this scenario does play out, we could see decrease in both lifespan and life expectancy.

A hopeful point is the fact that superbugs were created through unintended consequences and sloppy practices that people can avoid, once they are aware of the dangers. This is a case where everyday actions by many will be a better defense than relying on science to create ever-stronger drugs to fight resistant, ever-stronger bacteria. Not sharing towels, washing hands frequently, taking the entire antibiotic prescription, and not insisting on antibiotics when the doctor says they are unnecessary are all ways that each of us can help prevent the emergence of new superbugs.

Invasive Group A *Streptococcus* gets a lot of publicity because of its devastating and potentially disfiguring results. This kind of strep bacteria destroys fatty tissue and muscle, thereby gaining the nickname "flesh-eating bacteria." Usually the mode of transmission is an untreated skin wound. The wound becomes infected with strep, and tissue death occurs. Antibiotics can stop the infection, but any tissue that died will not grow back.

One in 10 people carries the bacteria responsible for meningococcal meningitis or **bacterial meningitis.** The bacteria are transmitted by close contact between people, which is why outbreaks are known to happen in places such as college dorms. Some people have enough of an immune deficiency that the bacteria get into the bloodstream,

Bacterial meningitis is an infection that can affect the brain and is potentially fatal.

affect the brain, and produce the symptoms associated with bacterial meningitis. These symptoms include severe headache, stiff neck, fever, frequent vomiting, and a rash. Fewer than 5 percent of victims will die. If the infection spreads, a condition called *septicemia* results, and the death rate can rise to around 20 percent or higher.

Bacterial meningitis and septicemia are very serious. When young people move into a college dorm or other setting where they come into close contact with a large number of people, they are at higher risk of exposure to the bacteria. Vaccination is the best method of prevention. In addition, it is important to be aware of the symptoms so that medical attention can be sought before the symptoms get worse. Early medical attention with antibiotics can mean the difference between life and death.

NEED TO KNOW

Bacterial diseases are common, although of all the types of bacteria only a relatively small number cause disease. Antibiotics treat bacterial infections. Bacterial meningitis is a life-threatening infection that sometimes breaks out in close living quarters like college dormitories. Fever, a stiff neck, vomiting, and a rash are symptoms of it. People can be vaccinated against bacterial meningitis.

➤ Viral Infections

Viruses are mysterious organisms. They are very simple—a strand of RNA or DNA wrapped in a protein coat. Viruses have the capability of invading the body and using the person's own cells as genetic material to replicate. This process baffles scientists, and because of its complexity, it has been difficult to medically intervene and rid the body of viruses in the way that antibiotics rid the body of bacteria. So the quality of the individual's immune response system, which can destroy the virus, is usually the key to dealing with viral infections. Examples of viral infections are the common cold, influenza, mononucleosis, herpes, and hepatitis. (Sexually transmitted viral infections will be covered later in the chapter.)

COMMON COLD

Over 100 different viruses can cause what we term the *common cold*. Over 50 percent of colds are caused by rhinoviruses, which are viruses that are in the nose. It makes sense that the symptoms of a cold are a runny nose, nasal congestion, a sore throat, and sometimes a headache and fever.

Most adults have two to three colds each year. There is no cure for the common cold, and since a healthy immune response system is very effective in eliminating the virus, the symptoms last about a week and tend to be self-limiting. Because most cold viruses are transmitted by the hands, the most effective way to prevent the spread of colds is to wash one's hands frequently and cover the mouth when sneezing or coughing.

INFLUENZA

Influenza, or the flu, spreads from person to person through coughing or sneezing. Shaking hands with an infected person is also a common mode of transmission; if

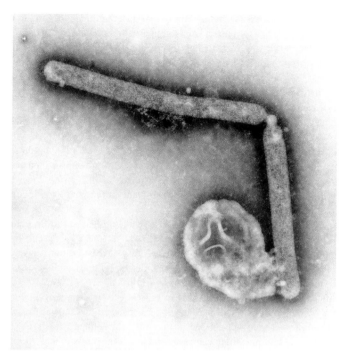

A virus as seen through a high-powered microscope.
Centers for Disease Control and Prevention (CDC)

people cough into their hand or wipe their nose, they can easily pass on the virus when they touch someone else. Influenza is similar to the common cold, but the symptoms are usually more severe. The incubation period for influenza is usually one to three days, and the symptoms include headache, tiredness, body aches, fever, and chills. There is no cure for the flu. A person's natural immune response will be helped if the flu sufferer gets plenty of rest and drinks lots of fluids.

There are three types of influenza: type A, type B, and type C. The most widespread is type A.

A sense of seriousness regarding influenza reached a fever pitch in spring 2009 when novel Influenza A, a subtype called H1N1 virus, was detected in humans. Mexico reported the first cluster of infections, followed soon after by the United States. H1N1 spread rapidly throughout the rest of the globe. Within a few months of its first detection, the World Health Organization officially classified H1N1 as a pandemic. With approximately 17,000 deaths attributed to H1N1, the pandemic did not turn out to be as serious as originally feared. In August 2010 the H1N1 pandemic was declared officially over.

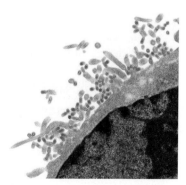

This electron-microscope view shows an influenza virus (yellow) budding from a host cell. The host cell nucleus is black.
© Science Photo Library RF/Getty Images

The *H* and *N* in the virus's name refer to two different kinds of proteins: hemagglutinin (allows the virus to attach to cells) and neuraminidase (in part responsible for releasing new viruses from cells). There are 16 types of hemagglutinin and 9 types of neuraminidase, and we can identify viruses by their specific protein makeup. For instance, the H3N2 virus was responsible for the Hong Kong flu epidemic in the late 1960s. Some but not all of these protein combinations are capable of causing human influenza.

Influenza A spreads from person to person. Symptoms of Influenza A are typical of other human flus: fever, cough, runny nose, aches, fatigue, and chills. Typically infected persons are contagious from one day before symptoms arise to about a week after symptoms subside. The best way to prevent Influenza A infection is the same protocol for preventing other forms of influenza: Cover the nose and mouth when sneezing or coughing, wash hands often, and avoid contact with sick people when possible.

If you do become infected with Influenza A, it is important to do your part to help prevent passing it on to others. The CDC advises that people with influenza-like symptoms stay home from work or school until at least 24 hours after they are free of fever or signs of a fever (such as chills or fatigue) without using fever-reducing medications like acetaminophen or ibuprofen.

Flu vaccinations are an effective way to prevent the flu. The best time to get the vaccine is between October and mid-November because it takes about two weeks for the vaccination to develop protection against influenza. Influenza should be taken seriously because complications can result, including pneumonia and, in rare cases, paralysis.

MONONUCLEOSIS

Mononucleosis is a common viral infection that as many as 95 percent of adults in the United States will contract by the time they are 40 years old. Epstein-Barr virus is the pathogen that causes mononucleosis. It is found in the saliva of the infected person and may be spread through direct contact, which is why it is nicknamed the "kissing disease."

Mononucleosis has a long incubation period. Approximately 30–50 days after exposure, the person can experience a fever, sore throat, swollen glands in the back of the neck, and fatigue. Symptoms can last anywhere from a week or two to several months. Although most people experience mono only once, it is possible for the virus to lie dormant and reactivate later, resulting in another episode of symptoms. As with influenza, treatment includes rest to help the immune system.

HERPES 1 (ORAL HERPES)

The most common types of this virus are **herpes simplex virus 1 (HSV 1)** and herpes simplex virus 2 (HSV 2). HSV 1, or oral herpes, will be discussed here, and HSV 2, or genital herpes, will be discussed in the section "Sexually Transmitted Infections."

Herpes simplex virus 1 (HSV 1) infections are common incurable oral infections, and cold sores around the mouth and lips are the most typical symptom.

The classic HSV 1 symptom is a cold-sore lesion on or near the mouth. The sores will appear for a week or two and then subside. The virus will then lie dormant and can reactivate at almost any time. The first outbreak of cold sores is usually the worst and most painful. HSV 1 is not dangerous unless one has a compromised immune system, and the infection spreads and affects the nervous system. Medications are available to reduce the severity of the symptoms, but no medications exist that actually rid the body of the virus. To prevent the spread of herpes, limit saliva contact with an infected person, cover cold sores if possible, and wash hands often.

HEPATITIS

Hepatitis is a generic term meaning "inflammation of the liver." There are several types of the disease, categorized as A, B, or C, depending in part on the mode of transmission. Hepatitis A can be present in the feces and is normally contracted through eating food prepared by someone who is infected and did not wash his or her hands after using the bathroom. Hepatitis B and C are contracted through contact with infected blood via transfusions, dirty needles, or sexual intercourse.

Since hepatitis affects the liver, a key symptom is a yellowing of the skin and eyes called *jaundice*. Other symptoms include brown urine, diarrhea or light-colored stool, fever, loss of appetite, stomach pain, nausea, and fatigue. These symptoms usually begin about four weeks after exposure, can last for a long time, may be quite intense, and are not usually self-limiting but do impair functioning. Hepatitis C victims can carry the virus the rest of their lives. Hepatitis is largely preventable. If restaurant workers wash their hands before touching food, risk of hepatitis A for customers is extremely low. Drugs are available to treat hepatitis, and vaccinations are available for hepatitis A and B. Also, the FDA recently approved a new drug, Incivek, that shows much promise in curing liver disease caused by hepatitis C.

Hepatitis B and C, which are the bloodborne forms of hepatitis, can be successfully prevented by using what are termed "universal precautions." All health care workers and many other workers are required to learn these precautions.

Figure 11.3 lists the universal precautions. After reviewing the list, you can easily see that the main effort is to protect the portal of entrance—the skin and nose—from contact with blood products or body fluids. Adhering to universal precautions reduces risk by blocking the portal of entrance through use of masks, gloves, and protective clothing. If implemented correctly, these precautions will significantly limit one's risk of bloodborne diseases.

EBOLA

Because of the 2014 pandemic in West Africa and the few cases in the United States, most people have heard of Ebola. Ebola is a very dangerous disease with the average fatality rate being 50 percent, meaning that 50 percent of the people contracting Ebola will die. However, unless you are in a certain area of the world, such as West Africa, Ebola is a very hard disease to catch.

Hepatitis is a generic term for an infection that causes inflammation of the liver.

FIGURE 11.3   UNIVERSAL PRECAUTIONS

1. **Using gloves** to provide a barrier between the hands and potentially infectious body fluids or items contaminated with body fluids. Wash hands immediately after removing gloves.

2. **Wearing** face protection such as masks to prevent droplets of potentially infectious body fluids from being inhaled.

3. **Wearing** protective body clothing such as disposable laboratory coats when there is potential for body fluids to be splashed onto the body.

4. **Washing hands** thoroughly if there is contact with body fluids.

5. **Washing surfaces** that have been exposed to body fluids.

6. **Avoiding injuries** caused by potentially contaminated needles and any other sharp instruments.

7. **Placing** all used gloves and disposable items exposed to body fluids in a specially designated hazardous-materials container.

Bloodborne diseases such as hepatitis B or HIV are best prevented by limiting exposure to potentially infectious body fluids, including blood, through following universal precautions. These precautions include three main practices: wearing a barrier between exposed skin and body fluids; washing hands; and placing exposed materials in a specially designated hazardous-materials receptacle.

Article
11.2

The Ebola virus is the cause of the disease. It is not new. Ebola has been diagnosed since 1976, and there have been numerous outbreaks mostly in remote villages in Africa. The virus is transmitted to people from animals, particularly those in the wild, and once a human is infected the virus can be transmitted person to person. But, for a person to contract the Ebola virus from another person he or she needs to come into contact with the blood of the infected person, meaning that he or she has to be in close contact and have exposed skin come into contact with the body fluids. So, medical workers dealing with Ebola patients are at risk if they don't follow correct procedures—covering all exposed skin, masks, and gloves. The medical workers contracting Ebola in the United States did not follow proper protocols and they were infected. Since the medical care system in the United States is high quality, the infected workers were isolated and hydrated and survived. Ebola cannot be transmitted through coughing or sneezing—it is not an airborne virus.

So, in the midst of the outbreak Americans were at minimal, if any, risk. Yes, Ebola is scary, but unless one is traveling in areas where the virus is common (e.g., remote villages in West Africa), calling the risk minimal is probably an overstatement.

Despite the fact that the Zika virus was first isolated in the late 1940s, most people had not heard of the Zika virus before the widespread media reporting in 2015 about Brazilian women giving birth to children with birth defects and the birth defects being due to maternal infection with the Zika virus. Generally, Zika virus infections tend to be mild with fever, rash, joint pain, and headache lasting a few days to a week. The mode of transmission for the Zika virus is the mosquito. There are no vaccines or medications currently available to prevent or treat Zika infections. The best way to prevent infections is to avoid areas in South and Central America where the infections are most common. These areas should be especially avoided if one is pregnant or planning on becoming pregnant. Other preventive measures include covering exposed skin and using insect repellents when traveling to areas where the virus is commonly found.

✔ NEED TO KNOW

Options for treating viral diseases are limited. A healthy immune system and frequent hand washing are the best defenses against viruses such as influenza. Avoiding contact with herpes sores is perhaps the best low-risk behavior to prevent a herpes 1 infection. Mononucleosis has been referred to as the kissing disease and the risk of getting it is increased by deep kissing with an infected person. However, many people get mononucleosis just through close person-to-person contact. Symptoms include sore throat, swollen glands, and extreme fatigue. Finally, to avoid contracting bloodborne diseases such as HIV and hepatitis, one should follow universal precautions. Universal precautions are based on three main practices: wearing a barrier between exposed skin and body fluids; washing hands; and placing exposed materials in a specially designed hazardous-materials receptacle.

➤ Fungal Infections

Fungi are pathogens capable of a wide range of infections, from minor annoyances like athlete's foot and ringworm to serious, life-threatening lung infections such as histoplasmosis.

Athlete's foot is caused by coming into contact with fungal spores commonly found on locker-room floors (hence *athlete's foot*). Skin from an infected person is shed, and a barefoot person stepping on the infected skin runs a risk of also becoming infected. The key symptoms of athlete's foot are redness, itching, and cracking of skin, usually between the toes. Normally, applying a topical antifungal medication will clear up the infection quickly. Prevention efforts include wearing flip-flops when walking on floors used by many barefooted people, especially in locker rooms, and keeping the feet dry.

Ringworm is a fungal infection normally confined to the scalp. The infection appears as a red circle on the scalp, and because it is raised, it looks like a worm. Direct physical contact with an infected person or animal is the chief method of

Self Assessment
11.2

developing the infection. Ringworm is highly contagious and can affect both children and adults. Once diagnosed, ringworm can be successfully treated with topical antifungal medications.

NEED TO KNOW

Serious fungal infections are rare. Most fungal infections are confined to the skin with typical symptoms being redness, itching, and in some cases blisters. Common fungal infections can be treated with antifungal medications, many of which are available over-the-counter. The best way to prevent these common infections is to limit contact with fungal spores, which basically means avoid contact with infected skin. Also, wearing flip-flops or shower shoes in public bathing facilities will limit exposure to spores on the public shower or bathroom floor. Finally, since fungal infections thrive in moist areas, keeping feet clean and dry will help prevent athlete's foot, the most common fungal infection.

➤ Sexually Transmitted Infections

Sexually transmitted infections (STIs) are common diseases caused by bacteria or viruses. Pathogens can be transmitted through sexual activities such as vaginal intercourse, anal intercourse, or oral sex. The common STIs include chlamydia, gonorrhea, syphilis, herpes 2, and human papillomavirus (HPV).

CHLAMYDIA

Chlamydia is a type of bacteria found in infected body fluids from the penis or vagina. The bacterium is transmitted during sexual contact. Symptoms typically appear 7–30 days after exposure. They usually include a discharge from the penis, vagina, or rectum; cramps or pain in the lower abdomen in women; burning or itching around the opening of the penis; pain in the testicles; and painful urination. Many people with chlamydia do not have symptoms, but they can still spread the disease. Women who are asymptomatic might not be aware of the chlamydia infection until they experience pelvic inflammatory disease (PID). However, vaginal discharge with odor or bleeding between cycles can indicate infection, and medical attention is required. Antibiotics can successfully treat chlamydia.

GONORRHEA

Gonorrhea, another sexually transmitted bacterial infection, is similar to chlamydia. The symptoms are virtually the same. However, symptoms usually appear sooner than for chlamydia, two to seven days after exposure. Untreated gonorrhea in women can lead to pelvic inflammatory disease. Vaginal discharge with odor or bleeding between cycles could indicate infection, and medical attention is required. Gonorrhea can be successfully treated with antibiotics.

Pelvic inflammatory disease (PID) is a serious complication of untreated chlamydia and gonorrhea. When the disease is not treated, the bacteria can find their way to the cervix, uterus, fallopian tubes, and eventually the lower pelvic cavity. The symptoms of PID include lower abdominal pain and abnormal vaginal discharge, fever, pain in the right upper abdomen, painful intercourse, and irregular menstrual bleeding. PID causes more than 100,000 women per year to become infertile. Another possible complication of PID is ectopic pregnancy, where the fertilized egg implants in the fallopian tube or the ovary (see Chapter 5).

PID can be difficult to diagnose because the symptoms can be similar to those of many other diseases. Antibiotics can be used to treat PID, but any damage to pelvic structures will remain.

SYPHILIS

Syphilis is another sexually transmitted infection. Unlike chlamydia and gonorrhea, the signs and symptoms are dependent on which stage of syphilis the person is experiencing.

The first stage of syphilis is called the *primary stage.* An infectious, painless lesion or sore called a *chancre* appears at the point of sexual contact. The chancre will most likely appear 10–90 days after exposure and remain for an average of 21 days, after which it will disappear naturally. Unfortunately, the disappearance of the chancre doesn't mean the person is cured. It indicates he or she is moving into the *secondary stage* of the disease.

During the secondary stage, the bacteria spread, and a rash appears all over the body. This rash can look like a sunburn or take the form of wartlike bumps and white patches in the mouth. In addition to the rash, an infected person might also have a fever, swollen glands, sore throat, patchy hair loss, headaches, weight loss, and malaise. The rash and other symptoms can last two to six weeks and will disappear.

If untreated during the primary and secondary stages, the bacteria will become even more disseminated and will damage body organs. This state is termed the *latent stage,* and most often it has no symptoms. A person can be in the latent stage for years before there are symptoms of organ damage, such as paralysis, blindness, and heart damage. This damage marks the last stage of syphilis, termed the *tertiary stage.*

The bacteria can be eliminated with antibiotics. At any stage in the infection, a person can receive the antibiotics and be cured. However, if organ damage occurs, it will not be reversed by antibiotic treatment.

HERPES 2 (GENITAL HERPES)

Herpes simplex virus 2 (HSV 2) is the sexually transmitted form of herpes. Approximately 2–12 days after exposure, a person develops small sores or lesions

Article
11.3

Pelvic inflammatory disease (PID) is a serious, painful condition often related to untreated chlamydia or gonorrhea.

Herpes simplex virus 2 (HSV 2) is an incurable viral infection; it is usually sexually transmitted, and lesions around the point of sexual contact are the most common symptom.

around either the external reproductive organs or the mouth, depending on the point of sexual contact and infection. These sores can be quite painful and will normally last for a week or two before disappearing. However, like herpes 1, when the sores disappear, it doesn't mean that the person is cured; rather, the virus has gone into dormancy and can reactivate at any time. There are medications that can limit the intensity or severity of the symptoms, but there is no cure—once infected, always infected. About 16 percent of Americans between the ages of 14 and 49 are infected with herpes 2. Women with herpes 2 infections have a higher risk of cervical cancer and run the risk of not being able to vaginally deliver a baby, especially if there are active sores.

HUMAN PAPILLOMAVIRUS

Human papillomavirus (HPV) is responsible for a condition commonly called *genital warts.* HPV is transmitted sexually, and the warts appear either externally or internally on the genitals between six weeks and eight months after exposure. In some instances people have the infection but never develop warts, leaving them unaware they have an STI. Approximately 79 million Americans are infected with HPV and approximately 50% of sexually active people will be infected with HPV at some point in their lives. Women infected with HPV are at higher risk of cervical cancer. As with herpes 2, they may have difficulty with a vaginal delivery of a baby, depending on whether the warts are in the vagina. Genital warts are treated by applying medications to the warts (causing the warts to fall off), freezing the warts with liquid nitrogen, using electrical heat (cauterizing), or laser therapy.

Article
11.4

A vaccine is available to protect against HPV. Gardasil provides protection against four types of HPV, including two that are responsible for the majority of cases of cervical cancer. It is believed that most of the HPV infections that lead to cervical cancer are acquired shortly after women become sexually active. The Centers for Disease Control and Prevention (CDC) recommend that all 11- and 12-year-old girls be vaccinated with Gardasil. The objective is to reduce cervical cancer, and if vaccination begins early, then the incidence of cervical cancer could be significantly reduced in the next 20–30 years.

Two controversies arise from the CDC recommendation of Gardasil. First, the vaccine must be administered in three separate injections with a cost of around $350. Second, many ethical issues are raised in administering the vaccine to 11- and 12-year-olds. Some parents believe the vaccine is too new to recommend widespread use, because not all its side effects may yet be known. And some parents believe administering the vaccine may somehow encourage girls to have sex earlier than they would otherwise, because they feel it is safer. Despite these issues, since HPV can lead to more serious conditions, the vaccination is becoming common practice for girls and women.

PREVENTION OF SEXUALLY TRANSMITTED INFECTIONS

Sexually transmitted infections can be prevented in a number of ways. First, abstinence is the lowest-risk preventive behavior. Second, use of condoms greatly reduces rates of transmission. Condoms are not 100 percent protection against STIs, but they do provide a barrier that blocks the portals of entry and exit.

✓ NEED TO KNOW

Sexually transmitted infections (STIs) are preventable. High-risk sexual choices can result in high risk for an STI. Condoms offer some protection. Pain upon urination, urethral or vaginal discharge, sores around the genital area, and pelvic pain all can be signs of an STI and require medical attention. Infertility can result from untreated STIs. A new vaccine offers some protection against the HPV virus, which is a leading cause of cervical cancer.

HIV AND AIDS

HIV and **AIDS** represent two ends of the same viral infection. Because this disease has such important life-and-death dynamics and is such a politically charged issue, we will discuss it independently of the common sexually transmitted infections.

The human immunodeficiency virus (HIV) is both the cause of acquired immunodeficiency syndrome (AIDS) and an infection itself. The term **HIV positive** is used for a person who has been shown to carry the virus but appears to have no symptoms; people whose infections have progressed to the point where they show symptoms are said to have AIDS. If the disease progresses, the person begins to experience fever, weight loss, swollen lymph glands, and white patches in the mouth.

HIV is transmitted through body fluids such as blood, semen, vaginal secretions, and breast milk of HIV-infected women. Once in the body, HIV attacks the immune system's T cells (described in the "Immune System" section earlier in this chapter). HIV changes the way T cells function so that over time, the T cells stop sending messages to B cells to produce antibodies to fight infections. As the immune system becomes increasingly deficient because of a lack of antibodies, the infected person is susceptible to what are termed *opportunistic diseases* such as Kaposi's sarcoma (a skin lesion) and PCP (pneumocystis pneumonia).

Self
Assessment
11.3

The most common modes of transmission of HIV are dirty needles, anal intercourse, and high-risk sexual practices where tissue is torn, allowing contaminated blood to enter another person's body. It can take between six weeks and six months after exposure for someone to test positive for HIV. People who feel fine despite being HIV positive can still pass the virus on to others.

Through medical interventions, people can live productive lives despite HIV infection. There are medications available that, if used at the appropriate time, can limit the reproductive capability of HIV and greatly prolong an infected person's life. If these drugs are not used, then most likely the infection will progress to AIDS.

HIV is the human immunodeficiency virus. **AIDS** is the end-stage disease caused by HIV.

HIV positive is the term for a person who has the HIV infection but doesn't exhibit any symptoms yet.

HIV is a relatively difficult disease to get. It breaks down the human immune system over time. Most HIV infections are a result of sexual relations with an infected person or from sharing needles when using drugs. Fortunately, being infected with HIV is not the death sentence it was years ago—but still, to take advantage of the life-saving medical interventions, a person should be diagnosed early.

➤ Bioterrorism

Bioterrorism was once a term used primarily in science-fiction movies. In recent years, with highly publicized "weapons of mass destruction" and the anthrax deaths after September 11, 2001, bioterrorism has become a concept that is now well integrated into our consciousness. It refers to the use of lethal pathogens in terrorism. The diseases of most concern in a bioterrorist context are anthrax, botulism, pneumonic plague, and smallpox. Figure 11.4 provides a clinical overview of the bioterrorist agents responsible for those diseases.

Anthrax is a bacterial disease most associated with cows. When humans are infected by inhaling anthrax spores, they experience flulike symptoms, and after a brief time period when they think they are recovering, they lapse into respiratory failure and shock. Unless there is medical intervention with high-powered antibiotics, death is likely.

Botulism is a bacterial foodborne disease. Because we have such strict food preparation standards, botulism has not been a serious problem. As a terrorist weapon, the organism would infect a person, and after incubation, dizziness, weakness, and paralysis would result. Unless botulism antitoxins are administered, the disease can be lethal.

Pneumonic plague is also caused by bacteria. A few days after exposure, the victim can spike a high fever and have a cough, chest pain, nausea, and vomiting. In the advanced form, skin sores will appear. Unless antibiotics are administered, respiratory failure and death can result.

Smallpox was once thought to be eradicated—meaning that enough of the total world population had been immunized to stamp out all infections. But in a bioterrorist context, the smallpox virus can be disseminated through the air. If people breathe in the smallpox virus, they can develop it. Symptoms include fever, vomiting, headache, and skin sores. Unlike the bacterial diseases, there is no cure for smallpox. The quality of the individual's immune response is the key to surviving smallpox. There is a smallpox vaccine that is derived from the virus, but because the disease was thought to have been eradicated, only a small supply of the vaccine is available.

Experts disagree on the extent of the threat of bioterrorism. Many of the diseases discussed here are caused by organisms that are hard to deliver to infect large numbers of people. But that doesn't mean that the organisms can't be manipulated to become easier to deliver and even more lethal. Bioterrorism should be considered a real threat.

Dealing with bioterrorism requires a comprehensive plan with involvement from every segment of American society. In an October 2007 Homeland Security

FIGURE 11.4 BIOTERRORIST AGENTS: WATCH FOR THESE SYMPTOMS

Disease	Signs & Symptoms	Incubation Time (Range)	Person-to-Person Transmission	Isolation	Diagnosis	Postexposure Prophylaxis for Adults	Treatment for Adults
Anthrax *Bacillus anthracis*							
A. Inhalation	Flu-like symptoms (fever, fatigue, muscle aches, dyspnea, nonproductive cough, headache), chest pain; possible 1–2 day improvement then rapid respiratory failure and shock. Meningitis may develop.	1 to 6 days (up to 6 wks)	None	Standard Precautions	Chest x-ray evidence of widening mediastinum; obtain sputum and blood culture. Sensitivity and specificity of nasal swabs unknown—do not rely on for diagnosis.	Prophylaxis for 60 days: Ciprofloxacin* 500 mg PO q 12h Or Doxycycline 100 mg PO q 12h Alternative (if strain susceptible and above contraindicated): Amoxicillin 500 mg PO q 8h *In vitro studies suggest that Levofloxacin 500 mg PO q 24h Or Gatifloxacin 400 mg PO q 24h Or Moxifloxacin 400 mg PO q 24h could be substituted	Inhalation anthrax Combined IV/PO therapy for 60d Ciprofloxacin 500 mg q 12h Or Doxycycline 100 mg q 12h. AND 1 or 2 additional drugs (vancomycin, rifampin, imipenem clindamycin, chloramphenicol, clarithromycin, and if susceptible penicillin or ampicillin)
B. Cutaneous	Intense itching followed by painless papular lesions, then vesicular lesions, developing into eschar surrounded by edema.	1 to 12 days	Direct contact with skin lesions may result in cutaneous infection.	Contact Precautions	Peripheral blood smear may demonstrate gram positive bacilli on unspun smear with sepsis.		Cutaneous anthrax Ciprofloxacin 500 mg PO q 12h Or Doxycycline 100 mg PO 12h
C. Gastrointestinal (GI)	Abdominal pain, nausea and vomiting, severe diarrhea, GI bleeding, and fever.	1 to 7 days	None	Standard Precautions	Culture blood and stool.	Recommendations same for pregnant women and immunocompromised persons	Recommendations same for pregnant women and immunocompromised persons
Botulism botulinum toxin	Afebrile, excess mucus in throat, dysphagia, dry mouth and throat, dizziness, then difficulty moving eyes, mild pupillary dilation and nystagmus, intermittent ptosis, indistinct speech, unsteady gait, extreme symmetric descending weakness, flaccid paralysis; generally normal mental status.	Inhalation: 12–80 hours Foodborne: 12–72 hours (2–8 days)	None	Standard Precautions	Laboratory tests available from CDC or Public Health Dept; obtain serum, stool, gastric aspirate and suspect foods prior to administering antitoxin. Differential diagnosis includes polio, Guillain Barre, myasthenia, tick paralysis, CVA, meningococcal meningitis.	Pentavalent toxoid (types A, B, C, D, E) 0.5 ml SQ may be available as investigational product from USAMRIID.	Botulism antitoxins from public health authorities. Supportive care and ventilatory support. Avoid clindamycin and aminoglycosides.
Pneumonic Plague *Yersinia pestis*	High fever, cough, hemoptysis, chest pain, nausea and vomiting, headache. Advanced disease: purpuric skin lesions, copious watery or purulent sputum production; respiratory failure in 1 to 6 days.	2–3 days (2–6 days)	Yes, droplet aerosols	Droplet Precautions until 48 hrs of effective antibiotic therapy	A presumptive diagnosis may be made by Gram, Wayson or Wright stain of lymph node aspirates, sputum, or cerebrospinal fluid with gram negative bacilli with bipolar (safety pin) staining.	Doxycycline 100 mg PO q 12 Or Ciprofloxacin 500 mg PO q 12h	Streptomycin 1 gm IM q 12h; Or Gentamicin 2 mg/kg, then 1.0 to 1.7 mg/kg IV q 8h Alternatives: Doxycycline 200 mg PO load, then 100 PO mg q 12h Or Ciprofloxacin 400 mg IV q 12h
Smallpox variola virus	Prodromal period: malaise, fever, rigors, vomiting, headache, and backache. After 2–4 days, skin lesions appear and progress uniformly from macules to papules to vesicles and pustules, mostly on face, neck, palms, soles, and subsequently progress to trunk.	12–14 days (7–17 days)	Yes, airborne droplet nuclei or direct contact with skin lesions or secretions until all scabs separate and fall off (3 to 4 weeks)	Airborne (includes N95 mask) and Contact Precautions	Swab culture of vesicular fluid or scab, send to BL-4 laboratory. All lesions similar in appearance and develop synchronously as opposed to chickenpox. Electron microscopy can differentiate *variola* virus from varicella.	Early vaccine critical (in less than 4 days). Call CDC for vaccinia. Vaccinia immune globulin in special cases—call USAMRIID 301-619-2833.	Supportive care. Previous vaccination against smallpox does not confer lifelong immunity. Potential role for Cidofovir.

Source: Adapted with permission from Bioterrorism Wallchart developed by North Carolina Statewide Program for Infection Control and Epidemiology (SPICE). Copyright 2003 by University of North Carolina at Chapel Hill. Photos: (first) Arthur E. Kaye/CDC; (second) James H. Steele/CDC; (third) Dr. Marshal Fox/CDC; (fourth) Dr. George Lombard/CDC; (fifth) CDC; (sixth) CDC.

Presidential Directive (HSPD-21), a national strategy for preparedness was presented. This strategy includes four major components: biosurveillance, countermeasure stockpiling and distribution, mass casualty care, and community resilience.

Biosurveillance measures include focused national and international activities to monitor disease occurrence and distribution for those diseases that are likely to be a part of bioterrorism in both animal and human populations. Countermeasure stockpiling and distribution involves ensuring that appropriate vaccines and drugs are available in the case of a real or potential bioterrorism event. Mass casualty care is the mobilization of public health and medical systems to treat those affected by a bioterrorism disease outbreak. Finally, community resilience is activities that communities and social networks can undertake to lessen the risk and damage done in such outbreaks.

HSPD-21 is key to both prevention and intervention activities to both protect citizens from effects of bioterrorist activities and to mobilize public health and medical sectors to deal with a bioterrorist event. The odds are something will eventually happen, and the impact of that event will be directly related to the degree of preparedness of the affected nation, with the United States being a key target. The need for a comprehensive plan that addresses the four major components is paramount and requires cooperation from institutions and individuals.

NEED TO KNOW

Manipulating lethal organisms for the purpose of bioterrorism is a real threat. Although there is very little that individuals can do to physically protect themselves, paying attention to Homeland Security warnings and threat levels are key to identifying people or groups who may be involved in harming others through biology. A bioterrorism event is likely to happen at some point. The severity of such an event will be directly related to how well the critical components of HSPD-21 are implemented. We all have a role to play in prevention of the bioterrorism threat, especially in helping our respective communities be resilient.

ARTICLES

11.1 "Adolescents at Risk: The Case for Meningococcal Vaccine." *Journal of Adolescent Health.* Challenges associated with early diagnosis of meningococcal disease are discussed.

11.2 "Where Does Ebola Come From?" *The Atlantic.* An examination of the role of eating bats, washing bodies, and lack of doctors in relationship to Ebola outbreaks.

11.3 "Genital Herpes: A Hidden Epidemic." *FDA Consumer.* An examination of the infection rate of genital herpes and why it is considered a hidden epidemic.

11.4 "Getting to Know Human Papillomavirus (HPV) and the HPV Vaccines." *Journal of the American Osteopathic Association.* A practical article on the spread of HPV and availability of HPV vaccines.

SELF-ASSESSMENTS

11.1 Do You Know How to Wash Your Hands?
11.2 Personal Infectious Disease Record
11.3 Sexually Transmitted Infections Quiz

Website Resources

American Medical Association **www.ama-assn.org/ama**
American Public Health Association **www.apha.org**
Centers for Disease Control and Prevention **www.cdc.gov**
Infectious Disease Society of America **www.idsociety.org**
MedlinePlus (NIH) **www.nlm.nih.gov/medlineplus/infectiousdiseases.html**
Medscape (WebMD) **www.medscape.com/infectiousdiseaseshome**
National Foundation for Infectious Diseases **www.nfid.org**
National Institute of Infectious Diseases **www.nih.go.jp/niid**
World Health Organization **www.who.int/topics/en**

Knowing the Language

Understanding the Content

1. Describe the communicable disease process using the following terminology: *pathogen, reservoir, mode of transmission, portal of entry, portal of exit, incubation, prodromal stage, acute stage,* and *recovery.*
2. What are the main mechanisms for fighting disease?
3. What is MRSA and why are most people at risk for it?
4. Why can PID be a problem associated with chlamydia and gonorrhea?
5. What is HPV and why should women be concerned about it?
6. What is the difference between HIV, HIV positive, and full-blown AIDS?
7. What are the main bioterrorism agents of concern?

Exploring Ideas

1. Why should we be so concerned about superbugs, and whose role is it to prevent the spread of these pathogens?
2. Should Gardasil be required for all girls beginning at ages 11 or 12? If so, why? If not, why not?
3. Should there be mandatory HIV testing to determine the extent of HIV infection? Why or why not?
4. What has been done since September 11, 2001, to prevent a bioterrorism event? Is America ready?

Selected References

American Public Health Association. *Control of Communicable Disease in Man* (17th ed.). Washington, DC: American Public Health Association, 2000.

Brown J. *Don't Touch That Doorknob.* New York: Warner Books, 2001.

Centers for Disease Control and Prevention. *Healthy People 2020,* 2020. **www.healthypeople.gov/.**

Centers for Disease Control and Prevention. Human Papilloma Virus. **www.cdc.gov/std/hpv/stdfact-hpv.htm** February 18, 2016.

Fauci AS. Emerging infectious diseases: A clear and present danger to humanity. *JAMA* 292 (15): 1887–1888, 2004.

Garrett L. The lessons of HIV/AIDS. *Foreign Affairs* 84 (4): 51–65, July/August 2005.

Garrett L. Probable cause. *Foreign Affairs* 84 (4): 3–23, July/August 2005.

Harrison LH, Dwyer DM, Maples CT, et al. Risk of meningococcal infection in college students. *JAMA* 281 (20): 1906–1910, May 26, 1999.

Karlen A. *Man and Microbes.* New York: Putnam, 1995.

Khazan, O. Where Does Ebola Come From? *The Atlantic.* July 29, 2014. **www.theatlantic.com/health/archive/2014/07/where-does-ebola-come-from/375206/**

Miller J, Engelberg S, Broad W. *Germs.* New York: Simon & Schuster, 2001.

Presidential Commission for the Study of Bioethical Issues. Ethics and Ebola. Washington, DC: Bioethics Commission, 2015.

Preston, R. *The Hot Zone.* New York: Random House, 1994.

The White House. Homeland Security Presidential Directive/HSPD-21. Released October 18, 2007. **www.whitehouse.gov/news/releases/2007/10/print/20071018-10.html**

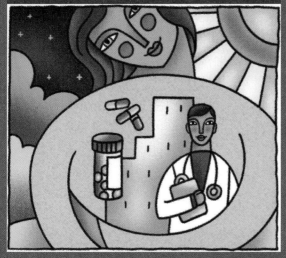

*When it comes to your
health, I recommend
frequent doses of that
rare commodity—
common sense.*

— Vincent Askey, M.D.,

President, American

Medical Association

© Imagezoo/Getty Images

Chapter 12

THE U.S. HEALTH CARE SYSTEM

In this chapter, we describe the U.S. system of health care.
Because of the growing interest in treatment options beyond
those of mainstream Western medicine, a review of complementary medicine is also included. We finish with an overview on the emerging concept of integrative medicine.

Chapter 12 | THE U.S. HEALTH CARE SYSTEM

EACH OF US has some familiarity with the U.S. health care system because we've all been patients. Most of you also have a family member or friend who works in health care. Yet, basic information on how our system works and the impact of health care reform are only background noise for many of you, as parents or family watch over your medical needs. The fact is you've had no compelling reason to understand the health care system. But the time is coming when you will. In contrast, a few of you already face responsibility for your health care. Perhaps you are no longer covered as a dependent on a parent's health insurance plan or you are attending college as an older student.

As the current or soon-to-be decision maker for your own health care, you need a basic knowledge of the system to use it effectively. Frankly, the U.S. system is complex and continually changing. For the uninformed, it can be confusing and downright overwhelming. In this chapter we present the fundamentals of how the system works. We explain the key players in conventional Western medicine, review the realm of complementary medicine, and end with a profile of the blended system known as *integrative medicine*. The aim is to help prepare you to be your own advocate.

As a side note, we also provide a glimpse into potential occupations. Many of you will eventually work in health care—either directly as a health care professional or indirectly in a health-related business. Among all jobs in the U.S. economy, those in the health care sector are expected to be among the fastest growing over the next decade.

➤ Organization of Our Health Care System

COMPONENTS AND LEVELS OF CARE

The U.S. system of health care is a multilevel, market-based network of individuals and organizations that provide and underwrite medical services. Our current system began as a simple two-party arrangement between a family doctor and a patient. The patient would either go to the doctor's office for care, or the doctor would make a "house call" (go to the patient's home). Patients paid doctors directly, and those payments were sometimes bartered—goods or services (for instance, food from a farmer) instead of money. Over the decades, this straightforward practice of medicine evolved into a complex health care system. Today, in addition to the general practitioner or family doctor, there are a myriad of physician specialists and allied health professionals, a multitude of high-tech instruments and specialized facilities for medical tests and procedures, and a wide array of third-party health care insurers.

Contemporary health care is described as being at one of three levels: primary, secondary, or tertiary. **Primary health care** involves diagnosis and treatment of common illnesses such as acne, influenza, high blood pressure, or depression. A family practice physician usually provides primary care; thus, he or she is known as the *primary care provider.* Your primary care provider orders standard tests such as urinalysis, blood tests, and X-rays to aid in diagnosis and treatment.

Primary health care is the diagnosis and treatment of simple, routine illnessess.

Health problems that are less common, more complex, or persistent may require **secondary health care.** This is the realm of the specialist. There are several approaches to finding a specialist, but the typical route is a referral from your primary care provider. For example, a patient may visit his or her primary care physician to treat migraine headaches. If the migraines persist despite the primary care physician's best efforts, then the physician will likely refer the patient to a neurologist, a doctor who specializes in treating nervous system disorders.

The tests and therapies provided by secondary care may solve the health problem. But if they do not, then **tertiary health care** can come into play. Tertiary care is the most complex set of medical services, involving many types of health care specialists and taking place at a medical center or specialized clinic. If, for instance, the neurologist is unsuccessful in helping the migraine sufferer, then the patient will likely be referred to a clinic at the closest medical school. The Mayo Clinic and Cleveland Clinic are examples of two nationally prominent medical centers providing tertiary care.

MAJOR CHALLENGES: CONTROLLING COSTS AND REDUCING ERRORS

In terms of highly trained health professionals and cutting-edge medical technology, the United States is one of the top countries in the world. Yet, despite recognized excellence in medical resources, significant weaknesses exist in our health care system. First, the American approach to health care is the most expensive in the world. Continuation of spiraling costs will have dire consequences. Experts contend that policy changes are needed sooner rather than later. Second, the rate of preventable medical errors that result in illness, disability, or death is unacceptably high. What's being done to reduce medical mistakes? As consumers and citizens, these two major challenges warrant our attention.

Health Care Costs

The major cost categories for health care are hospitals, physician and related clinical services, prescription drugs, and nursing home care. Predictably, hospital care and physician/clinical services account for over half of annual health care costs. Highly trained medical professionals justifiably earn high salaries, and state-of-the-art specialty equipment is extremely expensive to develop, manufacture, and maintain. The main concern is the *rate of rise* in the cost of health care. Health care spending in recent decades has exceeded overall growth in the U.S. economy. Put another way, for individuals and families, increases in the cost of health insurance and out-of-pocket medical expenses have consistently outpaced inflation and growth in workers' earnings.

Factors such as medical litigation, the aging population, and treatment for those without insurance contribute significantly to increasing health care costs. Today,

Secondary health care is the use of specialists for more complex or unusual conditions.

Tertiary health care is the utilization of complex medical services and networks in order to diagnose and treat the most challenging medical conditions.

physicians routinely carry malpractice insurance; high-risk specialists like obstetricians and surgeons pay malpractice premiums of over $100,000 per year. The costs
that physicians must bear to practice medicine are ultimately passed on in patient
fees. A second factor pushing health care costs higher is the "graying" of America—
those aged 60 and older comprise the fastest-growing segment of our population.
Older individuals require more health care services simply due to their age; consequently, as this proportion of the population increases, so do the total expenditures
for medical care.

A third factor that has contributed to rising health care costs is the large number
of uninsured people. In 2015, about one out of eight Americans had no health care
insurance. Since the Affordable Care Act took effect in 2014, the rate of uninsured
individuals has dropped from a high of 18 percent in 2013 to about 12 percent in
2015. Hopefully this progress can continue.

For those without insurance, the availability of low-cost or free care to treat
routine medical problems or conduct preventive screening is minimal. Limited
services are provided through state, county, and city public health departments and
benevolence organizations. Consequently, most uninsured individuals do not seek
medical care unless it is absolutely necessary. Then, they are treated at emergency
rooms, and the resulting high costs are underwritten with tax dollars.

By providing coverage to those who are uninsured, the Affordable Care Act may
significantly rein in rising health care costs. It will take a decade before we know
the impact on controlling costs (see the section on health care reform in Chapter 13).
In the foreseeable future we should continue to view health insurance as a necessity,
not an option. Without it, medical care is not affordable. Information on how to
select a health insurance plan is presented in the next chapter (see the section on
understanding health insurance in Chapter 13).

Article
12.1

Medical Errors

We've read about the tragic cases. A woman dies from an overdose during chemotherapy. A man has the wrong leg amputated. An eight-year-old dies during "minor"
surgery due to a drug mixup. Then there are the population numbers. In 1999, a
national study by the prestigious Institute of Medicine reported that up to 100,000
Americans die in hospitals each year as a result of medical errors. In 2013, new
findings indicated that a more accurate estimate is 400,000 deaths per year! This
puts preventable medical errors as the number three killer in the United States—
third only to heart disease and cancer.

The scope and size of the problem are huge. Consider that hospital patients
represent only a small proportion of the total number of people at risk. More
medical care and increasingly complex care are provided in outpatient surgical centers, medical clinics, physicians' offices, and nursing homes. Retail pharmacies and
home care are also settings for medical errors. The message is stark: health care
is not as safe as it should be.

As a result of national attention, significant steps have been taken to create safety
systems within health care organizations from top to bottom. For example, many
hospitals have gone to electronic patient records in which all medications are
recorded and noted when administered. This minimizes errors due to illegible hand-
writing, paper records, and different personnel across shifts. Yet, despite reforms to
improve health care services, progress has been slow. Fundamental change takes
time and commitment by all stakeholders.

Article
12.2

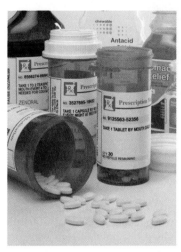

Receiving the wrong drug or the right drug at the wrong dose are examples of preventable errors.

© Don Farrall/Getty Images

Knowing that preventable medical errors are *not* a rare occurrence should reinforce our commitment to being active, engaged partners in our own treatment and medical management. Tips on preventing medical errors, especially those related to medicines and hospital stays, are presented in the next chapter (see the sections "Prescription and OTC Medicines" and "Medical Tests and Procedures" in Chapter 13).

Regarding the U.S. health care system, there are two clear messages for the individual consumer: (1) have adequate health insurance, and (2) be vigilant for medical errors. At the societal level, Americans should support policies to provide health care that is cost-effective, safe, and available to everyone.

✓ NEED TO KNOW

The U.S. health care system is a complex, market-based network of individuals and organizations. Medical care is provided at three levels: primary, secondary, and tertiary. Controlling health care costs and reducing medical errors are major challenges. In the American system both health insurance and vigilance are fundamental to receiving quality health care.

➤ Western Medicine

Western medicine is the predominant form of health care in the United States. *Western medicine,* also known as *conventional medicine* or *biomedicine,* is the science-based medicine to which most of us are accustomed. The term *Western medicine* reflects its origins; that is, it was largely developed in Europe and North America (the Western world). These mainstream health care professionals adhere to strict educational and licensing criteria. As consumers of health care, we need to have some familiarity with how doctors and allied health care professionals are trained and credentialed.

When the call goes out over the plane's intercom, "Is there a doctor on board?," you can be sure the attendant is calling for a physician, not a college professor. Yet, general knowledge about health care doctors other than physicians and dentists—such as podiatrists, optometrists, and clinical psychologists—is fairly limited. In each case, these doctors can function as independent health care practitioners and must be licensed to practice. A brief review of the training, specializations, and overlap among these mainstream health care doctors is provided.

There are two types of **physicians:** the M.D. (doctor of medicine) and the D.O. (doctor of osteopathic medicine). Both M.D.'s and D.O.'s are trained to use all the tools of modern health care including the vast array of medical tests, drugs, and surgery to diagnose and treat illnesses and injuries. There are more than 900,000 active physicians. Thirty-two percent are women and that number is rising; 48 percent of recent medical school graduates are female. D.O.'s comprise 8 percent of active physicians and that number is rising too: 22 percent of recent graduates were from schools of osteopathic medicine.

M.D.'s and D.O.'s are much more similar than different. The main distinction is that osteopathic medicine places special emphasis on the body's musculoskeletal system, preventive medicine, and holistic care. As a result, D.O.'s are more likely than M.D.'s to be primary care doctors and practice family medicine, internal medicine, pediatrics, or obstetrics/gynecology. D.O.'s are often referred to as *osteopaths,* which is a shortened term for *osteopathic physician.*

Physician Education

Medical education typically extends 7–11 years beyond the undergraduate degree. This is divided between 4 years of medical school and 3 to 7 years of postgraduate medical education (referred to as *residency*). Most of the first 2 years of medical school is spent in laboratories and classrooms taking core science courses such as anatomy, biochemistry, physiology, microbiology, pathology, and pharmacology as well as courses in human behavior, medical ethics, and medical law. During years three and four, students learn to take medical histories, examine patients, and diagnose illnesses under the supervision of physicians in hospitals and clinics. Students learn acute, chronic, rehabilitative, and preventive care in broad areas of medicine such as internal medicine, surgery, psychiatry, obstetrics/gynecology, pediatrics, and geriatrics.

Physician Specialties and Board Certifications

Following medical school, almost all physicians enter a residency in a major hospital or medical center. A residency is graduate medical education in a specialty that takes the form of paid on-the-job training. Residencies and additional training commonly last from 3 to 7 years. This advanced training prepares doctors for board certification in a specialty. This process is overseen by the American Board of Medical Specialists, which comprises 24 specialty boards, ranging from anesthesiology to radiology.

Board certification is not just a topic of interest among physicians—it's also relevant to consumers who want quality health care. Simply put, it's best to select a doctor who is board certified whenever possible. Board certification attests to the highest level of training in a specialty area. A few familiar medical specialties are highlighted in Table 12.1. These can be broadly grouped as primary care specialties, medical specialties, and surgical specialties. In most cases, we are referred to medical and surgical specialists by our primary care doctor. The eye specialist (ophthalmologist) and skin specialist (dermatologist) are two whom many of us have already visited. And, we may

A **physician** is either a doctor of medicine (M.D.) or a doctor of osteopathy (D.O.). Nearly all physicians trained and licensed in the United States have three or more years of residency training following graduation from medical school.

TABLE 12.1 EXAMPLES OF PHYSICIAN SPECIALTIES

PRIMARY CARE	MEDICAL SPECIALTIES	SURGICAL SPECIALTIES
Family Medicine	Dermatology	Colon & Rectal Surgery
Internal Medicine*	Emergency Medicine	Neurological Surgery
Pediatrics*	Ophthalmology	Orthopedic Surgery
Obstetrics & Gynecology	Otolaryngology (ear/nose/throat)	Plastic Surgery
	Psychiatry	Thoracic Surgery
	Urology	Vascular Surgery

*Within both internal medicine and pediatrics, physicians can pursue additional training in subspecialties such as cardiovascular disease, pulmonary disease, oncology, infectious disease, and endocrinology.

Source: American Board of Medical Specialties.

have been seen by an emergency medicine physician when we went to the ER (emergency room/department) after an accident or for a severe sudden-onset illness. You can determine if a physician is board certified at: **www.certificationmatters.org/.**

Primary Care Physicians

Article
12.3

The **primary care physicians** are our family or personal doctors. Most specialize in family medicine, internal medicine, pediatrics, or obstetrics/gynecology. They are skilled at diagnosing and treating common medical problems. Equally important, they know when to refer us to a medical or surgical specialist.

Doctors specializing in internal medicine (internists) focus on the primary care of adults, particularly the diagnosis and (nonsurgical) treatment of diseases of the internal organs. They solve diagnostic problems in which multiple illnesses and diseases may be occurring at the same time. They advise people on disease prevention, women's health, substance abuse, and mental health, as well as common problems of the eyes, ears, skin, nervous system, and reproductive organs. Although their focus is on the internal organs, they do treat the whole person. (Do not confuse *internists* with *interns*, who are doctors in their first year of residency training.)

Just as internists specialize in adult medicine, pediatricians are the primary care specialists in the medical care of infants, children, and adolescents. Obstetricians and gynecologists are trained in the medical and surgical care of the female reproductive system and associated disorders. They are also trained and often serve as primary care physicians for women.

The aim is to have a primary care physician with whom you've established a relationship over a period of years—a doctor who knows you well, provides ongoing medical care, refers you to specialists as needed, interprets results, and generally

A **primary care physician** is the front-line doctor (an M.D. or D.O.) who spends most of his or her time diagnosing and treating common and routine illnesses and diseases. Most specialize in family medicine, internal medicine, pediatrics, or obstetrics/gynecology.

advises you on medical matters. In addition to being board certified, it's important to select a primary care doctor who is a good communicator and with whom you feel comfortable. A solid patient–doctor relationship is based on confidence and trust.

✓ **NEED TO KNOW**

Twenty-first-century physicians (M.D.'s and D.O.'s) are highly trained specialists with three or more years of training beyond medical school. Adults should have a primary care physician who is a family medicine specialist or an internist. Women may elect to rely on their obstetrician/ gynecologist as their primary doctor. Infants, children, and adolescents should be seen by a pediatrician or family medicine specialist. To receive the best medical care, consumers should seek out physicians who are board certified. Finally, it's important to select a primary care doctor who is a good communicator and with whom you feel comfortable.

Breaking It Down Doctors and Drug Companies: Who's in Control?

An anonymous woman tries to disentangle a shopping cart from an interlocked row of carts outside a suburban store. She is frustrated and angry. She becomes even more exasperated when another shopper enters the frame, calmly unhooks a cart, and glides smoothly on her way. Watching this TV commercial unfold, it might look like the woman is experiencing little more than a normal bout of tension or stress. But the folks at the drug company Eli Lilly know better. This woman may need a powerful antidepressant because she is suffering from a severe form of mental illness known as PMDD. "Think it's PMS? It could be PMDD," intones the voiceover.

Not everyone agrees with the drug company's assessment. This example was taken from the book *Selling Sickness: How the World's Biggest Pharmaceutical Companies Are Turning Us All into Patients.* Authors Roy Moynihan and Alan Cassels argue that the pharmaceutical industry is no longer focused on selling cures for disease, but rather on marketing drugs to the masses. They provide persuasive evidence that the big drug companies now influence all facets of medication use—research, approval, marketing, and the doctors and their patients.

Selling Sickness is just one of many books to delve into this remarkable entanglement of capitalism, medicine, and culture. When the arthritis pain drugs Celebrex and Vioxx were recalled from the market because of reports that they increased the risk of heart disease, troubling questions arose. Were these drugs prematurely pushed through the approval process in the rush to get them to market? The intrusion of drug companies into the practice of medicine has been described as scandalous and fraudulent. Even those who are sympathetic to the drug companies recognize that the situation is—at the very least—troubling and problematic. Consumers should be alert and concerned.

(continued)

A few statements of fact: Many prescription drugs are truly life-saving and life-sustaining in curing or managing specific diseases and illnesses. Compelling evidence from years of research has shown drug therapies are effective and safe. Examples include the use of antibiotics to treat infections, antihypertensives to lower high blood pressure, and synthetic insulin to manage type 1 diabetes. The downside—drugs are often expensive and have side effects.

So what's the problem? Through strategic and systematic corporate sponsorship, drug companies have undue influence in the promotion and sales of prescription drugs. For starters, a large proportion of research at medical schools is funded by drug companies. Less noticeable because it's omnipresent is the benefactor role of drug companies in the lives of doctors. Such support pervades medical school, residency training, continuing education, as well as clinical practice. Drug companies sponsor educational and social events from luncheons for medical students to lavish seminars for physician specialists. And routinely, drug reps bestow small gifts or favors when visiting physicians to present new products.

But of all the inroads to influence, perhaps the most far-reaching is direct marketing to the public. Through slick "awareness-raising" campaigns, the drug industry has capitalized on the American illusion that we can have it all—eternal youth, sexual desire, enhanced intellect, and continual happiness—by taking a pill.

This has led to the creation or exaggeration of conditions such as PMDD (premenstrual dysphoric disorder, a severe form of premenstrual syndrome), motivational deficiency disorder, adult attention-deficit disorder, social anxiety disorder, female sexual dysfunction, and erectile dysfunction. Doctors are no longer just subliminally conditioned to prescribe drugs. They are now confronted by patients who saw an advertisement and subsequently ask for, and sometimes demand, the new drug.

The goal of for-profit companies is to increase sales, often aggressively within the limits of the law. In their ambition, drug companies have steadily pushed the envelope to broaden the base of potential clients beyond those who are sick to the healthy too. This has required new corporate strategies aimed at creating markets for their products. Moynihan asks, "Is the goal of pharma [the drug industry] a disease for every pill?"

In today's world, many factors influence how doctors prescribe drugs to their patients. We must remember doctors are human too and not immune from influences inherent in their training and practice. The sway of drug companies is another reason to select your doctor with care. Find one who accepts you, not only as a patient, but as a partner in your health care. And before asking for that new medicine you saw advertised, do your homework on its targeted medical condition. You may be just fine without it.

DENTISTS

Nearly every reader has visited a dentist within the last year or two. In America, we are fortunate to have regular access to dentists to help ensure good oral health. **Dentists** prevent, diagnose, and treat problems with teeth and with mouth tissue. They

A **dentist** is a doctor of dental surgery (D.D.S.) or dental medicine (D.M.D.), whose practice includes problems with teeth and gums and other aspects of oral health.

commonly remove tooth decay, fill cavities, interpret X-rays, straighten teeth, and repair or replace damaged or diseased teeth. They also perform corrective surgery on gums and supporting bones to treat gum diseases. They provide instruction on oral hygiene including diet, brushing, flossing, and the use of fluorides, as well as administer anesthetics and write prescriptions. There are more than 200,000 active dentists.

As with medical school students, most students who are admitted to dental school hold an undergraduate degree. Dental school is typically four academic years. During the last two years, students treat patients in dental clinics, under the supervision of licensed dentists. Most dental schools award the degree of doctor of dental surgery (D.D.S.). The rest award an equivalent degree, doctor of dental medicine (D.M.D.).

A major difference between the education of a physician and a dentist is the extent of postgraduate education. For medical school graduates, a three-year residency is standard. In contrast, most dental school graduates go straight into practice after graduation. Most become general practitioners, handling a variety of dental needs. Only about one in eight new graduates enrolls in postgraduate programs to prepare for a dental specialty. Orthodontists who straighten teeth with braces or retainers constitute the largest group of specialists. Oral and maxillofacial surgeons, who operate on the mouth and jaws, and periodontists, who treat gums and bone supporting the teeth, are two other types of specialists.

PODIATRISTS

A **podiatrist** is to the foot what a dentist is to the mouth. The podiatrist—or doctor of podiatric medicine (D.P.M.)—specializes in the prevention, diagnosis, and treatment of foot and ankle disorders. A podiatrist makes independent judgments, prescribes medications, and performs surgery. The foot may be the first area to show signs of serious conditions such as diabetes or heart disease. In this role, podiatrists often become a vital link in the patient's health care team.

Although podiatry has been a recognized medical practice for nearly a century, the profession remains poorly understood. Most foot and ankle problems are treated by primary care physicians or orthopedic surgeons (M.D.'s/D.O.'s). Although podiatrists are foot and ankle specialists, there is substantial overlap in medical care of foot injuries by physicians and podiatrists. Because there are only about 15,000 podiatrists nationwide, many Americans simply do not have access to podiatric care.

The medical training to become a podiatrist is similar to that for an M.D. or D.O. The curriculum leading to a D.P.M. is four years long. The first two years are classroom instruction and laboratory work; they are followed by two years of supervised clinical rotations. Graduation from podiatric medical school is followed by a two-year residency in a hospital-based program.

OPTOMETRISTS

Doctors of optometry (O.D.'s) are health care professionals for the eye. The primary function of **optometrists** is correcting what are known as *refractive errors*. A refractive

A **podiatrist** is a doctor who holds a doctor of podiatric medicine (D.P.M.) degree and whose practice focuses on medical problems of the foot and lower leg.

An **optometrist** holds an O.D. degree and is primarily trained to evaluate refractive errors and prescribe corrective glasses or contacts.

error is due to the eye not bending light correctly, resulting in a blurred image. Refractive errors are the most common eye disorders, and they include nearsightedness, farsightedness, and astigmatism. Optometrists prescribe corrective lenses both in the form of glasses and contact lenses. In addition they counsel people regarding their visual needs and associated surgical and nonsurgical options related to their occupations, avocations, and lifestyle.

Optometric Education

A four-year curriculum leads to the O.D. degree. Nearly all O.D.'s enter the workforce immediately following graduation. A small percentage complete an optional one-year residency in a specific area of practice.

Optometrist versus Ophthalmologist

Both optometrists and ophthalmologists are referred to as "eye doctors." Indeed, there is overlap in the services they perform. But there are differences as well. An ophthalmologist is a physician, with eight or more years of education beyond college (medical school, and at least four years of specialty training), who performs a full range of eye-related medical care, including surgery. In comparison, an optometrist has four years of education beyond college (four-year professional degree in optometry) and mainly examines eyes, prescribes corrective lenses, and advises on nonsurgical management of certain eye problems. As a final note, let's consider the optician. An optician is a technician licensed to fit and dispense eyeglasses and contact lenses according to a written prescription from an ophthalmologist or optometrist. The training and certification of opticians vary from state to state.

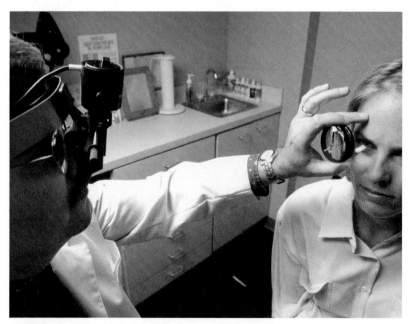

Optometrists use glasses or contact lenses to correct refractive errors of the eye.
© liquidlibrary/PictureQuest

Clinical psychologists are mental health practitioners. They work closely with physicians, often referring patients to each other. Clinical psychologists constitute the largest specialty group within the broad field of psychology. Clinical psychologists help people with mental/emotional illness adjust to life. They also assist medical and surgical patients in dealing with illnesses or injuries. For example, in physical rehabilitation centers, clinical psychologists can be found treating patients with spinal cord injuries, chronic pain or illness, stroke, and neurological conditions.

Clinical psychologists work with individuals of all ages from infants to older adults, as well as families, groups, and organizations. They use a wide range of assessments and interventions to promote mental health and to alleviate discomfort and maladjustment. Interventions are directed at preventing and treating emotional conflicts, personality disturbances, and psychopathology. Common interventions include psychotherapy, psychoanalysis, behavior therapy, marital and family therapy, group therapy, biofeedback, cognitive retraining, social learning approaches, and environmental consultation and design. Many clinical psychologists are also involved in research, teaching and supervision, program development and evaluation, and public policy.

Doctoral Education in Clinical Psychology

A doctoral program in clinical psychology—leading to either a Ph.D. or Psy.D. degree—takes five to seven years and requires substantial coursework in personality and psychopathology and a one-year internship. The American Psychological Association accredits clinical psychology doctoral programs. All states require a license to practice clinical psychology.

Clinical Psychologist versus Psychiatrist

As between optometrists and ophthalmologists, overlap exists between clinical psychologists and psychiatrists. The main difference is that psychiatrists are physicians who can order medical tests to assist in diagnoses and prescribe medications for treatment. Although the clinical psychologist's training is firmly rooted in psychology and the psychiatrist's in medicine, both are experts in mental health and, in fact, often work together on health care teams in hospitals and clinics.

✓ NEED TO KNOW

Along with the familiar physician (M.D., D.O.), a number of other doctors provide health care services. In addition to the dentist (D.D.S., D.M.D.), there are the doctoral-level professions of podiatrist (D.P.M.), optometrist (O.D.), and clinical psychologist (Ph.D., Psy.D.). Understanding the similarities and differences among these three professions versus the physician specialists of orthopedist, ophthalmologist, and psychiatrist, respectively, is important in making decisions about health care needs related to the foot, the eye, and the mind.

A **clinical psychologist** holds a Ph.D. or Psy.D. in clinical psychology and provides psycho-socio-behavioral therapies to help people adjust to or overcome emotional problems or mental illnesses.

In Western medicine, complex illnesses are treated and managed by medical teams led by physicians. The health care team may include many different allied health care professionals depending on the patient's particular needs. There are over 50 allied health professions, ranging from audiologists (hearing) and prosthetists (artificial limbs) to technologists trained in specializations from medical imaging to surgery. As a side note, many of you will eventually work in health care—as doctors, allied health care professionals, or employees in a health-related business. As job growth in health care is projected to remain strong, you may want to investigate these career paths. Four allied health professionals with whom you—as a patient—are likely to interact are the registered nurse, physician assistant, physical therapist, and registered dietitian. Let's take a closer look at their training and roles.

Registered Nurses

Registered nurses (R.N.'s) constitute the largest health care profession, with about three million active R.N.'s. Most work as staff nurses, providing health care services to patients under the direction of physicians and other health care practitioners. Round the clock, nurses are the true front-line caregivers. In the hospital or clinic, when a doctor orders a treatment or test, it's the nurse who typically administers or supervises the procedure. Basic duties include checking vital signs, dressing wounds, administering treatment and medications, educating and reassuring patients, and providing support to patients' family members. Additionally, R.N.'s record medical histories and symptoms, help perform diagnostic tests and analyze results, and assist with patient follow-up and discharge. In some cases, R.N.'s direct health screenings, immunization clinics, blood drives, and public seminars on various medical conditions.

There are three main paths to becoming an R.N.: a bachelor of science degree in nursing (B.S.N.), an associate degree in nursing, and a diploma. Over 750 colleges offer the bachelor's degree (typically a four-year program), about 1,000 community and junior colleges offer the associate degree (two to three years), and about 100 hospital-based programs award the diploma (about three years). Generally, licensed graduates of any of the three types of educational programs qualify for entry-level positions as staff nurses. Accelerated B S.N. programs also are available for people who have a bachelor's or higher degree in another field.

Some R.N.'s choose to become advanced practice nurses by obtaining a master's degree in one of four areas—as a nurse practitioner, clinical nurse specialist, nurse anesthetist, or nurse midwife. Nurse practitioners provide basic preventive health care to patients and increasingly are serving as primary and specialty care providers in medically underserved areas. Clinical nurse specialists provide direct patient care and expert consultations in a particular nursing specialty (related to a disease, a body organ or system, or a patient population). Nurse anesthetists administer anesthesia, monitor the patient's vital signs during surgery, and provide postoperative care. Nurse midwives provide primary care to women, including gynecological exams, family planning advice, prenatal care, assistance in labor and delivery, and neonatal care.

A **registered nurse (R.N.)** is a graduate of a nursing school (diploma, associate degree, or undergraduate degree) who has passed the licensing exam for the R.N. credential.

Physician Assistants

Physician assistants (P.A.'s) are health professionals licensed to practice medicine with a physician's supervision. There are more than 90,000 active P.A.'s. They can have significant autonomy in medical decision making and provide a broad range of diagnostic and therapeutic services. P.A.'s can take medical histories, perform physical exams, order and interpret laboratory tests, diagnose and treat illnesses, counsel patients, assist in surgery, and set fractures. In nearly all states they can prescribe medicines under the supervision of an M.D. or D.O.

P.A. training requires completion of a two- to three-year master's program, offered at about 180 universities. All programs emphasize primary care. Nearly all successful applicants already have a bachelor's degree. P.A.'s often have prior experience as registered nurses, while others come from varied backgrounds, including the military corps/medics and allied health occupations such as respiratory therapists, physical therapists, and paramedics. Many P.A.'s obtain additional training in a primary care specialty—family medicine, internal medicine, pediatrics, or obstetrics and gynecology. Others may opt for specialty fields, such as cardiovascular surgery, orthopedics, or emergency medicine.

Physical Therapists

Under the guidance of a physician, physical therapists (P.T.'s) provide treatments to restore function and improve mobility following surgery or recovery from injuries or disease. Their patients range from accident victims with fractures and injuries to the spine and head to people with disabling conditions such as low back pain, arthritis, stroke, and cerebral palsy. P.T.'s most commonly provide care in hospitals, clinics, and private offices. There are about 200,000 P.T.'s working in the United States. Throughout most of the rest of the world, physical therapists are known as *physiotherapists.*

There are about 230 programs awarding the doctor of physical therapy (D.P.T.). Nearly all programs require applicants to have an undergraduate degree with a core set of science courses. D.P.T. programs are three years with clinical internships interspersed throughout. P.T.'s can enter the workforce as generalists and treat patients with a wide range of conditions, or they can specialize in areas such as pediatrics, geriatrics, orthopedics, sports medicine, neurology, and cardiopulmonary rehabilitation.

Registered Dietitian Nutritionists

Registered dietitian nutritionists (R.D.N.'s) are food and nutrition experts who typically work in one of four areas: clinical, community, management, or consultant dietetics. Clinical dietitians provide nutritional services for patients in

A **physician assistant (P.A.)** is a health care professional trained to provide routine primary care to patients under the supervision of a physician.

A **physical therapist (P.T.)** is a health care professional who holds a degree in physical therapy and generally works in rehabilitation medicine helping patients restore musculoskeletal function.

A **registered dietitian nutritionist (R.D.N.)** is a food and nutrition expert who holds a degree in dietetics and has passed the national R.D.N. exam.

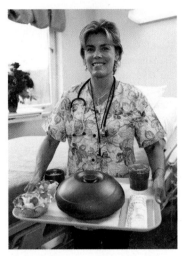

Many R.D.N.'s work for hospitals and nursing care facilities to ensure that the nutritional needs of patients are met.

© Stewart Cohen/Photodisc/Getty Images

institutions such as hospitals and nursing care facilities. They confer with doctors and other health care professionals to coordinate medical and nutritional needs for patients. Over half of all full-time R.D.N.'s work as clinical dietitians. Community dietitians work in public health clinics, home health agencies, and HMOs, where they counsel individuals and groups on nutritional practices to prevent disease and promote health. Management dietitians oversee large-scale meal planning and preparation in places such as school and company cafeterias. Consultant dietitians work on a contract basis for individual clients or organizations such as wellness programs, sports teams, supermarkets, and nutrition-related businesses.

To be eligible for the R.D.N. exam, the primary route today is enrolling in a B.S. or M.S. program that includes clinical practice hours. There are about 300 programs nationwide. R.D.N.'s translate the science of nutrition into practical solutions across the lifespan in disease prevention and health promotion, as well as medical nutrition therapy. There are about 90,000 active R.D.N.'s. Many pursue additional graduate training to prepare for advanced clinical positions, to work in public health, or to go into research. Given the current diet-related health problems faced by Americans, the value of an R.D.N. in advising patients and working with other health care professionals to coordinate medical care has never been greater.

For additional information on these and other types of allied health care professions, see the websites at the end of the chapter. Related to both consumer information and career prospects, it should be noted that competition is keen, and educational standards are continually increasing for allied health care professional preparation programs. As with doctors, the job opportunities in allied health careers are excellent.

✓ **NEED TO KNOW**

A patient's needs may require the expertise of a health care team that includes one or more physicians and a mix of allied health care professionals. The team approach is particularly important in diagnosing, treating, and managing complex illnesses. As a consumer, it's important to understand how these supporting professionals contribute to patient care. The training and roles of allied health care professionals—such as nurse, physician assistant, physical therapist, and dietitian—are varied and multifaceted and continue to evolve over time.

➤ Complementary Medicine

In addition to conventional or Western medicine, there is another category of health care known as **complementary medicine.** Many diverse practices based on principles quite different from those of Western medicine are included under the umbrella heading of complementary medicine. Two examples are chiropractic and acupuncture. When non-mainstream practices are used *together with* conventional medicine, they are *complementary*. If a non-mainstream practice is used *in place of* conventional medicine, it's considered *alternative.* True alternative medicine is unusual. Most individuals who use non-mainstream approaches use them along with conventional treatments.

OVERVIEW

The foundation of Western medicine is the scientific method—the discovery and accumulation of knowledge through systematic and rigorous research. In contrast, complementary practices are often rooted in culture-specific traditions and medical customs passed down across generations. These practices, also referred to as *traditional medicine,* are still widely used in parts of Asia, Africa, and Latin America. Fundamental differences between Western medicine and complementary medicine are summarized in Table 12.2.

The Western medicine approach involves the diagnosis and treatment of illness within a biomedical framework using highly trained specialists and advanced

TABLE 12.2	COMPARISON OF BASIC PRINCIPLES: WESTERN MEDICINE VS. COMPLEMENTARY MEDICINE
WESTERN MEDICINE	**COMPLEMENTARY MEDICINE**
Rooted in the scientific method and guided by empirical evidence from research	Often rooted in traditional medicine based on ancestral practices
Illness has a physical cause due to pathogens, environment, lifestyle, genetic factors, aging	Illness is due to an imbalance in the person or between the individual and others
Diagnosis of illness is based on established signs and symptoms that occur across patients	Illness is different in each person; evidence is case-based
Focus is to heal via outside intervention as with drugs and/or surgery	Focus is on helping the body's capacity for self-repair
Use of specialists and advanced technology to diagnose and treat illness	Based on metaphysical premises that may not be testable

Complementary medicine is a group of diverse medical and health care systems, practices, and products that are non-mainstream but are used together with Western or conventional medicine.

technology. Western medicine focuses on curing illness and disease through drugs and surgery, based on objective scientific evidence. In contrast, complementary medicine is generally case-based rather than research-based and often has spiritual or metaphysical underpinnings not readily testable by the scientific method. Illness is thought to be caused by an imbalance within the individual or between the individual and others, and treatment is directed toward assisting the body's innate capacity for self-repair and restoration of balance.

Thus, the very nature of complementary medicine—where interpretation of similar symptoms, diagnosis of illness, and prescribed treatments may vary widely from one patient to the next—makes these practices difficult if not impossible to study using the scientific method. Standard research methods typically involve studying hundreds of subjects with the same illness to test the effectiveness of a given treatment.

Western medicine is evidence-based and the bedrock of health care in the 21st century. Yet, complementary medicine is routinely used by significant segments of our population. Some complementary practices are beneficial for certain patients. More than 30 percent of American adults report using some form of non-mainstream practices on a regular basis. Our openness to these practices is reflected in increasing expenditures for complementary medicine. About half of these costs are paid out of pocket because insurance companies do not authorize payment for many complementary therapies.

As strong as Western medicine is, it cannot answer all our questions about health and disease. Even the foremost medical researchers agree on this point. And, conversely, as unproven as complementary medicine appears to those who understand the world through science, the fact remains that some non-mainstream therapies help people get better. With this in mind, let's remain open to the possibility that complementary medicine offers beneficial treatments, yet always examine specific practices based on their own merits and evidence. As consumers of health care, our challenge is to do our homework on the effectiveness and safety of a non-mainstream practice *before* making a decision about treatment.

In 1998 the National Institutes of Health created the National Center for Complementary and Integrative Health in response to the growing interest in non-mainstream medicine and the need for an objective resource for information and guidance on these diverse practices. The primary objectives of the Center are twofold: to investigate non-mainstream healing practices in the context of rigorous science and to disseminate authoritative information to the public and professionals. Most complementary health approaches fall into one of two groups—natural products or mind and body practices.

NATURAL PRODUCTS

Natural products use specific compounds, foods, or special diets—derived from natural sources—to treat an illness or disease. Examples include using aloe to treat a burn or consuming ginger to alleviate nausea. These therapies are referred to as biologically based because the use of the compound or food is believed to have a positive physiological effect in treating a given medical condition. Of all categories within complementary medicine, natural products or biologically based therapies may be the broadest, with several hundred treatments including but not limited to the use of plant-based products (herbals or botanicals), animal-based products (e.g., probiotics), and vitamins and minerals.

The vast majority of therapies involve the ingestion of a specific compound. About one in five American adults uses natural products. Echinacea, ginseng,

TABLE 12.3   POPULAR NATURAL MEDICINES USED BY AMERICANS

NATURAL PRODUCT	COMMON CONDITION TREATED	EVIDENCE
Echinacea	Prevent/treat colds, flu, infections	Mixed
Garlic	Prevent/treat infections	Mixed
Ginger	Prevent/treat nausea & vomiting	Promising
Ginkgo	Memory loss, variety of illnesses	Mixed
Ginseng	Reduce susceptibility to illness	Mixed
Glucosamine	Joint pain, osteoarthritis	Mixed
Fish oils (omega-3 fatty acids)	Circulatory disorders	Good
Peppermint oil	Digestive disorders	Mixed
Soy	Menopause hot flashes, high cholesterol	Promising
St. John's wort	Depression	Mixed

Sources: MedlinePlus, **nlm.nih.gov/medlineplus/druginformation.html;** and the National Center for Complementary and Integrative Health, **nccih.nih.gov/health/herbsataglance.htm.**

ginkgo, garlic, and glucosamine are among the most popular. The top 10 natural medicines, their typical uses, and level of evidence are summarized in Table 12.3. Note that for half of the natural remedies, evidence of effectiveness is mixed or uncertain; that is, some studies have found positive effects while others show no benefit. For ginger, glucosamine, and soy, the level of evidence to treat specific conditions is promising, but more research is needed. Finally, there is good evidence that fish oils lower cardiovascular risk and St. John's wort is effective in treating mild to moderate depression. However, not a single natural product among the 10 most popular has compelling evidence to support its use.

Several key points are important to keep in mind when thinking about using a biologically based therapy. These products are chemically active and can interact with other compounds, foods, and drugs. For this reason, it would be wise to first discuss the pros and cons of any natural product with your doctor, especially if you are on medications, including birth control pills, or have a chronic health condition. Also, be aware that nearly all natural products are classified as dietary supplements, not as drugs (see the section on dietary supplements in Chapter 2). Consequently, the purity, effectiveness, and safety of the compound must always be questioned. As a reminder, conventional medicines—both over-the-counter and prescription—go through a rigorous drug approval process by the FDA before they go to market, but this is *not* the case for dietary supplements, so it is buyer beware.

In the United States, herbalists and practitioners of other biologically based therapies have no standardized training or certification, and most are not medically qualified. Hundreds of natural products have been studied. For nearly all, evidence of effectiveness is negative or insufficient; for a few, evidence is mixed or promising. General contraindications are pregnancy and lactation. Additional precautions should be taken by people on medications or with chronic health conditions. Any natural product promoted as a treatment should be thoroughly investigated for proof of effectiveness and safety.

Mind and body practices include a large and diverse group of procedures or techniques administered or taught by a trained practitioner or teacher. A few of the most common practices will be briefly described in the following paragraphs. Remember, though, that the education or professional preparation for many practitioners, particularly of less well-known practices, is highly variable. In general, requirements are much less rigorous and systematic than for professionals of Western medicine. In many cases, no practice standards or credentialing exist.

So, what are some examples of mind and body practices in the realm of complementary medicine? Yoga and tai chi are popular movement practices. Less familiar movement pattern or postural awareness regimens include the Alexander technique and the Feldenkrais method. Common body-manipulative practices include chiropractic adjustment, therapeutic massage, and acupuncture. Meditation is perhaps the best-known mind practice. Less well known are creative therapies that use art, dance, or music as a means to treat people with communication or psychological disorders. Another mind-based practice is spiritual healing in which practitioners and in some cases laypeople use purposeful focused intention to help cure another person; faith healing and intercessory prayer are examples, respectively.

Meditation

Meditation is one of the oldest and most widely practiced mind–body therapies. Meditation and its different forms evolved from Eastern religions. During meditation one focuses on breathing or on a mantra (a single word or syllable) and is taught to disregard other thoughts and emotions. Classes or short courses are widely available to learn the technique. Meditation is a self-administered tool for mental and physical relaxation. It should be practiced daily to fully accrue its benefits.

For many people, meditation enhances general well being. However, systematic reviews show little scientific evidence demonstrating therapeutic effectiveness for any specific health condition. Most proponents practice meditation simply as a lifestyle choice, because meditation imparts a sense of relaxation and self-awareness. Aspects of meditation are closely related to other mind–body therapies including deep breathing, progressive muscle relaxation, and yoga.

Acupuncture

In the Western world, **acupuncture** is the best known of the traditional Chinese medicine treatments. Acupuncture is the practice of inserting small needles into carefully selected points along the body's energy pathways. Needles are positioned just under the skin or deeper into the muscle and then either manually rotated or electrically stimulated. Acupuncture treatment is based on the belief that by adjusting the body's *qi*, or vital energy, healing can occur.

Acupuncture has been thoroughly studied as a treatment for two conditions: low back pain and nausea/vomiting. Systematic reviews of multiple studies indicate acupuncture is more effective for relief of low back pain than no treatment or sham (pretended) treatment. Moreover, when acupuncture is added to conventional therapies, it relieves pain and improves function better than conventional therapies alone.

Acupuncture is a complementary medicine procedure used in or adapted from traditional Chinese medicine in which specific body areas are pierced with fine needles to treat a variety of illnesses.

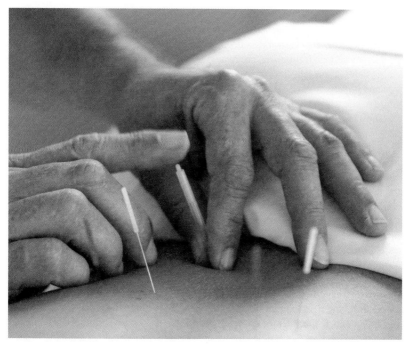

An acupuncturist carefully places needles in the body.
© Thinkstock/Punchstock

Multiple studies have also assessed whether acupuncture can be used to reduce nausea and vomiting (typically postoperative or following chemotherapy). Overall results indicate that acupuncture can be effective, particularly on the first day.

Practitioners of acupuncture are known as *acupuncturists*. The National Certification Commission for Acupuncture and Oriental Medicine has been providing certification in acupuncture since 1985. There are more than 25,000 certified acupuncturists **(www.nccaom.org)**.

Manual Therapies

In the United States, the three most common types of manual therapies are osteopathic manipulative treatment, chiropractic adjustment, and therapeutic massage. In manual therapy, practitioners use their hands to manipulate the patient's soft tissues and musculoskeletal joints, including the spine. The techniques and uses of these manual therapies vary somewhat with the type of practitioner—osteopath, chiropractor, or massage therapist.

As described earlier in this chapter, the osteopath or D.O. goes through training similar to the M.D.—both are physicians (Western medicine). A difference is that osteopathic medicine emphasizes manipulative techniques as a key part of medical training and an important clinical skill, particularly in the diagnosis and treatment of musculoskeletal problems. In general, osteopathic manipulative treatment is broadly accepted as part of conventional Western medicine. In contrast, chiropractic adjustment and therapeutic massage are still considered alternative practices.

Chiropractic The health care philosophy of chiropractic is centered on the body's inherent recuperative abilities and embraces a holistic view of the patient's well-being. A **chiropractor,** also known as a doctor of chiropractic (**D.C.**), primarily works with people whose health problems are related to the body's muscular, nervous, and skeletal systems, especially the spine. Chiropractors believe that interference with these systems impairs normal functions, lowers resistance to disease, and can cause pain. Chiropractic was established in 1895 by D. D. Palmer and is now practiced worldwide.

The D.C. degree is awarded after completion of a four-year program at one of 18 accredited chiropractic programs. At least two years of undergraduate education is required for entry, although many enter with an undergraduate degree. All states have licensing boards for chiropractic, and many health insurance companies cover chiropractic care. There are over 75,000 chiropractors. Most people see a chiropractor for a back, neck, or pain-related problem. It's estimated that 1 in 10 American adults visited a chiropractor within the last year. Chiropractic is gaining acceptance among Western medicine practitioners, and some physicians refer patients to chiropractors for treatment of back pain.

Chiropractors take medical histories, conduct clinical exams, and often use X-rays. The most common treatment procedure is *chiropractic adjustment,* also called *spinal manipulation.* Manipulating the patient's joints, particularly the spine, is used to reduce pain and restore joint function. The procedure seldom causes discomfort, and people often report improvements in symptoms immediately following treatment. Chiropractors do not perform surgery or prescribe drugs but often recommend changes in lifestyle—in eating, exercise, and sleeping habits. As needed, chiropractors refer patients to M.D.'s or D.O.'s.

Many studies have been done on chiropractic and back pain. Findings are mixed—some show positive effects while others indicate no benefit. As is common in research on complementary practices, many studies are poorly designed, which limits interpretation. Moreover, back pain is difficult to study because the cause is often never known, and in most cases the condition resolves within weeks regardless of treatment. Overall the evidence supporting chiropractic adjustment as an effective treatment for back pain is not convincing. It is no more or no less effective than conventional treatments.

Therapeutic Massage Therapeutic massage, or massage therapy, is one of the most popular forms of complementary medicine. The central principle of therapeutic massage is that the body's soft tissues will function optimally when the circulatory and lymphatic systems are unimpeded. There are different types of therapeutic massage (for example, Swedish, shiatsu, neuromuscular). Most involve similar manual techniques such as stroking, kneading, and stretching, and these are often combined during a treatment session. Therapeutic massage is generally used to treat joint and muscle pain and to reduce high stress levels.

A client usually sees a therapist with a diagnosis—and often a referral—from a physician or with a self-diagnosis or symptom. Therapists take a brief medical history to rule out contraindications such as skin infections, acute inflammations, or recent injuries and may ask questions to better understand the diagnosis or health complaint.

A **chiropractor (D.C.)** typically works with people whose health problems are associated with the muscular, nervous, and skeletal systems, especially the spine. Chiropractic adjustment is a common treatment to relieve neck and back pain. The effectiveness of such treatment holds promise, but conclusive evidence is lacking.

During the session, the therapist requests feedback as to how much pressure is preferred. Palpation, or touch, is fundamental to therapeutic massage and allows the therapist to identify areas of muscle tension or fluid accumulation with appropriate amounts of pressure for each individual, while also conveying a sense of caring.

In the United States, considerable variability still exists from school to school regarding the length and amount of training and from state to state regarding licensing. However, the National Certification Board for Therapeutic Massage, established in 1992, has become the leading organization in setting professional standards and administering written competency exams—over 90,000 people have been certified. When provided by a qualified therapist, therapeutic massage appears to be beneficial for musculoskeletal pain and for anxiety and depression. The evidence is promising but not unequivocal. Direct risks are minimal.

OTHER COMPLEMENTARY PRACTICES

The two broad areas previously discussed—natural products and mind and body practices—capture most complementary approaches. However, some practices may not neatly fit into either of these groups—for example, the practices of traditional healers, Ayurvedic medicine, traditional Chinese medicine, naturopathy, and homeopathy. Each of these is an alternative medical system based on its own unified body of thought and practice, reflecting unique historical origins and underlying philosophies. To illustrate, we'll briefly review one practice—homeopathy.

Homeopathy

Homeopathy is based on the *law of similars*. This refers to the observation that medicines can produce in healthy people the same symptoms they cure in sick people. This concept—also known as *like cures like*—was derived from simple trial and error or empirical observations. Homeopathic treatment involves giving extremely dilute medicines to trigger the patient's innate ability to heal. Homeopathic medicines are natural remedies derived from animal, plant, and mineral sources and are sold as over-the-counter products.

Homeopathy was developed over 200 years ago in Europe by Samuel Hahnemann, a German physician. His followers immigrated to the United States in the mid-1800s and established the American homeopathic movement, which flourished for several decades. However, the tide turned in the first half of the 20th century. As medical science (Western medicine) grew, and more and more modern drugs were discovered, homeopathy lost its appeal.

Even though all formal degree programs were disbanded by 1950, homeopathy has persevered over the decades and still has its advocates. Seminars and courses continue to be offered by homeopathic interest groups. A resurgence of interest in homeopathy has occurred in recent years as part of the broader interest in self-care and alternative medicine. Because there is no federal licensure exam, the current practice of homeopathy is generally limited to medically licensed physicians (M.D.'s, D.O.'s) who use selected homeopathic remedies along with conventional medical treatments.

The scientific basis and medical effectiveness of homeopathy remain dubious. Although there may be instances in which like cures like, the concept does not qualify as a universal principle. A limited number of studies have evaluated homeopathic treatments. Few carefully controlled randomized studies have been conducted due to the lack of positive findings from smaller studies. Systematic reviews of homeopathic treatments find no conclusive evidence of effectiveness for any specific medical condition. Although the risk of serious side effects from using highly diluted homeopathic remedies appears low, there is no compelling theory or solid evidence to support their use.

DUE DILIGENCE

If you are considering using a non-mainstream medical treatment, it's very important to know how to get credible information. Most treatments under the heading of complementary medicine are unregulated. Misinformation, misleading claims, and outright hoaxes abound. The key is to sort the honest, credentialed practitioners from those who cannot help you—including well-meaning pretenders and modern-day quacks. Use the following tips to assess services and products found on the Internet:

1. Who runs the web page? Is it a credible professional (.org), educational (.edu), or governmental (.gov) group? Or a business set up to market a product (.com)? Generally, the .edu, .gov, and .org sites are more trustworthy than the .com sites.
2. Be wary of sites that diagnose illnesses or suggest a course of treatment. These services should be provided only by a doctor who knows the patient's medical history and has performed a physical examination.
3. Be suspicious of quasi-scientific statements that go against common sense or known health principles. Discount any treatments or products that make claims about miracle cures.
4. Don't rely on a single website for the final word. Always cross-check information on independent websites known to be reputable. For example, use the following websites as a starting point:

   National Center for Complementary and Integrative Health: **https://nccih.nih.gov**
   Quackwatch: **www.quackwatch.org**
   Office of Dietary Supplements: **ods.od.nih.gov**

Remember, to find bona fide treatment options for a troubling health problem, seek solid information. Be aware that advertisements can be disguised as health columns or news reports. Many are easy to spot; others are more sophisticated. Convincing claims or personal success stories are not a substitute for scientific evidence. As always, your best guide is accurate and trustworthy information.

INTEGRATIVE MEDICINE

Self
Assessments
12.1

Integrative medicine is the coordinated combining of practices or treatments from complementary medicine with those of Western medicine. It's based on an awareness and appreciation of the strengths and weaknesses of both. Integrative medicine is a growing movement. Medical schools no longer dismiss or ignore complementary medicine. Today more than 60 leading academic medical centers such as Harvard, Yale, Duke, Stanford, UCLA, Cleveland Clinic, and Mayo Clinic are members of

Integrative medicine seeks to restore and maintain health by first understanding the patient's unique condition and circumstances, and then coordinating the most appropriate treatments from both complementary approaches and mainstream health care.

Health & the Media Patent Medicines

So-called patent medicines (protected by a patent or trademark and available without a doctor's prescription) were common following the Civil War. The illustration here is an example of a patent medicine trade card—an early form of advertising that extended the reach of peddlers and medicine shows. At county fairs and frontier settlements, doctors and druggists—often with suspect credentials—engaged in aggressive selling. Many were talented entertainers capable of wowing audiences with enthralling oratory and theatrics. Ayer's Sarsaparilla could "improve the complexion, purify the blood, and make the weak strong." Quackery continues today. Many ads, across all media—print, radio, TV, and the Internet—still use unsubstantiated claims of healing and generalized health benefits. Satisfaction "guaranteed," of course.

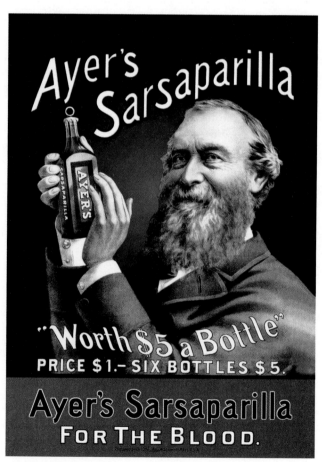

© Getty Images

the Academic Consortium for Integrative Medicine and Health. The Consortium's mission is to advance health care by educating medical students and physicians about integrative medicine and conducting research on non-mainstream practices to better determine which treatments are effective or hold promise.

Prominent physicians Ralph Snyderman and Andrew Weil succinctly describe the appeal of integrative medicine for patients:

> Most Americans would probably jump at the chance to consult a physician who is well trained in scientifically based medicine and who is also open-minded and knowledgeable about the body's innate mechanisms of healing, the role of lifestyle factors in influencing health, and the appropriate uses of dietary supplements, herbs, and other forms of treatment, from osteopathic manipulation to Chinese and Ayurvedic medicine. In other words, they want competent help in navigating the confusing maze of therapeutic options that are available today, especially in those cases in which conventional approaches are relatively ineffective or harmful.

As an example, low back pain is a widespread health problem, affecting up to one out of three adults in a given month. Conventional medicine is important in identifying serious, underlying problems such as a herniated disc, rheumatoid arthritis, infection, fracture, or cancer. If no underlying cause can be determined—which occurs in a large percentage of cases—conventional medicine has little to offer the patient. Yet, there is promising evidence that acupuncture can relieve pain and improve function. In a clinic that practices integrative medicine, the doctor would discuss acupuncture as a possible treatment and arrange for treatments if requested.

Article 12.4

Integrative medicine reaffirms the importance of the doctor–patient relationship, focuses on the whole person—not just a specific condition or disease—and makes use of all appropriate curative preventive approaches. The bottom line is that physicians practicing integrative medicine are not restricted to a particular dogma, Western or Eastern, but rather guided by a "get the patient better" philosophy.

Integrative medicine considers *all factors that influence health*. These include a person's body, mind, and spirit as well as his or her family, community, and society. This broad perspective recognizes the importance of cultural expectations, biotechnological advances, and public policies. All play significant roles in treating patients and shaping their lifestyle and health behaviors.

✓ NEED TO KNOW

Complementary medicine encompasses a multitude of diverse approaches to healing. These can be categorized into three groupings: natural products, mind and body practices, and other practices. Even though many Americans regularly use these non-mainstream practices, fundamental questions about the risks and benefits of many treatments are yet to be answered. Research is ongoing. Integrative medicine brings together practices from Western medicine and complementary medicine, based on good science and the needs of the patient. Integrative medicine is gaining acceptance at leading academic medical centers and may well become the mainstream medicine of the future.

ARTICLES

12.1 "Yes, Prevention Is Cheaper Than Treatment." *Newsweek*. Dr. Dean Ornish makes the case for moving preventive medicine to the forefront of the American health care system.

12.2 "Doctors Make Mistakes: A Commentary on Medical Errors." *The Huffington Post*. Doctors, hospitals, and patients all have a role to play in reducing medical mistakes.

12.3 "Treat the Patient, Not the CT Scan." *New York Times*. Technology cannot replace a doctor's clinical skills.

12.4 "Building the Precision Medicine Initiative National Research Cohort—The Time Is Now." National Institutes of Health. Personalized medicine of tomorrow is beginning today.

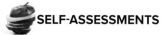

SELF-ASSESSMENTS

12.1 Understanding U.S. Medical Care

Website Resources

MEDICINE—M.D.'s AND D.O.'s

American Association of Colleges of Osteopathic Medicine **www.aacom.org**
American Board of Medical Specialties **www.abms.org**
American Medical Association **www.ama-assn.org**
American Osteopathic Association **www.osteopathic.org**
Association of American Medical Colleges **www.aamc.org**

DENTISTRY

American Dental Association **www.ada.org**
American Dental Education Association **www.adea.org**

PODIATRY

American Association of Colleges of Podiatric Medicine **www.aacpm.org**
American Podiatric Medical Association **www.apma.org**

OPTOMETRY

American Optometric Association **www.aoa.org**
Association of Schools and Colleges of Optometry **www.opted.org**

CLINICAL PSYCHOLOGY

National Register of Health Service Providers in Psychology
   www.nationalregister.org
Society of Clinical Psychology **www.div12.org**

NURSING

Accredited Nursing Programs **www.nlnac.org/Forms/directory_search.htm**
American Nurses Association **www.nursingworld.org**
Guide to Nursing Education and Careers **www.allnursingschools.com/faqs**

PHYSICIAN ASSISTANT

American Academy of Physician Assistants **www.aapa.org**
Physician Assistant Education Association **www.paeaonline.org**

PHYSICAL THERAPY

American Physical Therapy Association **www.apta.org**
Physical Therapist Education **www.apta.org/PTEducation/**

DIETETICS

Academy of Nutrition and Dietetics **www.eatrightpro.org**
Commission on Dietetic Registration **www.cdrnet.org**

COMPLEMENTARY MEDICINE

Academic Consortium for Integrative Medicine and Health
    www.imconsortium.org
American Chiropractic Association **www.acatoday.org**
American Massage Therapy Association **www.amtamassage.org**
Cochrane Reviews: Search for Complementary Medicine **cochrane.org**
MedlinePlus: Herbs and Supplements
    www.nlm.nih.gov/medlineplus/druginfo/herb_All.html
National Center for Complementary and Integrative Health **https://nccih.nih.gov**
National Certification Board for Therapeutic Massage and Bodywork
    www.ncbtmb.com
National Certification Commission for Acupuncture and Oriental Medicine
    www.nccaom.org
NCCIH: Herbs at a Glance **nccih.nih.gov/health/herbsataglance.htm**
Quackwatch **www.quackwatch.org**

GENERAL

Agency for Healthcare Research and Quality **www.ahrq.gov**
Explore Health Careers **explorehealthcareers.org**

acupuncture, 362
chiropractor, 364
clinical psychologist, 355
complementary medicine, 359
dentist, 352
integrative medicine, 366
optometrist, 353
physical therapist, 357
physician, 349

physician assistant, 357
podiatrist, 353
primary care physician, 350
primary health care, 345
registered dietitian nutritionist, 357
registered nurse, 356
secondary health care, 346
tertiary health care, 346

Understanding the Content

1. Define and provide examples of primary, secondary, and tertiary health care.
2. Identify and discuss two of the major challenges facing our current system of medical care.
3. Define and contrast Western medicine with complementary medicine.

Exploring Ideas

1. Western medicine is often referred to as evidence-based medicine. Explain what is meant by this statement. For example, consider the centrality of the scientific method, how physicians and allied health professionals are trained in comparison with non-mainstream practitioners, and the role of clinical trials in advancing medical knowledge.
2. Assume one of your parents has a recurring medical problem, and the doctors have been unable to effectively treat it. Your parent now wants to try a complementary medicine approach that was recommended by a neighbor. What advice would you give? List and explain the steps you would take to check out this practice or product.
3. Explain the concept of integrative medicine. How does it differ from Western medicine? What changes need to occur if integrative medicine is to become widely accepted?

Selected References

Ernst E, Pittler M, Wider B. *Desktop Guide to Complementary and Alternative Medicine: An Evidence-Based Approach* (2nd ed.). Philadelphia: Mosby, 2006.

Food and Drug Administration. How to spot health fraud. February 2010.
www.fda.gov/health fraud

Gawande A. *The Checklist Manifesto: How to Get Things Right.* New York: Henry Holt, 2010.

Gawande A. The cost conundrum. *The New Yorker,* June 1, 2009

Institute of Medicine. *Complementary and Alternative Medicine in the United States.* Washington, DC: National Academies Press, 2005.

Institute of Medicine. *Integrative Medicine and the Health of the Public Agenda.* Washington, DC: National Academies Press, 2009.

James JT. A new, evidence-based estimate of patient harms associated with hospital care. *Journal of Patient Safety* 9: 122–128, 2013.

Kaiser Family Foundation. Health care costs: A primer. 2012. **kff.org/health-costs/issue-brief/health-care-costs-a-primer**

Kohn L, Corrigan J, Donaldson M (eds.). *To Err Is Human: Building a Safer Health System.* Washington, DC: Institute of Medicine, National Academies Press, 2000.

Leape LL, Berwick DM. Five years after *To Err Is Human.* What have we learned? *JAMA* 293: 2384–2390, 2005.

Micozzi M. *Fundamentals of Complementary and Integrative Medicine* (5th ed.). St. Louis: Saunders, 2015.

Moynihan R, Cassels A. *Selling Sickness: How the World's Biggest Pharmaceutical Companies Are Turning Us All into Patients.* New York: Nation Books, 2005.

Rakel DP. *Integrative Medicine* (3rd ed.). Philadelphia: Saunders, 2012.

Snyderman R, Weil A. Integrative medicine: Bringing medicine back to its roots. *Archives of Internal Medicine* 162: 395–397, 2002.

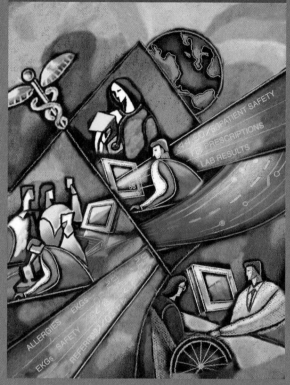

A hospital should also have a recovery room adjoining the cashier's office.

—Francis O. Walsh

© Kain Zernitsky/Getty Images

Chapter 13

HEALTH CARE DECISION MAKING

In Chapter 12, we described the structure of the U.S. health care system and types of medical care available. This leads us to the question, How can we effectively use such information to navigate the system? In this chapter, we address this question by reviewing recommendations on medical self-care, the patient–doctor relationship, and health insurance. We end this last chapter by revisiting two recurrent themes central to optimal health: health literacy and preventive health care.

Caring for Yourself

SIGNS AND SYMPTOMS

DIAGNOSING COMMON MEDICAL PROBLEMS

HANDLING MEDICAL EMERGENCIES

PRESCRIPTION AND OTC MEDICINES

BODY ART

Developing a Patient–Doctor Partnership

FINDING THE RIGHT DOCTOR

COMMUNICATING WITH YOUR DOCTOR

MEDICAL TESTS AND PROCEDURES

KEEPING MEDICAL RECORDS

Understanding Health Insurance

HEALTH INSURANCE TERMINOLOGY

PRIVATE HEALTH INSURANCE: FEE FOR SERVICE AND MANAGED CARE

PUBLIC HEALTH INSURANCE: MEDICARE AND MEDICAID

CHOOSING AN APPROPRIATE PLAN

HEALTH CARE REFORM

Striving for Optimal Health

STAYING INFORMED

PRACTICING PREVENTION

CHOICES we make can put us at risk of illness and injury, and significant medical expenses can result. Consider the case of Dave, a first-year college student. He attended a party and over a six-hour period consumed about 4 beers and 12 shots of whiskey. Toward the end of the evening, Dave passed out. His friends were scared when they noticed his very shallow breathing and a swollen area on his head where he had fallen and hit the floor. They took him to the emergency room at the local hospital.

Dave was semiconscious, slurring his words, and having difficulty answering questions. His friends told the emergency room doctors what happened. In order to ascertain the extent of Dave's intoxication and possible injury, the medical team performed a physical evaluation, gave him intravenous saline solution, ran blood tests, and performed a CT scan to determine if there was a serious head injury from the fall. The CT scan was normal, and it was determined that Dave would recover from his excessive drinking after his body processed the alcohol. The ER team observed him for several hours, and then he was released.

Dave was lucky that his friends realized he might be in serious trouble and got him help after he passed out. He was also fortunate not to have a permanent injury. But his luck ends there, for the cost of his "bad night out" is much more than a bruise, embarrassment, and a hangover. Medical care in the United States is very expensive. Dave's treatment cost $500 for the emergency room visit, $350 for physician services, $150 for IV saline solution, $250 for blood tests, $1,500 for the CT scan, and $250 for the radiologist to evaluate the CT scan—$3,000 total. Dave was on his parents' health insurance so some of the costs got covered. However, because of the nature of the emergency room visit, and with co-payments and deductibles, Dave's parents are still responsible for $1,000 of the bill. In this instance, Dave was semiconscious when he was injured, so he had no input regarding the care he received. The emergency room was morally and legally obligated to help him. However, it was also very costly and preventable.

Article
13.1

We do not always have a choice in the type of health issues we face in life. However, everyone faces many choices and decisions regarding health care. How much can we do on our own? How do we determine when we need to use the health care system? How do we go about finding the right doctor?

Then there are the financial reality questions about cost and health insurance. What are the health insurance options, and what particular type of plan is the right one for us? This chapter will help answer these questions. Key information and resources for making informed choices about self-care, medical care, and health insurance are provided to help you navigate the health care and insurance systems.

➤ Caring for Yourself

Medical self-care is the steps and actions you take to optimize your health and to self-treat common illnesses and injuries. When motivated consumers have access to clear, simple health information, many health problems can be prevented or treated

> **Medical self-care** is decisions and actions that an individual can take to cope with a health problem—in particular, informed steps that one can take without seeing a health care practitioner.

effectively and inexpensively without a visit to the doctor's office. Consequently, in this section we'll focus on medical self-care as it relates to self-recognition of emergent signs and symptoms, and making decisions about self-treatment or seeing a health care professional. There are two key aspects of self-care: First, we must be sensitive to signs and symptoms, and second, we need to know how to acquire the relevant information. A start to the process is to complete a Health and Well-being Questionnaire and make health decisions based on the results.

SIGNS AND SYMPTOMS

Self
Assessments
13.1

The terms *sign* and *symptom* are similar but not synonymous. A **sign** can be measured objectively, usually by a health care provider during a physical exam. For example, heart rate, respiratory rate, body temperature, and blood pressure are standard vital signs. Elevated blood pressure is a sign of possible heart disease. On the other hand, a **symptom** is a person's subjective perception, such as nausea or knee pain. Signs and symptoms are used together in recognizing and diagnosing medical conditions.

Being sensitive to signs and symptoms means listening to your body. Being attuned to changes in your body is central to medical self-care because you are the best judge of what is normal and routine for you and what is not. It's important to pay attention to your intuition or premonitions that something is not right. As mentioned in Chapter 11, *prodrome* is a medical term for patients' feelings or early symptoms indicating the onset of an illness. For example, most of us have a sense that we are coming down with a cold a day or two before the signs and symptoms are clearly recognizable. The true story of Carolyn Benivegna in "Breaking It Down" demonstrates the importance of knowing and listening to your body and following your intuition.

Breaking It Down When Diagnosis Is a Long and Winding Road

Carolyn, an extremely healthy and health-conscious middle-aged woman, became alarmed when her abdomen suddenly enlarged and she began experiencing bouts of constipation and bloated abdomen. She soon discovered that getting the correct diagnosis is not always a straightforward process. It can take a combination of luck and perseverance.

She first went to her primary care doctor. Because her symptoms seemed to be intestinal, Carolyn was referred to a specialist of the digestive system—a gastroenterologist. He ran tests to determine whether there was a bacterial infection. After ruling that out, he diagnosed her with irritable bowel syndrome. Irritable bowel

A **sign** is a result of injury or illness and can be measured objectively by a health care provider.

A **symptom** is a result of injury or illness that is subjectively perceived by the patient.

syndrome (IBS) consists of several symptoms at the same time; for example, abdominal pain, constipation, and abdominal swelling often occur together. Yet, this didn't seem right to Carolyn: "I guess I would have accepted this diagnosis had it not been for my enlarged abdomen. I swear to you, it looked like I was four to five months pregnant! I therefore insisted on more tests." The doctor ordered X-rays, which also found nothing. Carolyn was again assured she had irritable bowel syndrome and was encouraged to go on her scheduled monthlong trip to Europe. But she remained worried: "I couldn't wear any of my slacks or shorts because I couldn't get them buttoned. I *knew* something was radically wrong. I *insisted* on more tests."

Carolyn's doctor reluctantly scheduled a CAT scan (computerized axial tomography). This test showed an abnormal buildup of fluid in her abdomen. This finding suggested that Carolyn was indeed correct—she did *not* have IBS. Finally, a special blood test gave her a diagnosis: She had primary peritoneal cancer, a cancer involving the membrane that surrounds the organs in the abdomen and pelvis. In this case, the correct diagnosis was elusive because peritoneal cancer is closely related to ovarian cancer, yet Carolyn no longer had her ovaries (previously removed during a complete hysterectomy). Therefore, her doctors initially overlooked this type of cancer as a possible cause of her bloating and intestinal problems.

Carolyn's message is clear and direct: "I have learned that each of us must take *total* responsibility for our own health care." She knew her body well enough to realize that something serious might be wrong, and she pushed for more tests when she felt the doctor was missing something. The correct diagnosis was a direct result of her perseverance. Her actions led to getting life-saving treatment sooner rather than later. Carolyn's story is not typical, but it's not rare, either. The main point is not that the doctor misdiagnosed her illness, but rather that Carolyn and her doctor worked *together* to solve the mystery of her illness.

You know yourself—or should know yourself—better than anyone else. Pay attention to physical and mental changes and communicate with your doctor.

Source: Adapted from Johns Hopkins Pathology, Personal Stories: Carolyn Benivegna.

DIAGNOSING COMMON MEDICAL PROBLEMS

To adequately address the topic of common medical problems requires the power of the Internet. Several excellent online resources are available to help us identify appropriate next steps when interpreting signs and symptoms. Two resources that are highly reputable, time-tested, and designed for the layperson are the American Academy of Family Physicians website (**www.familydoctor.org**) and the *Merck Manual* online medical library (**www.merck.com/mmhe/index.html**). Both websites are comprehensive, regularly updated, and known for their ease of use.

The familydoctor.org website has a page that is organized alphabetically by symptoms—over 40 of the most common—from abdominal pain to urination problems (**familydoctor.org/online/famdocen/home/tools/symptom.html**). Clicking on any symptom generates a decision chart that provides guidance on a course of action. Decision charts are easy to follow and logically step through the decision-making process. For example, a decision chart for headaches is presented in Figure 13.1. Following the first column under the heading of symptoms, one can scan down and follow the Yes or No branches to a probable diagnosis (second column) and then to a self-care action (third column), such as "Use an over-the-counter medicine," "Call your doctor," or "Go to the emergency room." Embedded in the website's decision

FIGURE 13.1 A DECISION CHART FOR HEADACHES

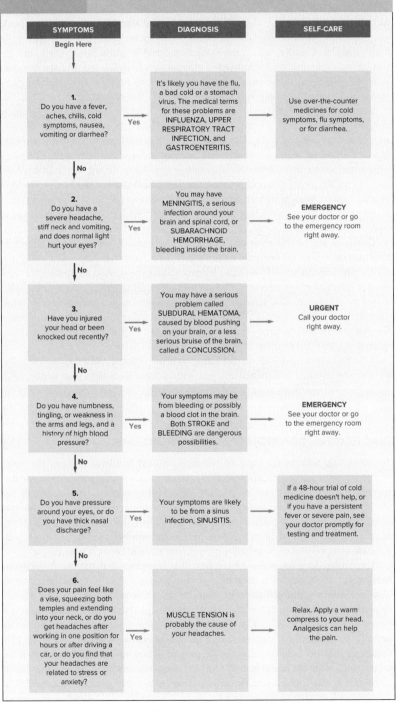

SYMPTOMS

Begin Here

1.
Do you have a fever, aches, chills, cold symptoms, nausea, vomiting or diarrhea?

Yes →

DIAGNOSIS

It's likely you have the flu, a bad cold or a stomach virus. The medical terms for these problems are INFLUENZA, UPPER RESPIRATORY TRACT INFECTION, and GASTROENTERITIS.

→

SELF-CARE

Use over-the-counter medicines for cold symptoms, flu symptoms, or for diarrhea.

No ↓

2.
Do you have a severe headache, stiff neck and vomiting, and does normal light hurt your eyes?

Yes →

You may have MENINGITIS, a serious infection around your brain and spinal cord, or SUBARACHNOID HEMORRHAGE, bleeding inside the brain.

→

EMERGENCY
See your doctor or go to the emergency room right away.

No ↓

3.
Have you injured your head or been knocked out recently?

Yes →

You may have a serious problem called SUBDURAL HEMATOMA, caused by blood pushing on your brain, or a less serious bruise of the brain, called a CONCUSSION.

→

URGENT
Call your doctor right away.

No ↓

4.
Do you have numbness, tingling, or weakness in the arms and legs, and a history of high blood pressure?

Yes →

Your symptoms may be from bleeding or possibly a blood clot in the brain. Both STROKE and BLEEDING are dangerous possibilities.

→

EMERGENCY
See your doctor or go to the emergency room right away.

No ↓

5.
Do you have pressure around your eyes, or do you have thick nasal discharge?

Yes →

Your symptoms are likely to be from a sinus infection, SINUSITIS.

→

If a 48-hour trial of cold medicine doesn't help, or if you have a persistent fever or severe pain, see your doctor promptly for testing and treatment.

No ↓

6.
Does your pain feel like a vise, squeezing both temples and extending into your neck, or do you get headaches after working in one position for hours or after driving a car, or do you find that your headaches are related to stress or anxiety?

Yes →

MUSCLE TENSION is probably the cause of your headaches.

→

Relax. Apply a warm compress to your head. Analgesics can help the pain.

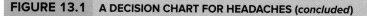

FIGURE 13.1 A DECISION CHART FOR HEADACHES *(concluded)*

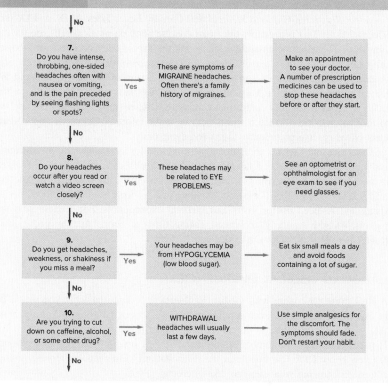

Pain in one area or multiple areas of the head sometimes is accompanied by other symptoms. There are many causes for headaches. For more information, consult your doctor. If you think the problem is serious, call your doctor right away. This tool is for general educational purposes only. It is not a substitute for medical advice. Always consult your family doctor with questions about your individual condition and circumstances.

Source: **FamilyDoctor.org.** Reprinted with permission from American Academy of Family Physicians.

chart are links to descriptions of the possible conditions that may be causing your symptoms.

The Merck website provides the online version of the *Merck Manual of Medical Information,* 2nd Home Edition. The *Merck Manual* has been a standard reference guide for physicians and pharmacists for over a century. The home edition is a plain-language version of the classic medical reference text for people with an interest in health care but no medical training. It is organized alphabetically into over 20 sections, including accidents and injuries, digestive disorders, ear-nose-throat disorders, infections, men's health issues, mental health disorders, and women's health issues. Nearly all sections have illustrated subsections on the biology of the particular topic along with specific descriptions of related illnesses and conditions including symptoms, diagnosis, and treatment.

Last, we would be remiss if we did not recommend *Take Care of Yourself: The Complete Illustrated Guide to Medical Self-Care* by James Fries, M.D., and Donald Vickery, M.D. This is arguably the finest concise book on medical self-care for the consumer. These physician-authors pioneered the use of decision charts in medical self-care. As was illustrated by Figure 13.1, a decision chart (or flow chart) is a graphical representation of a process that shows a start point, end points, and the logical steps and possible branches in between. Decision charts originated in the fields of business (quality control) and computer science (programming). As applied to medical self-care, decision charts help us make informed decisions about treatment based on interpretation of signs and symptoms.

Drs. Fries and Vickery are nationally recognized for their leadership in educating and empowering everyday folks about their own health care. *Take Care of Yourself* is one of the few books whose impact has been systematically evaluated in randomized studies. Use of this book in community and worksite studies improved health status and reduced doctor visits and medical expenditures. For readers who are parents, see the similarly acclaimed *Taking Care of Your Child* by pediatrician Robert Pantell along with Drs. Fries and Vickery.

HANDLING MEDICAL EMERGENCIES

A final point on coping with medical problems is to consider what you would do in case of an emergency such as a heart attack, a serious fall, or a poisoning. Does the 9-1-1 system operate in your location? Where is the closest emergency room? Is your doctor's phone number readily accessible or programmed into your phone? Do you know CPR (cardiopulmonary resuscitation)? Emergencies require prompt action, so knowing what steps to take is crucial.

If you do not know CPR, or if it has been a few years since you learned it, we strongly recommend that you take a course. A basic course includes information and practice on how to assist an unconscious or choking person—an infant, child, or adult—and how to use an automated external defibrillator (AED). Even better, take a first aid course that, in addition to CPR, teaches basic skills to treat wounds and bleeding, injuries to bones and joints, extremes of hot and cold, and poisoning, bites, and stings.

In any serious accident, assume the victim is in shock to some degree. Shock is a condition of general weakness caused by physical trauma such as loss of blood (internal or external bleeding) or extreme pain or fear. People in shock may feel faint, giddy, anxious, or restless. They may feel sick, may vomit, and may lose consciousness. To assist a person in shock, take the following steps:

- Lay the person down and raise the feet above the level of the head.
- Treat obvious wounds and loosen tight clothing.
- Minimize any movement if serious neck or spine injuries are suspected.
- Cover the person with a blanket or coat and keep him or her as comfortable as possible.
- Check pulse and breathing every few minutes.
- Stay with a person in shock, because constant reassurance is extremely important.

Remember, emergencies will occur. How well we deal with them depends largely on knowing what actions to take. For further information, refer to the Mayo

Clinic First Aid Guide or go to the *Merck Manual* website and click on the "Accidents and Injuries" section. (The URLs are in Website Resources at the end of this chapter.)

PRESCRIPTION AND OTC MEDICINES

Determining which **drugs** are distributed by prescription and which are over the counter (OTC) relates to the FDA drug approval process and the pharmaceutical company's application regarding how to make a drug available to the public. Generally speaking, most **prescription (Rx) drugs** have a potential for harm that is higher than nonprescription **over-the-counter (OTC) drugs.** Therefore, use of prescription medication must be prescribed by a licensed medical professional, and the drug itself must be dispensed by a pharmacist. Some prescription drugs contain controlled substances, such as codeine, and have the potential for dependence. Others may have a very narrow safety margin between the effective dose and a lethal dose, so they require careful physician and pharmacist oversight. Over-the-counter drugs need no physician or pharmacist oversight, and when taken as directed by consumers are safe and effective.

Many prescription drugs are produced in lesser strength and are available as OTC drugs. For example, the pain reliever Motrin (also known as ibuprofen) has a prescription-strength pill that is 600 mg per tablet. But it can also be purchased over the counter in a pill that has 200 mg per tablet. The decision to make available what was once a prescription drug in an over-the-counter form also has to do with brand name marketing, market share, and profits. Sometimes it may be less expensive to purchase the prescription form of the drug than the over-the-counter strength.

One last point regarding prescription and OTC medicines has to do with the concept of generics. Every drug has a generic or chemical name. It is usually long, convoluted, and hard to pronounce; that is why a simple, easy-to-remember brand name is developed—for example, cetirizine hydrochloride is marketed and sold as Zyrtec. Generic and brand name drugs are equivalent in terms of effect and are available in both prescription and OTC forms. But a generic version is usually significantly less expensive than the brand name version of the drug.

Article
13.2

The top prescription drugs in the United States for over a decade have been cardiovascular medicines to reduce high cholesterol (statins), to treat hypertension (antihypertensives), and to thin blood (anticoagulants). These drugs reduce the risk of stroke and heart attack. The best-selling prescription drug every year since 2000 has been Lipitor, a cholesterol reducer. Other top-selling prescription drugs include antibiotics, antidepressants, anti-ulcer drugs (for heartburn), and analgesics (for pain). In 2010, total prescription drug expenditures in the United States exceeded $307 billion, which was close to $1,000 per American.

A **drug** within the context of health care is a substance used in the diagnosis, treatment, or prevention of an illness or disease; a drug is also known as a *medicine* or *medication*. A **prescription (Rx) drug** can be sold only by a pharmacist when authorized by a written prescription from a medical practitioner. An **over-the-counter (OTC) drug** can be purchased without a doctor's prescription.

Finding the Right OTC Medicines

Unlike a medicine prescribed by a doctor, an OTC medicine is generally selected by the individual. The top three types of OTC medications are for colds and coughs, pain, and heartburn. The number of choices is surprisingly high and can be intimidating. Thankfully, all OTC medicines have standardized drug facts labels that use simple language and an easy-to-read format. This is required by the FDA so that consumers can more easily compare products and follow dosage instructions. An example of a drug label is presented in Figure 13.2.

A few precautions should be mentioned. If taking more than one OTC medicine, compare the active ingredients. You don't want to be taking multiple doses of the same medication in different products. Also, many common brands have multiple products—often different combinations of active ingredients. The brand packaging may be similar so it's wise to double check the label each time you purchase a product. Don't misuse OTC medicines by taking them longer or in higher doses than recommended. Don't hesitate to discuss your needs with a pharmacist. Pharmacists are trained and willing to assist you in finding the right medicine for your particular condition. If symptoms persist, see your doctor.

Everyone should keep a few basic medications and medical supplies on hand to deal with minor illnesses and accidents. A basic home pharmacy should include common OTC drugs such as pain and fever medications, cold and allergy medications, cough medications, and upset stomach medications. Each of these is briefly discussed below. In addition, your medicine kit should contain an antiseptic such as

FIGURE 13.2 EXAMPLE OF OTC DRUG FACTS LABEL

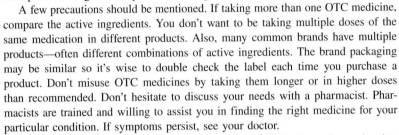

Drug Facts

Active ingredient (in each tablet)	*Purpose*
Chlorpheniramine maleate 2 mg...	Antihistamine

Uses temporarily relieves these symptoms due to hay fever or other upper respiratory allergies;
■ sneezing　■ runny nose　■ itchy, watery eyes　■ itchy throat

Warnings
Ask a doctor before use if you have
■ glaucoma　■ a breathing problem such as emphysema or chronic bronchitis
■ trouble urinating due to an enlarged prostrate gland

Ask a doctor or pharmacist before use if you are taking tranquilizers or sedatives

When using this product
■ you may get drowsy　■ avoid alcoholic drinks
■ alcohol, sedatives, and tranquilizers may increase drowsiness
■ be careful when driving a motor vehicle or operating machinery
■ excitability may occur, especially in children

If pregnant or breast-feeding, ask a health professional before use.
Keep out of reach of children. In case of overdose, get medical help or contact a Poison Control Center right away.

Directions

adults and children 12 years and over	take 2 tablets every 4 to 6 hours; not more than 12 tablets in 24 hours
children 6 years to under 12 years	take 1 tablet every 4 to 6 hours; not more than 6 tablets in 24 hours
children under 6 years	ask a doctor

Other information　store at 20-25° C (68-77° F)　■ protect from excessive moisture

Inactive ingredients　D&C yellow no. 10, lactose, magnesium stearate, microcrystalline cellulose, pregelatinized starch

Source: FDA (**www.fda.gov**).

hydrogen peroxide to clean minor cuts, bandages and adhesive tape to protect such wounds, and a thermometer to check body temperature.

Pain and Fever Medications

Inflammation (redness and swelling) and headache pain are the two most common types of pain. Medications that help relieve pain are called *analgesics.* Common analgesics include nonsteroidal anti-inflammatory drugs (NSAIDs) and acetaminophen. NSAIDs include four drugs: aspirin (common brand names are Bayer and St. Joseph), ibuprofen (Advil, Motrin), naproxen (Aleve), and ketoprofen (Orudis). NSAIDs, as the name indicates, also reduce inflammation (redness and swelling) if taken in substantial dosage. The common brand name for acetaminophen is Tylenol. Some products contain both aspirin and acetaminophen (Excedrin Extra Strength, Excedrin Migraine, Vanquish).

Side effects from OTC pain relievers aren't common for healthy adults who use these medications only occasionally. However, side effects can be a concern with long-term use. For example, NSAIDs can cause gastrointestinal problems, from upset stomach to bleeding in the digestive tract. In general, acetaminophen should be the first choice for pain and fever relief in children and adults because of its greater safety. Children with fever should not be given aspirin or products containing aspirin due to the risk of developing a potentially fatal condition called Reye's syndrome. If you use pain relievers often, talk to your doctor about which drug will be most effective for you.

Cold and Allergy Medications

Common OTC cold medications such as Actifed and Contac are generally combinations of three kinds of drugs: a pain and fever reducer (acetaminophen, aspirin, ibuprofen), a decongestant such as pseudoephedrine to shrink swollen nasal passages and reduce congestion, and an antihistamine such as chlorpheniramine to dry the nasal passages and block allergies. Decongestants may cause insomnia and antihistamines drowsiness, although individual responses vary widely.

For treating colds and flu, the most important drug is the pain and fever reducer, along with standard treatment such as drinking plenty of fluids (water, fruit juices, clear soups) and getting additional rest. To treat allergy symptoms, the primary drugs are the decongestants and antihistamines. Because the cold-flu-allergy illnesses often overlap, people sometimes inadvertently overdose on these drugs by taking several products without realizing that they contain some of the same ingredients. Be sure to read the labels and know the active drugs in each medication. To be more selective in treating symptoms, you may wish to use single drugs instead of the combination medications.

Cough Medications

There are three types of coughs: congested and productive, congested and nonproductive, and dry and nonproductive. Congested and productive means that the lungs have excess mucus, and coughing allows the person to spit up or expectorate the phlegm. Congested and nonproductive means that while extra mucus is present, coughing does nothing to remove it from the lungs. Finally, in dry and nonproductive coughs there is no congestion—hence, no expectorating.

OTC cough medications contain expectorants such as guaifenesin and/or antitussives such as dextromethorphan. Expectorants stimulate the flow of fluid in the lungs and aid in breaking up and removing the phlegm through coughing.

Antitussives suppress the cough center in the brain so the urge to cough is reduced.

Knowing the type of cough you have can indicate the type of cough medication you should use. With a dry and nonproductive cough, the main objective is to stop the cough, so a medication with an antitussive should help. A congested and productive cough might not need any treatment, since your body is already expectorating the phlegm on its own. Congested and nonproductive coughs might require an expectorant to make them productive. When in doubt ask the pharmacist, and you will be directed to the correct medication. Finally, if a cough lasts more than 10 days be sure to see a physician.

Upset Stomach and Constipation Medications

Dyspepsia, or upset stomach, is a common medical condition that can be treated using OTC antacids or acid reducers. When the stomach becomes too acidic, gas—both painful and unpleasant—is the result. Antacids are very effective at neutralizing the stomach acid, and the effects are felt almost immediately. Common antacids include calcium carbonate (Tums, Rolaids), sodium bicarbonate (Alka-Seltzer), bismuth subsalicylate (Pepto-Bismol), and magnesium (Maalox).

Antacids are designed to treat occasional dyspepsia. If a person has frequent dyspepsia or other common problems like heartburn or gastroesophageal reflux disease (GERD), reducing the amount of acid being secreted might be a better treatment option. These medications cause the acid-secreting cells in the stomach to decrease the amount they release. Common OTC acid reducers are Tagamet, Pepcid, Zantac, and Prevacid.

Difficulty in having a bowel movement or passing dry, hard stools is a very unpleasant but common condition called *constipation.* Most cases of constipation can be prevented by taking in the recommended amount of fiber in the diet, drinking plenty of water, and exercising. However, there are times when a person will want to treat constipation with laxatives.

There are two main options for OTC laxatives: bulk forming and bowel stimulating. Bulk-forming laxatives (Metamucil) are fiber. Once in the bowel the additional fiber creates a bulkier stool, and that facilitates a bowel movement. Bowel-stimulating laxatives (ex-lax, Feen-a-Mint, Correctol) contain chemicals that irritate the bowel wall and cause excessive fluid to be absorbed into the bowel. The combination of irritation and fluid results in cramping and the immediate need for a bowel movement (usually multiple bowel movements). Bulk-forming laxatives are generally safe, whereas too-frequent use of bowel-stimulating laxatives can result in weakening of the bowel wall and physical dependence on the laxative.

Reducing Prescription and OTC Medication Mistakes

Americans take more drugs per capita than people in any other nation. Based on personal experience, we know that most of us, our family members, and those we live with take one or more OTC or prescription medications on a regular or occasional basis. According to a recent estimate by the Institute of Medicine, in any given week 3 out of 10 U.S. adults take five or more different medications. These medications can be found in many different places—a counter, a table, or a drawer in bathrooms, bedrooms, or the kitchen. With so many drugs being taken by so many people, medication errors are not uncommon. To prevent mistakes, consider applying these tips on safe storage and use of medications.

- Keep medications in their original containers.
- Store as indicated regarding temperature, light, and humidity.
- Keep your medications separate from those of others in the household as well as from pets' medications and household chemicals.
- Turn on the light when you take your medication.
- Store medicines where children can't see or reach them.
- Periodically check expiration dates and discard and replace as appropriate.
- Don't take someone else's prescription medication.

These simple steps can reduce errors, minimize confusion, and lessen the likelihood of drug misuse.

Accessing Information on Prescription and OTC Medicines

The number of medicines available today is vast, numbering in the thousands. An Internet source that provides consumer information on both prescription and OTC medicines is the PDR Health website (**www.pdrhealth.com/drug_info**) sponsored by the publisher of the *Physicians' Desk Reference (PDR)* series. Updated annually, the *Physicians' Desk Reference* is the authoritative source for prescription drug information used by physicians and other health care professionals. The 2010 edition is over 3,000 pages! A companion volume is the *PDR for Nonprescription Drugs*. The PDR Health website translates information from these two PDR texts into nontechnical explanations about OTC and prescription drugs, including possible side effects and drug interactions. A second online source is the National Institutes of Health's MedlinePlus Drugs, Supplements, and Herbal Information web page, provided in cooperation with several pharmacy organizations (**www.nlm.nih.gov/medlineplus/druginformation.html**).

BODY ART

The decision to get a tattoo or body piercing is a personal one. From a health perspective, it's prudent to carefully balance the pros and cons and not rush a decision. Laws and regulating authorities for tattooing vary widely among and within states. Consequently, additional precautions should be taken. Risks associated with tattoos and piercings include bloodborne diseases, skin infections, skin disorders such as scarring, and allergic reactions. Also, a number of the dyes used in tattooing have not been studied, and little is known about their toxicity. Risks are reduced if you go to a reputable and licensed tattoo or piercing studio with trained employees who follow recommended procedures such as washing their hands, wearing gloves, using only sterile disposable needles and FDA-approved dyes, and autoclaving nondisposable instruments.

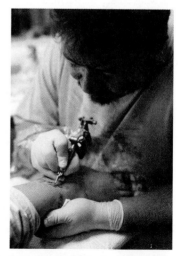

Laws regulating safe practices for body piercing and tattooing vary greatly from state to state.

© Photodisc/Getty Images

Under these conditions and with proper follow-up care, medical complications appear to be low.

It is not uncommon for people to grow dissatisfied with their tattoos. Several removal techniques are available—laser surgery, dermabrasion, surgical removal—but these require multiple visits, significant expense, and typically leave some scarring or skin imperfections. In short, investigate the risks and benefits, including advice from medical specialists in cosmetic surgery. If you proceed with some form of body art, be sure that the procedure will be done under the best of conditions and by an experienced professional.

✓ NEED TO KNOW

Medical self-care empowers people to make informed decisions and take actions to heal themselves, particularly with respect to common short-term illnesses. Knowing how to use the Internet for information on signs and symptoms, decision charts, coping with emergencies, and using medicines is key to effectively caring for yourself. Be especially vigilant if you are considering a tattoo or body piercing because state and local oversight vary widely.

➤ Developing a Patient–Doctor Partnership

Part of medical self-care includes knowing where to draw the line between dealing with an illness on your own and needing to see a doctor. When it comes to choosing your primary care physician, just any doctor won't do. In this section, we share strategies on finding the right doctor and developing a trusting patient–doctor partnership. Over time, your end of this partnership will encompass more than just showing up at your doctor's office with a list of symptoms. As an active participant in your health care, you may need to inform yourself about various medical tests and treatments and perhaps at some point prepare for a hospital stay. Moreover, it's certainly wise for you to maintain a complete personal medical record. We'll provide some guidelines on each of these points in the following paragraphs.

FINDING THE RIGHT DOCTOR

Self Assessment 13.2

Regardless of how many times you may move or switch health plans, you can always use the same approach to finding a primary care doctor. Typically your insurance plan includes a directory of primary care doctors from which to choose. The size of the pool of potential physicians depends on the size of the student health center or the type of health plan, but you will generally have some latitude in selecting a doctor. As discussed in Chapter 12, selecting a board-certified physician is wise. In the practice of modern medicine, having only an M.D. (doctor of medicine) or D.O. (doctor of osteopathy) degree without the additional training required for board certification is just not good enough, so it's best to check your potential doctor's credentials before you start seeing him or her. Also remember that a primary care physician is typically a family practitioner or internist, though women may have the additional option of choosing a gynecologist to be their primary care doctor.

Ask your family, friends, and coworkers for recommendations. Let them know that in addition to making sure the doctor is board certified, your aim is to find a doctor who shares your perspective about the patient–doctor relationship—that it is a partnership rather than a one-way relationship in which the doctor dispenses medical care to the patient. Another possible selection criterion is the gender of the doctor. It is natural for most people to want a doctor of the same gender. You may feel more comfortable and be better able to communicate frankly and openly with a doctor of the same gender.

In your initial office visit, you'll want to assess the manner or presence of the doctor and your comfort level with him or her. This is less tangible and involves impressions but is an important consideration. If you are not comfortable with a particular doctor, it doesn't mean he or she is not a good physician; rather the doctor may simply not be a good match for you. It may take several sessions with a doctor before you are able to decide whether he or she is the right doctor for you. To help with this process, ask yourself the following questions:

- Is this doctor a good listener?
- Does this doctor answer my questions completely and in terms I understand?
- Does this doctor ask for my input when options are available?
- Does this doctor use medicines conservatively?
- Does this doctor appear interested in me as a person and in my overall health?
- Does this doctor seem to give me quality patient time?
- Am I comfortable talking with this doctor, or am I intimidated or anxious?
- Do I have a high degree of trust and confidence in this doctor?

Answers to these questions will highlight how compatible you would be with the doctor. The more compatible you are, the more likely a meaningful patient–doctor partnership will be developed.

COMMUNICATING WITH YOUR DOCTOR

Both you and your doctor have responsibilities when it comes to making the most of an office visit and developing a solid partnership. Always remember that communicating with your doctor goes both ways. For an effective patient–doctor interaction to occur, we need to appreciate the larger health care delivery context in which doctors work. They are often overworked, behind schedule, and pressured to spend only a few minutes with each patient. Patients—in addition to being sick or having a medical concern—are often frustrated with traffic, parking, and paperwork and tired of waiting and being shuffled from one room to another. Is it so surprising that the doctor wants to immediately focus on your chief complaint, and you are less than articulate in describing the problem?

Many factors can hamper the patient–doctor visit. Intimidation, fear, and embarrassment are three common barriers to effective communication between patients and doctors. Doctors are esteemed for their intelligence and compassion. This high regard can be intimidating to some patients, particularly those with little knowledge about medical matters. Patients' fear of the unknown and the possible dire consequences of a troubling symptom or health condition can also interfere with logical thinking and clear communication. Other patients may be embarrassed to talk about highly personal or disconcerting issues that make them feel self-conscious or ill at ease. Your doctor is aware of these communication obstacles and will work to allay them. You too must be aware of them and strive to minimize such concerns and doubts by being forthright and trusting with your doctor.

As Drs. Fries and Vickery succinctly state in *Take Care of Yourself,* "You and your doctor need to be able to listen, explain, ask questions, understand each other,

Health & the Media Communicating with Your Doctor

It is understandable that patients can feel uneasy communicating with the doctor, yet the quality of this communication is critical to the success of the doctor–patient relationship. Most patients do not have mastery over medical language, diagnosis, and treatment, but that really isn't necessary. What is most important is to communicate effectively during the limited amount of time spent with the doctor. To get the most out of a visit to the doctor, educate yourself, be up-front, ask questions, and take a friend.

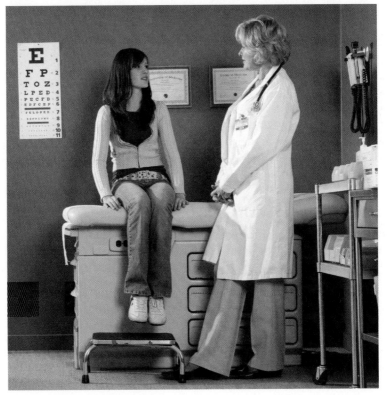

© Radius Images/Getty Images

and choose options wisely." As a patient, you need to prepare for the office visit by being ready to describe your symptoms, their timeline, and any self-care measures you have taken, including the use of OTC medications. Ahead of time, you may want to make notes listing symptoms and key questions for reference during your visit. You should be ready to name all prescription drugs and dietary supplements that you take and all allergies and chronic medical conditions that you have. Also, it's a good idea to take a writing pad to make notes during the visit. Even a few hours later, let alone a few days later, many people have difficulty recalling the details of what their doctor said.

Depending on the severity of the illness or the complexity of the health problem, you may want to have a family member or friend take you to the doctor—not only to drive or physically assist you if needed but also to facilitate communication with the doctor. Ask someone who can ably serve as your advocate—that is, a person who can ensure that your symptoms are clearly explained and that the doctor's course of treatment is understood. Two sets of ears are always better than one.

A final point concerns advance directives. Advance directives are documents (e.g., living will, power of attorney) that specify the type of medical care you want if you are too sick to express your wishes. Although people who are terminally or seriously ill are more likely to have advance directives, those in good health may also want to consider them in case of a catastrophic accident or sudden serious illness. Advance directives deal with a variety of issues—for example, whether to resuscitate or not, use of breathing machines and feeding tubes, and organ donation. Discuss the options for medical care under these special circumstances with your doctor. Once you establish advance directives, be sure to share them with your doctor as well as your family. Knowing your wishes ahead of time will avoid confusion later.

MEDICAL TESTS AND PROCEDURES

Your physician may want to conduct tests to help make a diagnosis. Many standard tests are done on blood and urine. For example, a CBC (complete blood count) is a routine test that provides information about white blood cells, red blood cells, and platelets. Abnormal variations in the number, type, size, and shape of cells may indicate an infection, anemia, or a host of other conditions. The basic urine test, or urinalysis, screens for urinary tract infections, metabolic disease, and kidney disorders by examining the urine physically, chemically, and microscopically. The results of such tests may lead your doctor to order more specialized tests to help in making a diagnosis. Dozens of clinical lab tests are available; a comprehensive listing and descriptions are available at Lab Tests Online (**www.labtestsonline.org**).

Your doctor may order a medical imaging test, too. From routine X-rays and ultrasound imaging to more complex CT (computed tomography) and PET (positron emission tomography) scans, these tests—which fall within the specialty of radiology—can provide important clues to abnormalities that exist or may be developing within the internal tissues and organs of the body. For example, MRI (magnetic resonance imaging) uses radiofrequency waves in a strong magnetic field to generate detailed pictures of soft-tissue structures around bones. Especially useful in diagnosing sports injuries, MRI can show even small tears in ligaments and muscles around the spine and major joints (knee, shoulder, hip, elbow). RadiologyInfo (**www.radiologyinfo.org**), developed by the American College of Radiology, is an excellent website to answer consumer questions about medical imaging and radiation therapies.

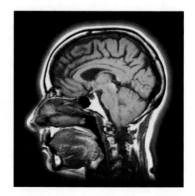

A magnetic resonance imaging (MRI) scan.

© Jim Wehtje/Getty Images

The more complex your illness or disease, the more likely your doctor will refer you to a specialist for an expert opinion. This in turn may lead to further testing or medical procedures requiring specialized hospital equipment and facilities. As described in Chapter 12, this sequence reflects the widening circle of medical care from primary care to secondary and tertiary care. Ideally, your primary care physician will receive copies of the results of all tests and procedures and continue to coordinate overall medical care. For example, you can discuss a specialist's diagnosis and treatment options with your primary care doctor. If you feel uneasy or uncertain regarding a recommendation for a major surgical or medical treatment, you should not hesitate to get a second opinion. Good doctors will understand your concern and not take offense. An excellent consumer resource that provides interactive health tutorials on common medical conditions is available at MedlinePlus (**www.nlm.nih.gov/medlineplus/healthtopics.html**).

There will be times when you, a family member, or a close friend must be admitted to a hospital. Many illnesses and injuries are successfully treated in hospitals. Indeed, many lives are saved. Yet, hospitals are also dangerous places; far too many errors occur resulting in unnecessary death and disability. Consequently, it's important to feel confident about the hospital of choice and to take reasonable precautions. Discuss this issue with your physician and ask questions about the hospital's experience in performing the particular treatment or procedure. Is it routinely done, and what is their safety record?

Once you are admitted to the hospital, consider the following tips to reduce the risk of medical errors:

- Carefully read and fully understand any consent form before signing.
- Find out why tests or treatments are being performed.
- Discuss the results of tests with your doctor.
- Know the purpose and side effects of all medications, whether given by mouth, injection, or intravenous (IV) administration.
- Be sure that all health care workers wash their hands before they have physical contact with you.
- Understand the follow-up treatment plan when you are discharged.

Remember, you have the right to be fully informed of all procedures, so never hesitate to ask questions or express concerns. If necessary, be persistent: Ask to speak to the supervisory nurse or discuss concerns with your doctor. If you will be incapacitated for a prolonged period, try to arrange to have a capable advocate oversee your care and ask questions on your behalf.

KEEPING MEDICAL RECORDS

Your current primary care doctor should have a complete medical file on you. However, if you are like most people, you probably have your health information scattered across multiple providers and facilities. For this reason alone, it's important to keep your own complete, updated, and easily accessible personal health record. Based on a national survey by the Harris Poll, only two in five adults keep personal or family health records, yet almost all of those who don't keep health records think it would be a good idea to do so. Simply put, it's an important task to take on, and you are in the best position to do it. In fact, it's necessary if you are to be a full partner in your health care.

A personal health record is a collection of key information about your health (or the health of someone you're caring for, such as a parent or a child) that you actively

maintain and update. It can contain any information that affects your health, including information that your doctor may not have, such as your exercise routines,
dietary habits, and over-the-counter drugs you routinely take. Keeping a personal
health record can reduce or eliminate duplicate procedures or processes, which saves
health care costs, your time, and the provider's time.

A straightforward approach to a personal health record is to organize paperwork
into categories such as the following:

1. *General information:* Include medical exam results, blood profiles, and other
   measures such as height, weight, waist circumference, and blood pressure.
   Organ donor authorization or living wills should also be kept here.
2. *Specific medical conditions:* Keep a separate file for these so they can be easily
   updated.
3. *Prescription drugs and dosages:* Keep a record of all prescription drugs, both
   those you take regularly and those you have taken for specific illnesses. Be
   sure to note any allergies or side effects.
4. *Insurance information and medical bills:* A separate file for health insurance
   and medical bills is necessary. Include a description of coverage, instructions
   and forms for filing, a ledger of payments for bills, and a log of phone calls
   and written communications on bills that require follow-up or resolution.

Regardless of how smart or healthy we may be, our memory alone is not adequate
for keeping a personal health record! So get your records together and start filing in
an organized fashion if you haven't already developed a system. Or set up your system
now and start using it with your next physician visit or medical test. Like any organizational system, it takes some time at first, but it will be well worth your while.

Electronic health record (EHR) systems are now commonly used by health professionals and agencies. An EHR is a single complete (electronic) record of a patient's
profile, diagnoses, allergies, and lab results that can be continually updated by *all*
clinicians involved in treating the patient. Connectivity would extend to labs, pharmacies, hospitals, and insurers as well as to the patient. EHR is a major information
technology initiative within both the federal government (HHS Health Information
Technology, **www.healthit.gov/providers-professionals/faqs/what-electronic-
health-record-ehr**) and the private sector (American Health Information Management
Association, **www.ahima.org**). The advantages seem clear—improved efficiency and
integration of medical services should result in better patient care and significant cost
savings. There is little doubt that EHR is spreading through the health care system.
The question is how long it will take for widespread adoption. In the meantime, be
sure to maintain your own medical records.

✓ **NEED TO KNOW**

One must be proactive to find a compatible primary care physician and to
develop an effective patient–doctor partnership. Understanding how to optimize patient–doctor communication and how to access basic information
about medical tests and procedures is our responsibility as active participants in our own health care. Taking precautions to minimize medical errors
in hospitals and keeping an updated personal medical record are other
actions that informed consumers can take to improve their health care.

➤ Understanding Health Insurance

The ideal way to access the services of our health care system and to receive quality care is by having "good" health insurance. However, just because one has health insurance doesn't mean that worries about health care are over. Unfortunately, health insurance is not user-friendly. It requires knowledge both to select the right plan and then to use it. A case in point—try to get a health insurance representative on the phone and you'll typically be routed through a prolonged queuing system. When you finally make contact with a live human, that person may seem disinterested and less than helpful. By educating ourselves about health insurance options and coverage, we can do much to minimize the pitfalls and barriers that appear to be so widespread. In this section, we'll provide practical tips on selecting and navigating the health insurance system.

HEALTH INSURANCE TERMINOLOGY

Insurance has its own language, and a common mistake consumers make is to assume they understand what a word means. Knowing the insurance language increases the likelihood of using the system more effectively and reducing health care costs. The insurance company is often called the *insurance carrier,* and the insured person is the *subscriber.* Subscribers pay **premiums,** usually on a monthly basis, to hold an insurance policy. The policy is based on the (insurance) concept of indemnity, which means "assumption of risk." In the case of health insurance, the insurance company assumes the majority of medical costs within limitations defined in the policy. Many insurance plans have **deductibles,** which is the amount of money a subscriber must pay for medical services (e.g., treatments, tests, doctor's visits) before the insurance company pays.

Exclusions are those services not covered by the insurance policy. Since insurance companies are for-profit businesses, health insurance policies often control costs by excluding coverage of certain treatments, drugs, or office visits. One important type of exclusion is known as *preexisting conditions.* These are specific diseases or conditions (e.g., heart disease, cancer, diabetes) that are known to exist when you sign up for your insurance. If you have preexisting conditions, your policy may not pay for related treatments for either a specific time or ever. It is critical to carefully read and compare differences in coverage of available policies before enrolling in a specific plan.

Generally, health insurance in the United States is either private or public. Private health insurance is the most common with about 50 percent of Americans receiving coverage through employer-sponsored plans and 9 percent through individually purchased plans. Public health insurance, which includes government-supported Medicare and Medicaid, provides coverage to a smaller proportion of Americans. Both types of health insurance—private and public—will be reviewed in the following sections.

A **premium** is the amount of money the subscriber pays to maintain the health insurance policy.

A **deductible** is the additional cost the subscriber pays per medical service before the insurance company pays.

There are two basic types of plans under the private health insurance umbrella: fee for service and managed care.

Fee for Service

A **fee-for-service (FFS) plan**—also known as a *traditional indemnity plan*—was the predominant type of health insurance in the United States into the latter part of the 20th century, though it makes up only a small percentage of policies today. There are two major components to FFS: basic and major medical. Basic health insurance is primarily hospital insurance, and major medical includes just about everything else—physicians, diagnostic testing, and medications. In both basic and major medical, a deductible must be met before the insurance begins paying for a person's medical bills. FFS plans cover a percentage of the remaining amount—typically 80 percent of the total costs. The policyholder is responsible for paying the deductible and the remaining 20 percent of the cost.

FFS has advantages. The chief advantage is the freedom to select physicians and medical care services. However, this freedom of choice comes, quite literally, at a high cost—consumers pay significantly more for medical care under the typical FFS plan than they do under a managed care plan. Approximately 1 percent of the health insurance market is fee for service.

Managed Care

There are two primary types of **managed care plans:** preferred provider organizations and health maintenance organizations.

Preferred Provider Organization Preferred provider organizations (PPOs) are groups of health care providers and hospitals that negotiate plans with an insurance carrier. The PPO agrees to charge the insurance company's subscribers reduced fees for their services. In exchange, the PPO-affiliated facilities and personnel get a higher volume of clients and quicker payment from the insurance company. PPO insurance policyholders can opt to go "out of network" and receive care from doctors and hospitals that are not part of their PPO. However, out-of-network services are much more expensive than in-network services.

The way most PPOs work is that a client selects a primary care physician (PCP) from a list of doctors in that particular network. The PCP will be the point of contact when medical care is being sought, providing primary care as well as coordinating any referrals to secondary care or diagnostic and treatment services. Patients can see their PCP as often as they want for a predetermined office visit co-payment. A co-payment—or simply "co-pay"—is a relatively small portion of the overall cost of the actual visit. For example, if a doctor charges $80 for an office visit, the co-pay for the patient might be only $20. The remaining $60 is paid by the insurance company.

A **fee-for-service (FFS) plan,** or traditional indemnity plan, allows subscribers the greatest choice of doctors and hospitals but at a greater cost.

Managed care plans such as PPOs and HMOs limit subscribers to specific networks of doctors and hospitals but provide medical care at lower costs.

When referred by their PCP to facilities for tests or to other in-network specialists, the patient is also charged reduced fees for those providers' services. If for some reason the patient does not get a PCP referral for secondary care or opts to go out of network, then the insurance company often still reimburses the patient for some of those costs, but not nearly as much as it does for in-network providers who were visited with a PCP referral.

A PPO is a cost-effective way to receive medical care. There are fewer out-of-pocket expenses than with an FFS plan. However, there is also less choice among doctors and treatment options. PPO administrators can be reluctant to approve payment of certain services, which means that a person with this type of insurance may need to be assertive to use the system effectively. PPOs are popular, accounting for about 58 percent of the health insurance market.

Health Maintenance Organization Health maintenance organizations (HMOs) are plans that allow access to primary, secondary, and tertiary care within a health network. There are many slightly varying models of the HMO, and in promotional materials an insurance company may refer to a staff model, group model, independent practice association model, or point-of-service plan. But regardless of the HMO model used, the basic approach is that the HMO, after premiums are paid, will provide all the medical care one "needs" for no additional charge or for a small co-pay.

For example, an HMO patient can be seen for a broad range of services from an office visit for a sore throat to tertiary care involving major surgery and pay only $10–$30 per visit or service beyond the normal monthly premium. These are by far the lowest-cost plans for consumers. The downside of HMOs is that in order to receive care at rock-bottom costs, the patient abdicates most decision making and control over choice in hospitals, testing clinics, doctors, and the like. HMOs are designed to save money, and they do this by rationing services. A patient may wait for a longer period of time to receive certain diagnostic tests in an HMO than in a PPO, and treatment options may be more limited than in other types of plans.

Brief explanations of the main types of HMOs follow:

- *Staff model HMOs* typically include a free-standing facility owned by the HMO where all the doctors and clinical professionals are salaried employees. It is a primary care version of one-stop shopping for doctor appointments, testing, and even filling of prescriptions.
- *Group model HMO* is a group of private practice doctors that contracts with a corporate HMO and agrees to serve HMO patients at a reduced rate. The HMO pays the group at the prenegotiated rate, and the group pays its own doctors. The group model HMO is a contract, not a facility. Other clinical services that an HMO patient may need are also negotiated with laboratories and pharmacies.
- *Independent practice association (IPA)* is another HMO structure whereby private practice physicians contract with the HMO to see HMO patients at a prenegotiated rate. Similar to the group model HMO, the IPA includes large numbers of private practice physicians.
- *Point-of-service (POS)* is a relatively new type of HMO structure. The POS allows members more choice in selecting providers and services because they have the option of going out of the network and seeing a physician of their choice, not the choice of the HMO. However, the co-pay is higher if an out-of-network physician is used.

HMOs are approximately 13 percent of the health insurance market.

Table 13.1 provides an overview of the various types of plans including what the plans offer, methods of cost control, and the advantages and disadvantages. The structures of these plans are constantly changing, and sometimes it is difficult to distinguish between an HMO and a PPO. Regardless, it is imperative that consumers know what plan they have and what is covered. When you select a health insurance plan, you are entering into a business agreement.

PUBLIC HEALTH INSURANCE: MEDICARE AND MEDICAID

Since the 1960s, the federal government has provided health care to two vulnerable groups of Americans—elderly people and low-income people. The program for older people (aged 65 and older) is Medicare, and it is funded completely by the federal government. There are two parts to Medicare: Part A covers hospitalizations and Part B covers medical expenses such as laboratory tests, physical therapy, and mental health services. Medical expenses are not entirely covered by either Part A or Part B. There are small premiums and deductibles and certain limitations in coverage. This can be a problem for older people of modest means. Because Medicare doesn't cover every expense, many recipients elect to purchase supplemental policies. Finally, Medicare Part C allows for private health insurance companies to provide Medicare services, and Medicare Part D is prescription drug insurance.

Medicaid, the other type of public health insurance, is for individuals whose income is below the poverty level. Medicaid is a joint federal–state program where each pays for half the program. Potential recipients must qualify for Medicaid to receive services. Like other insurance plans, both Medicare and Medicaid negotiate discounted rates of reimbursement with physicians and hospitals. With Medicaid in particular, reimbursements for providers tend to be quite low compared to what private-sector insurance companies pay for the same services—in fact, they are so low that many physicians will not accept Medicaid patients.

This reduced access to health care for Medicaid patients is problematic. It results in many low-income individuals having to use the emergency room for their care, which can cost 20 times as much as a physician's visit. Furthermore, because of limited access, some people wait too long to be seen. When they finally are evaluated, they may be so sick that they require hospitalization or other costly medical service.

Both Medicare and Medicaid have undergone many changes over the decades and will undergo even greater changes in the years ahead. These public health programs are well intentioned but no longer cost-effective. The graying of America, escalating health care costs, and the current tax system all contribute to the dilemma. The political debate will continue until a legislative solution is found. As voters we need to stay abreast of the issues and encourage legislators to explore options that are both cost-effective and provide health care access to all.

CHOOSING AN APPROPRIATE PLAN

Every American citizen must have health insurance or pay a fine. Health insurance can be a benefit of work or purchased through an insurance agent or through a health insurance exchange (see section on Health Care Reform). An unwise choice of a health insurance plan can have a significant negative financial impact. Simply put, choosing the wrong plan can quickly lead to excessive medical bills. This in turn can add to the emotional burden that one is already facing in dealing with a medical

TABLE 13.1 PRIVATE HEALTH INSURANCE: COMPARISON OF COMMON TYPES

TYPE OF PLAN	WHAT IT OFFERS	COST CONTROL METHODS	ADVANTAGES	DISADVANTAGES
Fee for Service (Indemnity)	Services from any doctor or hospital	None except screening for fraudulent claims	Choice of any doctor or hospital	Claim forms to file; preventive services not covered
Indemnity with Utilization Review	Services from any doctor or hospital	Prior approval required for hospitalization and some outpatient procedures	Choice of any doctor and access to any hospital after prior approval	Additional paperwork to get approval for some services; preventive services not covered
Preferred Provider Organization (PPO)	Services from any doctor or hospital, but at lower cost to those using network providers	Discounts negotiated with doctors and hospitals; prior approval required for hospitalization and some outpatient procedures	Higher rate of reimbursement when using doctors and hospitals in the network	Higher cost for services outside network; extra paperwork to get approval of some services; preventive services are not always covered
HMO—Staff/ Group Model	Services from hospitals under contract with HMO or salaried doctors at HMO medical centers	Primary care doctors at HMO medical centers manage services; hospital fees are discounted	Low co-payments; preventive care covered; no claim forms	Must use the HMO medical center doctors and hospitals
HMO—Independent Doctors (IPA)	Services from any hospital or independent doctor affiliated with HMO	Primary care doctors manage services; hospital and physician fees are discounted	Low co-payments; preventive care covered; no claim forms	Must use approved doctors and hospitals
HMO—Point of Service (POS)	Services from any doctor or hospital, but at lower cost to those using network providers	Within network, primary care doctors manage utilization of services; hospital and physician fees are discounted	Within network, lower co-payments; preventive care covered; no claim forms	Higher cost for services outside network; extra paperwork to get approval of some services

condition. Having the right plan for your needs can allow you to focus on getting better without the added stress of limited access or affordability.

Health insurance plans offered as an employee benefit often have fixed benefits because the insurance was prenegotiated on the part of the organization (employer). Most often, these plans are reasonably good; however, it is still important to fully understand the choices and the specific plan and its coverage.

There is no one-size-fits-all "best" insurance plan. What is best for an individual depends on a variety of factors including age, gender, personal health history, current health status, family situation, and financial means. These factors must be considered along with whether you are willing to pay more to have more control over your treatment or prefer to pay less and are willing to relinquish control. Here are some key issues to consider as you formulate questions to ask about health insurance plans.

Choice of Doctors

Does a particular doctor you already see accept the insurance you are considering? Or are there a large number of doctors in the network?

Facilities—Proximity and Quality

Is the insurance plan–sponsored hospital too far from your home to be convenient? The hospital or clinic might be nearby, but does it have a reputation for quality care? What is the quality of the outpatient and inpatient facilities? Will you have access to diagnostic tools like MRIs and CT scans?

Waiting Periods

Is there a waiting period if you have a preexisting condition such as asthma, diabetes, heart disease, or cancer? If there is a waiting period, can you afford to pay for treatment out of pocket in the interim? Make sure your treatments won't be excluded indefinitely before you sign up for a plan.

Health Screenings

How easy is it to get routine health screenings like cholesterol profiles, Pap smears, and mammograms? Does the plan let women go to a gynecologist for an annual exam without going through their primary care physician?

Other Features/Options

If you (or your spouse) are or may become pregnant, what type of prenatal coverage is available? If a family member needs long-term care, is convalescent care provided in the plan? Are dental and vision care covered?

Once a decision has been made regarding appropriate services, then cost becomes a major factor. Be sure you understand how much the premiums, deductibles, and co-pays are. For employer-sponsored plans, talk to a benefits officer and ask a lot of what-if questions. Create possible scenarios for yourself (and family), and see if the answers are acceptable. If they are acceptable, then most likely you have appropriate coverage. If not, you may want to add additional services to your coverage or purchase a different policy.

Prices of policies purchased on the open market as an individual or family are determined by age, previous medical conditions, family history, and results of a comprehensive physical exam. It is not inexpensive, but it is necessary. Remember that not knowing what is covered or how a policy works is not an acceptable excuse for avoiding a health care bill.

NEED TO KNOW

Private health insurance plans can be broadly categorized as fee for service or managed care. Fee-for-service plans provide maximum choice but can require significant out-of-pocket expenses. Managed care is generally offered as either a preferred provider organization (PPO) or a health maintenance organization (HMO). PPOs provide some choice in providers and facilities, yet keep out-of-pocket costs fairly low. HMOs provide comprehensive care within a specific network of doctors and facilities while minimizing out-of-pocket expenses. Medicare and Medicaid are government-funded programs that provide health care for elderly and low-income people, respectively. When choosing a health care plan, take the time to carefully study the available options and select the plan that best meets your needs.

HEALTH CARE REFORM

Article
13.4

Over $2.9 trillion is spent on health care in the United States each year. That's approximately 17 percent of the country's gross domestic product. The United States spends the most of any country in the world on health care, yet the United States ranks 28th in life expectancy and 29th in infant mortality. Some countries such as Sweden, Italy, and Japan spend half of what the United States does on health care, yet they have better outcomes. To make matters worse, health care costs are the leading cause of personal bankruptcy in the United States today.

Nearly everyone—policymakers, economists, and the general public—tends to agree that the high cost of U.S. health care is unsustainable and causes a myriad of problems. Some argue that this ever-increasing cost will be the next economic bubble to burst. Recognizing the problems that come from steadily increasing health care costs is not new. Presidents Nixon, Carter, and Clinton all wanted some degree of health care reform during their administrations but were unsuccessful in drafting legislation that was passed. Health care in America had its first major change in decades when, in 2010, President Barack Obama was successful in getting the Patient Protection and Affordable Care Act (PPACA) passed.

PPACA primarily is a series of reforms that will increase the number of Americans who have health insurance. Provisions of the law phase in over a 10-year period, so that by 2019 almost all Americans will be covered by some form of health insurance. As well, the law mandates some key health care items that now must be covered by health insurance policies.

Some of PPACA has already phased in. For example, before the legislation passed, companies could deny insurance coverage to individuals with preexisting medical conditions. That meant a person with asthma or a past history of cancer treatments might be able to purchase an insurance policy, but the insurance company would often refuse to pay for any tests, medication, or treatments for the very thing that needed the most monitoring in those individuals. The reason insurance companies operated in this manner was that most are for-profit companies in the United States. From a business perspective, insurance firms want to keep the pool of policyholders as healthy (and as unlikely to incur big medical bills) as possible to keep profits up. But what makes sense for businesses doesn't necessarily result in a good outcome for the general public. Not only were people with preexisting conditions at risk for great financial hardship due to being underinsured or uninsured, but their predicament also ultimately led to poor-quality care.

Now because of PPACA, adults who had been denied coverage because of preexisting medical conditions can get insurance from a high-risk insurance pool. Likewise, insurance companies can no longer revoke existing policies if people get ill, as the new law bans lifetime limits on policyholder coverage. Preventive services such as vaccinations and mammograms now must be fully covered, and small businesses will also be eligible for tax credits if they offer insurance to employees.

One PPACA change that directly impacts many college students came into effect in 2011. Parents may now keep children on the family health insurance through age 26. Previously, insurance companies could remove children from parents' policies as early as age 19. This added to the problem of so many uninsured Americans because most young adults either attend school or work at lower-paying jobs that often do not offer insurance.

The most sweeping change of PPACA is that it mandates that all Americans must have insurance by the end of the phase-in period or pay a penalty. The idea is that if insurance companies are being forced to cover more treatments with less exclusions, then everyone should take part in the system and buy policies. To aid in increasing the number of policies, in 2014 each state established health insurance exchanges so that it is easier for individuals to shop around. There will also be tax credits for people who make too much money to be eligible for Medicaid but are still low income. Table 13.2 displays the key changes of PPACA.

TABLE 13.2	**KEY PPACA CHANGES TO THE U.S. HEALTH INSURANCE SYSTEM**	
RULE	**PROBLEM IT ADDRESSES**	**PHASED IN**
Parents may insure children through age 26.	Many young adults went without insurance during college and/or early in their careers.	2011
Preexisting condition exclusions and lifetime policy expense caps are banned.	Those needing treatment often could not obtain it or went into bankruptcy paying for it without insurance.	2011
Preventive care must be included in policies.	Many of the least expensive old-style policies didn't cover basics such as mammograms or vaccinations.	2011
Health insurance exchanges are created.	Previously difficult to compare the cost and type of coverage among different insurance companies.	2014
There are penalties for not having health insurance.	The trade-off of increasing health insurance coverage is that everyone is required to get a policy.	2019

FIGURE 13.3   HOW PEOPLE GET HEALTH COVERAGE UNDER THE AFFORDABLE CARE ACT BEGINNING IN 2014

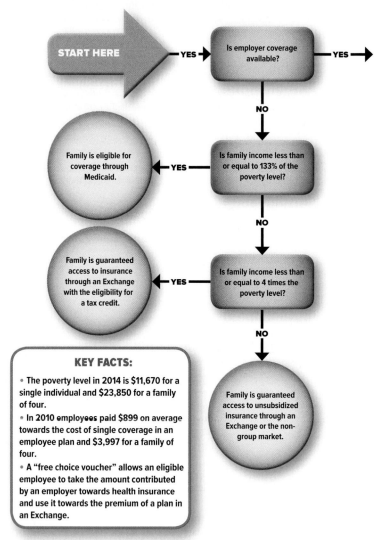

START HERE —YES→ Is employer coverage available? —YES→

NO ↓

Is family income less than or equal to 133% of the poverty level? ←YES— Family is eligible for coverage through Medicaid.

NO ↓

Is family income less than or equal to 4 times the poverty level? ←YES— Family is guaranteed access to insurance through an Exchange with the eligibility for a tax credit.

NO ↓

Family is guaranteed access to unsubsidized insurance through an Exchange or the non-group market.

KEY FACTS:

• The poverty level in 2014 is $11,670 for a single individual and $23,850 for a family of four.

• In 2010 employees paid $899 on average towards the cost of single coverage in an employee plan and $3,997 for a family of four.

• A "free choice voucher" allows an eligible employee to take the amount contributed by an employer towards health insurance and use it towards the premium of a plan in an Exchange.

NOTES

• Some states may have higher income eligibility levels for Medicaid.

• In some cases, children may be eligible for public coverage through Medicaid or CHIP while their parents are covered through an employer or an Exchange.

• Undocumented immigrants are ineligible for Medicaid and may not purchase coverage in an Exchange or receive a tax credit.

• In general, people are required to obtain coverage or pay a penalty, but those whose health insurance premiums exceed 8% of family income (after tax credits or employer contributions are taken into account) will not be penalized if they choose not to purchase coverage.

Source: "Visualizing Health Policy: Health Coverage Under the Affordable Care Act (ACA)"; Adapted with permission, Henry J. Kaiser Family Foundation, December 2012; **http://kff.org/ inforgraphic/visualizing-health-policy-health-coverage-under-the-affordable-care-act-aca/.**

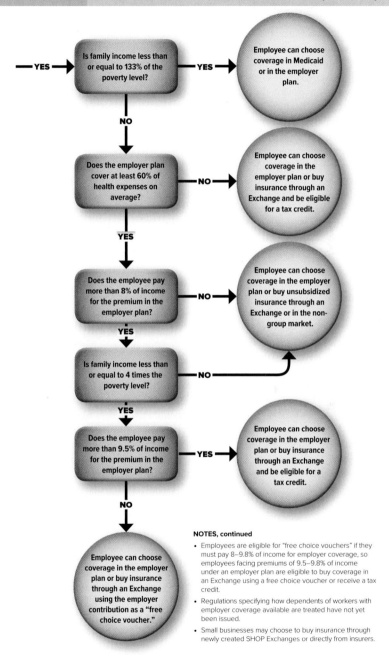

NOTES, continued

- Employees are eligible for "free choice vouchers" if they must pay 8–9.8% of income for employer coverage, so employees facing premiums of 9.5–9.8% of income under an employer plan are eligible to buy coverage in an Exchange using a free choice voucher or receive a tax credit.

- Regulations specifying how dependents of workers with employer coverage available are treated have not yet been issued.

- Small businesses may choose to buy insurance through newly created SHOP Exchanges or directly from insurers.

PPACA Controversies and Criticisms

PPACA attempts to correct some of the structural problems and inequities in our health care delivery system. If the Congressional Budget Office (CBO) is correct, implementing the law will result in two things: Americans will have better access to the health care delivery system, and there may be overall cost savings.

The issue of the cost of the law has been hotly contested, with estimates of federal savings varying by billions of dollars depending on which variables and time periods are examined. It is also possible that not every group will see the same savings across the board. For example, the government and low-income citizens could see overall health care expenditures decrease, while costs for the average, middle-income American might actually go up. Also, some doctors and hospitals do not accept Health Care Exchange plans and patients find out that health care coverage (insurance) and access are not one and the same.

One criticism of PPACA says that the act was passed too quickly. There is some merit to this complaint, for while the problem of increasing costs and restricted access grew larger for decades, the final law came together very quickly under a brief window where the U.S. House, Senate, and presidency were all held by a majority of Democrats. Many people felt the law was rushed through at a time when the country had other problems to address, such as the war on terrorism and a bad economy. Still others wonder if the cost-saving estimates will ultimately hold true.

The complaint that PPACA is socialized medicine is false. The majority of Americans have loudly stated they do not want socialized medicine—although it is less clear if the public understands what socialized medicine actually is. For example, older adults are quite happy with their Medicare. If one examines the structure of Medicare, it is very close to being a type of socialized medicine. Medicare covers all citizens over age 65, and the government sets the reimbursement rates for services and providers.

Many Americans like their interactions with our "old" health care system, warts and all. If you have insurance and can afford the premiums, you have a wide variety of choices, an array of services, and easy access to care. Those who get the best of care may not realize or be concerned that the system is unfair or problematic for others. But like it or not, the ever-increasing costs of the traditional system are considered unsustainable, which is what ultimately led to the passage of PPACA. Figure 13.3 lays out the steps to obtaining health insurance with PPACA.

✓ NEED TO KNOW

The Patient Protection and Affordable Care Act (PPACA) is the most significant attempt at health care reform since Medicare and Medicaid in the mid-1960s. PPACA will in some way affect every American, including young adults. For example, young adults can stay on their parents' health insurance until age 26. When PPACA is fully implemented, most Americans should have access to medical care. It is expected that there will be some changes to PPACA. To that end, it is important that citizens access valid and reliable information sources to understand how PPACA will affect them and to keep informed of the implementation of PPACA.

In Chapter 1, we set up a personal health roadmap directing you to selected destinations on fundamental health behaviors, medical conditions, and health care topics. Our aim has been to provide you with the knowledge, confidence, and motivation to explore a variety of paths in pursuit of a healthier life. As we come to the end of the last chapter, we're completing our journey by returning to the starting point. As seen in Figure 13.4, let's remember that our health is determined by a combination of interacting factors including genetics, behaviors, environments, policies and interventions, and access to health care. All factors can contribute to varying degrees based on an individual's circumstances and surroundings. However, for most Americans, health is largely determined by lifestyle choices and behaviors. The fact that each of us has the potential to significantly affect our own health may seem obvious to us today. In actuality, the necessary knowledge and resources to support this statement have been realized only within the last few generations.

We trust that you view the concept of health much differently now. At this point, defining health as simply the absence of disease and illness seems shortsighted and self-limiting. We hope you have gained an appreciation for health as a multidimensional concept directly related to your quality of life. And this includes your quality of life *right now and in the weeks and months ahead*. Striving for optimal health is not just about reducing chronic disease and disability in middle age and beyond; it's also about feeling good and functioning at a high level today. To this end, staying informed and practicing prevention go hand in hand with living a full and healthy life.

STAYING INFORMED

Staying informed is all about health literacy. As discussed in Chapter 1, *health literacy* means having the knowledge and skills to successfully access, analyze, and interpret relevant information to answer personal health questions. Common questions relate to seeking guidance on dealing with a health condition or changing a health behavior.

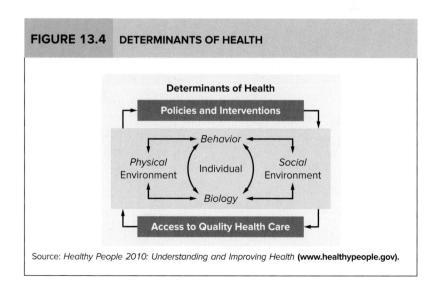

FIGURE 13.4   **DETERMINANTS OF HEALTH**

Source: *Healthy People 2010: Understanding and Improving Health* (**www.healthypeople.gov**).

Health literacy also encompasses a working knowledge of the health care system, which has been the focus of this and the previous chapter.

Self-directed learning, effective communication, and critical thinking—three threads of health literacy—have been emphasized throughout *iHealth*. It's important to continue to develop your skills in these areas beyond this course. Health literacy also assumes a mindfulness and a curiosity that motivate continual learning. Hopefully, this mind-set is present or will develop with time. Recommended Internet sites on general health information for the consumer are listed at the end of the chapter.

PRACTICING PREVENTION

As shown in Figure 13.5, health care encompasses four areas: acute care, chronic care, palliative care, and preventive care. The majority of all health care involves treatment of acute illnesses and injuries and control of chronic diseases. Acute care is predominant among younger adults, while chronic care is more common among middle-aged and older adults. Palliative care is an emerging area of care that focuses on improving the quality of life of people who have a serious or life-threatening disease by controlling pain and providing comfort.

Preventive care, the fourth area of care, has historically received little emphasis because most medical systems are designed to treat and cure illness, not prevent it. The tide is turning, though. The value of *keeping* people healthy—rather than treating them *after* they develop disease—has become clear. Preventive medicine makes sense in several ways—it's less costly, it contributes to a more productive workforce, it reduces human suffering, and it generally improves overall quality of life. Preventive care comprises healthy behaviors, regular wellness exams, and consulting a doctor about relevant medical and lifestyle strategies for your individual situation.

Responsibility for preventive health care ultimately rests with each individual. Selecting a prevention-minded doctor and a health insurance plan that encompasses

FIGURE 13.5 **HEALTH CARE EMPHASIS AREAS**

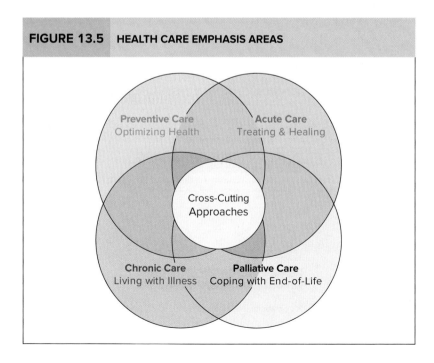

TABLE 13.3 TEN ACTION STEPS TO BEING HEALTHY

1. Focus your efforts on things that matter; inform yourself about risks and benefits.
2. Don't smoke or use tobacco products.
3. Eat a balanced diet and handle foods safely.
4. If you drink alcoholic beverages, keep your intake moderate.
5. Exercise regularly.
6. Achieve and maintain a healthy weight.
7. Protect yourself against AIDS and other sexually transmitted infections.
8. See your doctors for scheduled screening and preventive maintenance.
9. Always separate drinking and driving.
10. Use safety devices—such as seat belts, helmets, safety glasses—every time.

Source: Adapted from *Make 2008 the Healthiest Year Yet,* American Council on Science and Health (**www.acsh.org/publications/pubID.1648/pub_detail.asp**).

prevention are important choices. Following through by undergoing age- and gender-appropriate screening tests according to evidence-based guidelines is an important habit to establish. These tests are listed under "Adult Health Resources" on the website of the Agency for Healthcare Research and Quality (**www.ahrq.gov/ppip/adguide**). Yet, as discussed throughout this book, perhaps the most important steps are those we take every day—our personal actions, especially those related to eating, exercising, sexual behavior, drug use, and managing stress.

Many of you now have a better appreciation for the challenges involved with changing a health behavior. It's generally much more complex than people realize, particularly today when social conditioning and environmental design often favor health-compromising behaviors. Developing healthy behaviors requires planning and strategies. Conceptual frameworks and examples have been provided to help you implement positive lifestyle changes.

Always remember that health is more than just physical health—it's a multidimensional concept encompassing physical, emotional, intellectual, social, and spiritual elements. Striving for optimal health is an active, ongoing process. Fundamental health-promoting actions are listed in Table 13.3. As you chart your own course toward better health, tailor your own list and map out a plan. Implement positive actions, maintain other healthy behaviors, and resolve to stay on track. Good health habits provide a strong foundation for a full life. Making informed decisions about health care and practicing prevention further strengthen this foundation.

NEED TO KNOW

Our health is determined by a combination of factors from the realms of heredity, lifestyle, environment, and health care policy and access. All factors can contribute to varying degrees based on a person's circumstances and surroundings. However, for most Americans, our health is largely determined by our own lifestyle choices and behaviors. We each chart a course that either strengthens or weakens our health. Staying informed and practicing prevention are two key elements in striving for optimal health.

connect Resources

ARTICLES

13.1 "Health Disparities: A Case for Closing the Gap." *Healthreform.gov.* A government report highlights the problems that led to health care reform.

13.2 "Are You Ready for a World Without Antibiotics?" *The Guardian.* Resistant bacteria are becoming such an important issue that the era of antibiotics might just be coming to a close.

13.3 "Abuse of Prescription and Over the Counter Medications." *Journal of the American Board of Family Medicine.* Abuse of both prescription and over-the-counter medications is becoming a major problem in the United States.

13.4 "America, the Doctor Will See You Now." *Time.* The Patient Protection and Affordable Care Act (PPACA) is one of the most significant pieces of legislation ever passed. PPACA has many moving parts so the implementation will be challenging. This article highlights those challenges.

SELF-ASSESSMENT

13.1 Health and Well-Being Questionnaire
13.2 Finding the Right Doctor

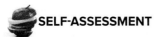 Website Resources

GENERAL

Agency for Healthcare Research and Quality **www.ahrq.gov**
Food and Drug Administration **www.fda.gov**
Joint Commission on Accreditation of Healthcare Organizations
    www.jointcommission.org
Kaiser Family Foundation **www.kff.org**

COMMON MEDICAL PROBLEMS

American Academy of Family Physicians (Search by Symptom)
    familydoctor.org/online/famdocen/home/tools/symptom.html
Merck Manual of Medical Information, 2nd Home Edition
    www.mercksource.com/pp/us/cns/cns_merckmanualhome.jsp

HANDLING MEDICAL EMERGENCIES

CPR and First Aid Courses (Contact Your Local Chapter)
• American Heart Association **www.americanheart.org**
• American Red Cross **www.redcross.org**
• National Safety Council **www.nsc.org**
Mayo Clinic First Aid Guide **www.mayoclinic.com/health/FirstAidIndex/**
    FirstAidIndex

PRESCRIPTION AND OTC MEDICINES

MedlinePlus Drug Information **www.nlm.nih.gov/medlineplus/
druginformation.html**
National Council on Patient Information and Education **www.talkaboutrx.org**
PDRhealth (*Physicians' Desk Reference*)
www.pdrhealth.com/drugs/drugs-index.aspx

FINDING THE RIGHT DOCTOR

American Board of Medical Specialties **www.abms.org/Who_We_Help/Consumers**
Specialty Boards, American Osteopathic Association
**www.osteopathic.org/inside-aoa/development/aoa-board-certification/
Pages/specialty-subspecialty-certification.aspx**

MEDICAL TESTS AND PROCEDURES

Lab Tests Online **www.labtestsonline.org**
MedlinePlus Health Surgery Tutorials
www.nlm.nih.gov/medlineplus/surgeryvideos.html
RadiologyInfo **www.radiologyinfo.org**

UNDERSTANDING HEALTH INSURANCE

Agency for Healthcare Research and Quality (Choosing a Health Plan)
www.ahrq.gov/patients-consumers/care-planning/plans/index.html
America's Health Insurance Plans (AHIP)
www.ahip.org/Issues/Individual-Market-Health-Insurance.aspx
Patient Protection and Affordable Care Act (PPACA) **www.healthreform.gov**

STAYING INFORMED

Centers for Disease Control and Prevention (CDC) **www.cdc.gov**
Columbia University's Health Q & A **www.goaskalice.columbia.edu**
healthfinder® **www.healthfinder.gov**
Healthline **www.healthline.com**
Mayo Clinic **www.mayoclinic.com**
MedlinePlus **medlineplus.gov**

PRACTICING PREVENTION

Adult Health Resources **www.ahrq.gov/ppip/adguide**

Knowing the Language

Understanding the Content

1. What are signs, symptoms, and decision charts?
2. What are three common types of OTC medications that should be available in every home?
3. What characteristics would you like to see in a primary care physician?
4. What is a personal health record? What information should it include?
5. What are the two main types of private health insurance? Contrast and compare.

Exploring Ideas

1. A key to effective medical self-care is knowing how much to do on your own and knowing when to contact your doctor. Think of two instances in which you were sick and sought medical care. Apply the signs and symptoms in each instance to the self-care resources (**familydoctor.org, mercksource.com**) and see what steps are recommended. Are the steps similar to or different from how you proceeded when you were sick?
2. Our current health care system offers several levels of care to diagnose and treat a vast array of illnesses and injuries from the simplest to the most complex. As a patient, how can one efficiently access and utilize medical care? What health care suggestions about finding a doctor or using a hospital would you give to a friend who is moving to the United States from another country?
3. Typically, young adults can choose from many different health plans. Assume a 25-year-old had two major medical costs in a year: $1,700 for an emergency room visit to check on a possible concussion and $450 incurred from a visit to his primary care physician to treat an infection (including blood tests and Rx drug). To what degree would these charges be covered by your health plan versus different plans of two friends? Compare bottom-line costs by incorporating insurance premiums and deductibles.

Selected References

Agency for Healthcare Research and Quality. Choosing a Health Plan. **www.ahrq.gov/patients-consumers/index.html**

Agency for Healthcare Research and Quality. Healthcare Cost and Priority Populations. **www.ahrq.gov/health-care-information/priority-populations/index.html**

Agency for Healthcare Research and Quality. Medical Expenditure Panel Survey. **www.ahrq.gov/data/mepsix.htm**

Agency for Healthcare Research and Quality. 20 Tips to Help Prevent Medical Errors. **www.ahrq.gov/consumer/20tips.htm**

America's Health Insurance Plans. Questions and Answers about Health Insurance: A Consumer Guide. August 2007.

Aspden P, Wolcott J, Bootman J, et al. (eds.). *Preventing Medication Errors.* Washington, DC: Institute of Medicine, National Academies Press, 2007.

Center on Budget and Policy Priorities. More Americans, including more children, now lack health insurance. August 31, 2007. **www.cbpp.org/8-28-07health.htm**

Consumer Healthcare Products Association. Statistics on OTC Use. 2011. **www.chpa.org/MarketStats.aspx**

Drug Topics. Voice of the Pharmacist. **drugtopics.modernmedicine.com/**

Fries JF, Vickery DM. *Take Care of Yourself: The Complete Illustrated Guide to Medical Self-Care* (9th ed.). Cambridge, MA: Da Capo Press, 2009.

Harris Interactive. Two in Five Adults Keep Personal or Family Health Records and Almost Everybody Thinks This Is a Good Idea. August 10, 2004. **www.harrisinteractive.com/news/allnewsbydate.asp?NewsID=832**

Kaiser Family Foundation. *Health Care and the Middle Class: More Costs and Less Coverage.* July 24, 2009. **www.kff.org/healthreform/7951.cfm**

Koh HK, Sebelius KG. Promoting prevention through the Affordable Care Act. *New England Journal of Medicine,* September 13, 2010.

Kokoska M, Eisenberg L, Stack B, et al. Health care for all? A single or multiple payer system. *Otolaryngology—Head and Neck Surgery* 143: 16, 2010.

MayoClinic.com. Tattoos: Risks and precautions to know first. February 16, 2008. **www.mayoclinic.com/health/tattoos-and-piercings/MC00020**

Mills, P. The Development of a New Corporate Specific Health Risk Measurement Instrument, and Its Use in Investigating the Relationship Between Health and Well-being and Employee Productivity. Environmental Health: A Global Access Science Source. January 28, 2005. **www.ehjournal.net/content/4/1/1**

National Coalition on Health Care. Health Insurance Cost. 2009. **www.nchc.org**

National Conference of State Legislatures. Managed Care, Market Reports and the States. June 2013. **www.ncsl.org/research/health/managed-care-and-the-states.aspx**

Ornish D. *The Spectrum: A Scientifically Proven Program to Feel Better, Live Longer, Lose Weight, and Gain Health.* New York: Ballantine, 2007.

Ornish D. Yes, prevention is cheaper than treatment. *Newsweek,* April 24, 2008. **www.newsweek.com/id/133751/**

Pantell RH, Fries JF, Vickery DM. *Taking Care of Your Child: A Parent's Illustrated Guide to Complete Medical Care* (8th ed.). Cambridge, MA: Da Capo Press, 2009.

United Health Foundation. Communicate with Your Health Care Team. **www.unitedhealthfoundation.org**

U.S. Department of Health and Human Services. Medicare. **www.medicare.gov**

U.S. News & World Report. America's Best Health Plans 2009. **health.usnews.com/sections/health/health-plans/index.html**

AUTHOR BIOSKETCHES

Phillip B. Sparling is a Professor of Applied Physiology and Health Behavior in the College of Sciences at Georgia Institute of Technology (Georgia Tech). He received his undergraduate degree from Duke University and master's and doctorate from the University of Georgia. In addition to being a teacher and researcher at Georgia Tech for three decades, he has been a Fulbright Scholar at the University of Cape Town Medical School in South Africa, a Senior Scientist at the Centers for Disease Control and Prevention (CDC) in Atlanta, and a Visiting Research Professor in the School of Population Health at the University of Queensland in Australia. He has published some 75 peer-reviewed articles in scientific and medical journals. Dr. Sparling is a Fellow of SHAPE America, the American College of Sports Medicine, the Society of Behavioral Medicine, and the National Academy of Kinesiology. His current work focuses on real-world projects that enable individuals and communities to change lifestyle behaviors to prevent and control chronic diseases.

Kerry J. Redican is a Professor of Public Health and is extensively involved in the Master of Public Health program in the Virginia Maryland College of Veterinary Medicine at Virginia Tech. He is also a Professor of Biomedical Sciences in the Virginia Tech Carilion School of Medicine. His education includes a bachelor's degree from California State University at Long Beach, M.S.P.H. from the UCLA School of Public Health, Ph.D. from the University of Illinois at Champaign–Urbana, and M.P.H. in health administration from the University of North Carolina at Chapel Hill. As a faculty member at Virginia Tech for over three decades, he has been actively involved in development, implementation, and evaluation of health education programs in schools and communities. He is a coauthor of four textbooks and has over 70 publications in health journals. Dr. Redican is a Fellow of the American School Health Association and has served on the Board of Directors of the American Association for Health Education. He is currently President-Elect of the Virginia Public Health Association.

INDEX

Page numbers in boldface indicate key term definition. Page numbers followed by *t* indicate material in table, *f* indicate material in a figure or an illustration. Numbers followed by *a* indicate material covered in an online *iHealth* article; the number indicates the chapter number and sequence in which the online article can be found.